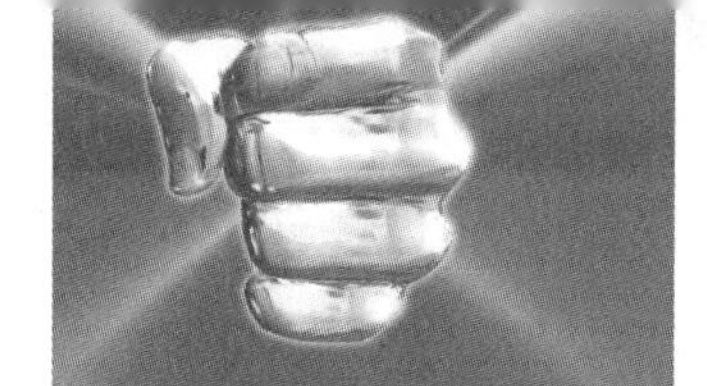

Crush Step 3

2nd Edition

The Ultimate USMLE Step 3 Review

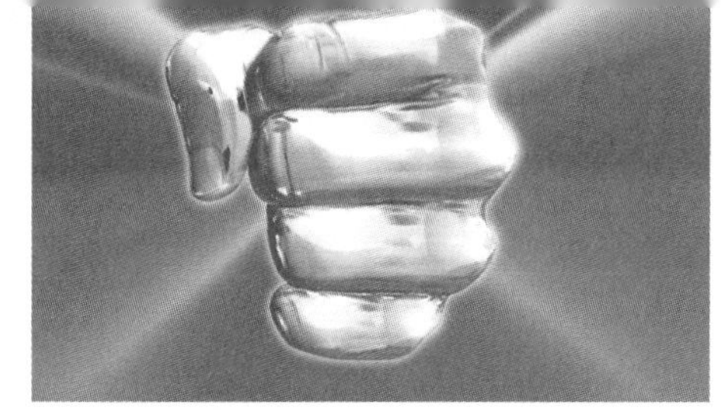

Crush Step 3

2nd Edition

The Ultimate USMLE Step 3 Review

Adam Brochert, MD
Staff Radiologist
Memorial Health University Medical Center
Savannah, Georgia

HANLEY & BELFUS, INC. / Philadelphia
An Affiliate of Elsevier

HANLEY & BELFUS, INC.
An Affiliate of Elsevier

The Curtis Center
Independence Square West
Philadelphia, Pennsylvania 19106

Note to the reader: Although the information in this book has been carefully reviewed for correctness of dosage and indications, neither the author nor the publisher can accept any legal responsibility for any errors or omissions that may be made. Neither the publisher nor the author makes any warranty, expressed or implied, with respect to the material contained herein. Before prescribing any drug, the reader must review the manufacturer's current product information (package inserts) for accepted indications, absolute dosage recommendations, and other information pertinent to the safe and effective use of the product described.

Library of Congress Control Number: 2003114342

Crush Step 3, 2nd edition ISBN 1-56053-607-1

Printed in the United States of America

Last digit is the print number: 9 8 7 6 5 4 3

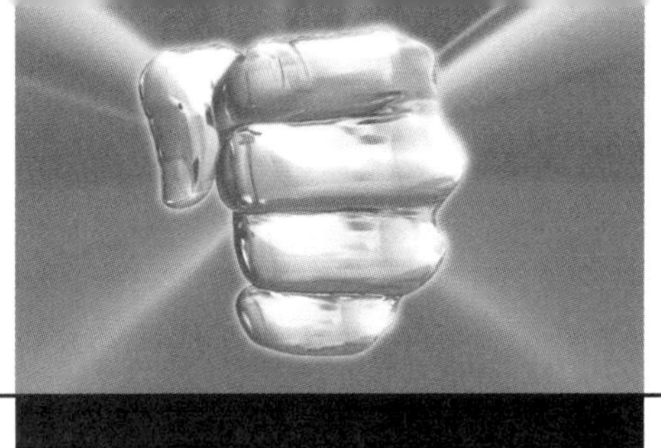

Contents

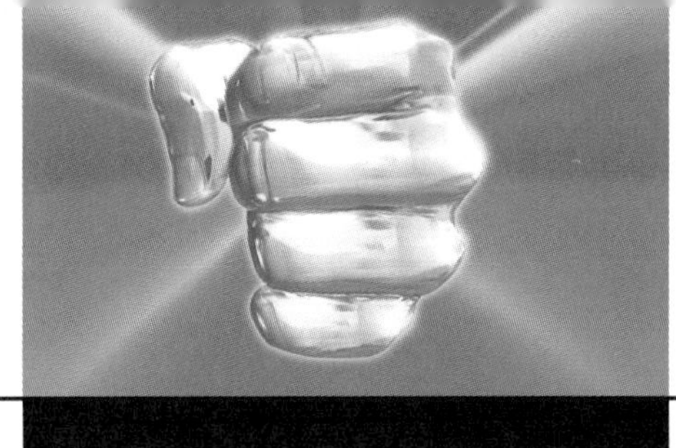

Introduction

This book was written because I felt there was not a good, quick, high-yield review book for the USMLE Step 3. If you're interested in this book, you are probably a busy house officer with little free time. This book is designed for you. You already know how to take USMLE exams and (hopefully) feel somewhat comfortable with the types of things you will be asked—otherwise, you'd be re-studying for Step 1 or 2 right now! Step 3 covers a lot of information, and this book was written to touch on important concepts in a brief enough format to allow it to be read quickly. If you know all the concepts in this book, you should do much better than just pass: you should Crush Step 3!

Step 3 has the same level of difficulty as Steps 1 and 2, but the questions are more relevant to the day-to-day management of patients in both inpatient and outpatient settings. Step 3 stresses the things that a general practitioner should know. Knowing how to diagnose, manage and treat common diseases is stressed. In addition, common emergencies must be recognized.

Knowing how to manage exotic or rare conditions is low-yield. Usually, when the examiners ask about a rare disease, they simply want you to recognize it from a classic presentation.

The topics on Step 3 are broad-based and cover all subspecialties. Most of the exam contains standard multiple choice questions with fairly long passages. The final segments of the exam are clinical-case scenarios in which the examinee "sees" a patient in the clinic or emergency room. In this section of the test, you can get results from a history and physical, order lab and radiologic tests, perform interventions, and assess how those interventions have affected the patient.

It is extremely important that the examinee practices the case-scenario format using the practice CD distributed with the registration materials by the USMLE. Without prior familiarity, this section of the exam could easily be flunked by the examinee simply due to lack of ability to use the program effectively. Only after spending an hour or so with the practice CD will this part of the exam test your clinical knowledge (as opposed to your computer skills!).

Studying for Step 3 can seem like an overwhelming task—in a sense, anything is fair game. Given the time constraints of residents, most need a concise review of the commonly tested topics. It is my hope that *Crush Step 3* will meet your needs in this regard.

I have compiled a list of "ten commandments" for taking the Step 3 exam that should prevent you from missing easy points:

1. It is just as important to know when something is normal or only needs observation as it is to know when to jump in and be a hero. If the patient is not "crashing" in front of

your eyes, always consider delaying intervention and taking the conservative, "wait and see approach" if you're not certain of the diagnosis (surgery residents, are you paying attention?). However, when a patient is truly crashing in front of you, take action! In other words, get the crash cart, intubate, put in a chest tube, etc. (psychiatry residents, are you paying attention?).

2. A presentation may be normal (especially in pediatrics and psychiatry) and need no treatment
3. If you're going to take the time to study for Step 3, study outside your field. In other words, if you're a medicine resident, don't study medicine for Step 3; study everything else. After six months to a year as a resident within a specific specialty, you probably know what you need to know for Step 3 purposes in that field. Those who are transitional residents probably have the best Step 3 prep from their experience (but probably haven't mastered a specific field).
4. You need to know common cut-off values for the treatment of common conditions. In other words, what glucose level defines diabetes, what blood pressure defines hypertension, when do you treat hypercholesterolemia, etc. This book provides the info you need in this regard.
5. Subspecialties are fair game. We've all heard about or experienced the exam with "a million" dermatology or orthopedic questions. You never know what field may be stressed in a particular exam administration.
6. Be a patient advocate. Don't yell at your patient, don't harshly judge them, don't refuse to be their doctor if they don't want treatment or tell you they're going to take some tree root for their cancer. Protect them when you can, and respect their autonomy. Work with them and ask them "why" whenever their actions puzzle you.
7. Don't be afraid to consult a specialist if you've made a diagnosis that you know is not commonly treated by a general practitioner. For example, if you think a patient may have a ruptured aortic aneurysm, look for an option that discusses consulting a vascular surgeon.
8. If the passage is very long, consider reading the question at the end first. The question can sometimes be answered without reading the passage, or you may save time when you read the passage because you know what important points to look for.
9. Never forget health maintenance. If a 35-year-old woman presents with a migraine headache and hasn't seen a doctor in 10 years, the correct answer of what to do next may be a Pap smear because of routine health maintenance!
10. Don't even think about taking the exam before you have practiced the format for the computer-based case simulations using the compact disc provided by the USMLE when you sign up for the exam.

I wish you the best on the exam and in all your future endeavors.

Adam Brochert, MD

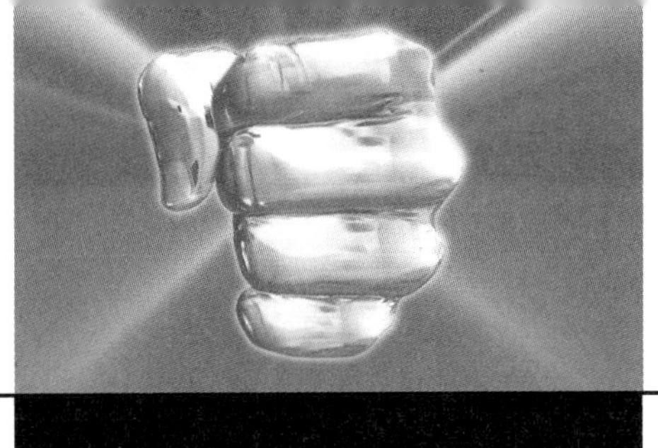

Computer-based Case Simulations (CCS)

The most important thing regarding this section of the exam is being prepared to use the software. I cannot stress enough how important it is to practice the CCS format with the compact disc that is sent with the USMLE information booklet when you register for the exam. If you are not familiar with this part of the exam, it doesn't matter how much medicine you know - your score on this section will suffer. You can also visit the official USMLE web site (www.usmle.org), which has sample items as well. If you don't have a computer, find someone's you can use. Plan to spend at least a few hours getting comfortable with all the features. Try clicking on every possible button/option and get familiar with short-cuts (know that you can type "CXR" instead of "perform chest x-ray" when trying to order a chest x-ray). You never know when you might want to use a certain feature, and familiarity with the program will prevent time from being a major factor.

If you have a good reason for ordering a test, don't start any potentially risky treatment until you have the results back:

EXAMPLE 1: A man presents with severe chest pain and your main differential concerns include a heart attack, unstable angina, and aortic dissection. You order an EKG and a chest x-ray. If the EKG comes back with inverted T waves, don't start heparin or aspirin before you get the results of the chest x-ray, as the patient may have an aortic dissection (widened mediastinum on chest x-ray), and you have now increased the risk of a life-threatening hemorrhage.

EXAMPLE 2: A man presents with a classic transient ischemic attack and his neurologic deficits have already started improving. You order a head CT just in case. Don't start aspirin therapy until you get the results of the CT back, as the patient may have an intracranial hemorrhage.

Don't forget to order a pregnancy test on any reproductive age female before ordering any treatments or tests that are potentially harmful to a fetus, such as teratogenic drugs or x-ray tests.

If you feel confident that you are giving the right treatment, give it a chance to work. The examiners may try to trick you into thinking you've made the wrong diagnosis.

EXAMPLE 1: A man presents with classic depression. You prescribe fluoxetine. He calls the next day to say he doesn't feel any better. Of course he doesn't, because antidepressants take 1–4 weeks to work. Do nothing and maintain the patient's initially scheduled follow-up appointment.

EXAMPLE 2: A man has classic appendicitis. You order an appendectomy. Two hours after surgery, the man says he is still hurting. Of course he is, he just had surgery (though in this case, you should consider increasing the man's pain medication dose).

Always make sure the patient has follow up, whether it is in 30 minutes or 3 months.

Consider giving outpatient instructions as a written order (e.g., write an order to "avoid aspirin" for a patient whom you have finished treating for a gastrointestinal bleed). You'd be amazed at some of the orders the software can recognize (another reason practicing with the software helps tremendously).

Don't forget the basics: IV access, oxygen, EKG monitoring, pulse oximetry monitoring, IV fluids, keeping the patient NPO or ordering a special diabetic diet, vital signs, repeat physical exam, ask how the patient is doing since the last time you saw him or her, the ABCs (airway, breathing, circulation), and review the old chart if available (or even the current chart if you can't remember what has happened in the 5 minutes since the case started).

Don't forget health maintenance. Example: If it is mentioned in the history and physical that a woman hasn't had a Pap smear in 5 years, order one.

Start every case with a complete history and physical exam, regardless of the chief complaint or scenario.

Don't be afraid to order a consultation if you know the condition would not be treated by a general physician, but don't be surprised when the consultant says, "treat the patient as you see fit." You may be the one performing an emergency abdominal aortic aneurysm repair (just write the order and it shall be done).

You never know how long the case will last. Don't get too frustrated if the case ends before you've had a chance to do/order everything you wanted to. Alternatively, don't screw around just because you've made the diagnosis. The examiners may want to see how you manage a condition after diagnosis.

When considering follow-up, think in terms of the real world. If somebody has osteoarthritis and you make the diagnosis and give initial treatment, you may not need to see the patient for 3 or 6 months if there are no other active problems.

Don't forget to terminate orders that are no longer appropriate and always transfer the patient to the proper level of care. As patients get better, discharge them or move them from ICU to the regular floor, stop their oxygen or IV fluids, etc.

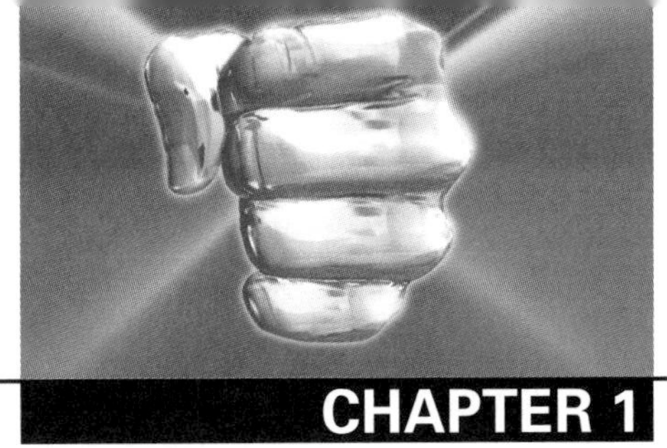

CHAPTER 1

Pediatrics

SCREENING AND PREVENTIVE CARE

Height, weight, blood pressure, developmental/behavioral assessment, history/physical examination, and anticipatory guidance (counseling/discussion about age-appropriate concerns) should be done at every pediatric visit. Also, remember the following:

1. **Metabolic/congenital disorders.** All states screen for hypothyroidism and phenylketonuria at birth (must be done within the first month). Most states screen for galactosemia and sickle cell disease.

   ➤ **CASE SCENARIO:** A newborn screening test is positive for phenylketonuria. What should you do next? Order a confirmatory test to make sure that the screen gave you a true positive.

2. **Anticipatory guidance.** Keep the water heater < 110–120°F; use car restraints; put the baby to sleep on his or her **back** (on the side is a less desirable second choice) to help prevent sudden infant death syndrome (SIDS); do not use infant walkers, which cause injuries; watch out for small objects that the baby may aspirate; do not give cow's milk before 1 year of age; introduce solid foods gradually, starting at 6 months; supervise children in a bathtub or swimming pool; and keep chemicals out of reach.

3. **Height, weight, and head circumference.** Head circumference (HC) should be measured routinely in the first 2 years; height and weight should be measured routinely until adulthood. All three are markers of general well-being. The pattern of growth along plotted growth curves tells you more than any raw number. If a patient has always been low or high compared with peers, the pattern is generally benign. If a child goes from a normal curve to an abnormal one, the pattern is much more worrisome. The classic situation involves parents who bring in a child with delayed physical growth/puberty: you must know when to reassure them and when to investigate further after looking at a plotted growth curve (see figure on next page).

   Note: Increased HC may mean hydrocephalus or tumor; decreased HC may mean microcephaly from **t**oxoplasmosis, **o**ther infections [congenital syphilis and viruses], **r**ubella, **c**ytomegalovirus, and **h**erpes simplex virus (TORCH) infection or other congenital anomaly.

   ➤ **CASE SCENARIO:** What should you suspect as the cause of obesity? Obesity usually is due to overeating and lack of exercise. Less than 5% of cases are due to organic causes (e.g., Cushing syndrome).

   ➤ **CASE SCENARIO:** What is the most common cause of failure to thrive? Defined as growth below the 5th percentile for age, failure to thrive most commonly is due to **psychosocial or functional** problems (watch for child abuse or neglect). Organic causes should have specific clues to trigger your suspicion.

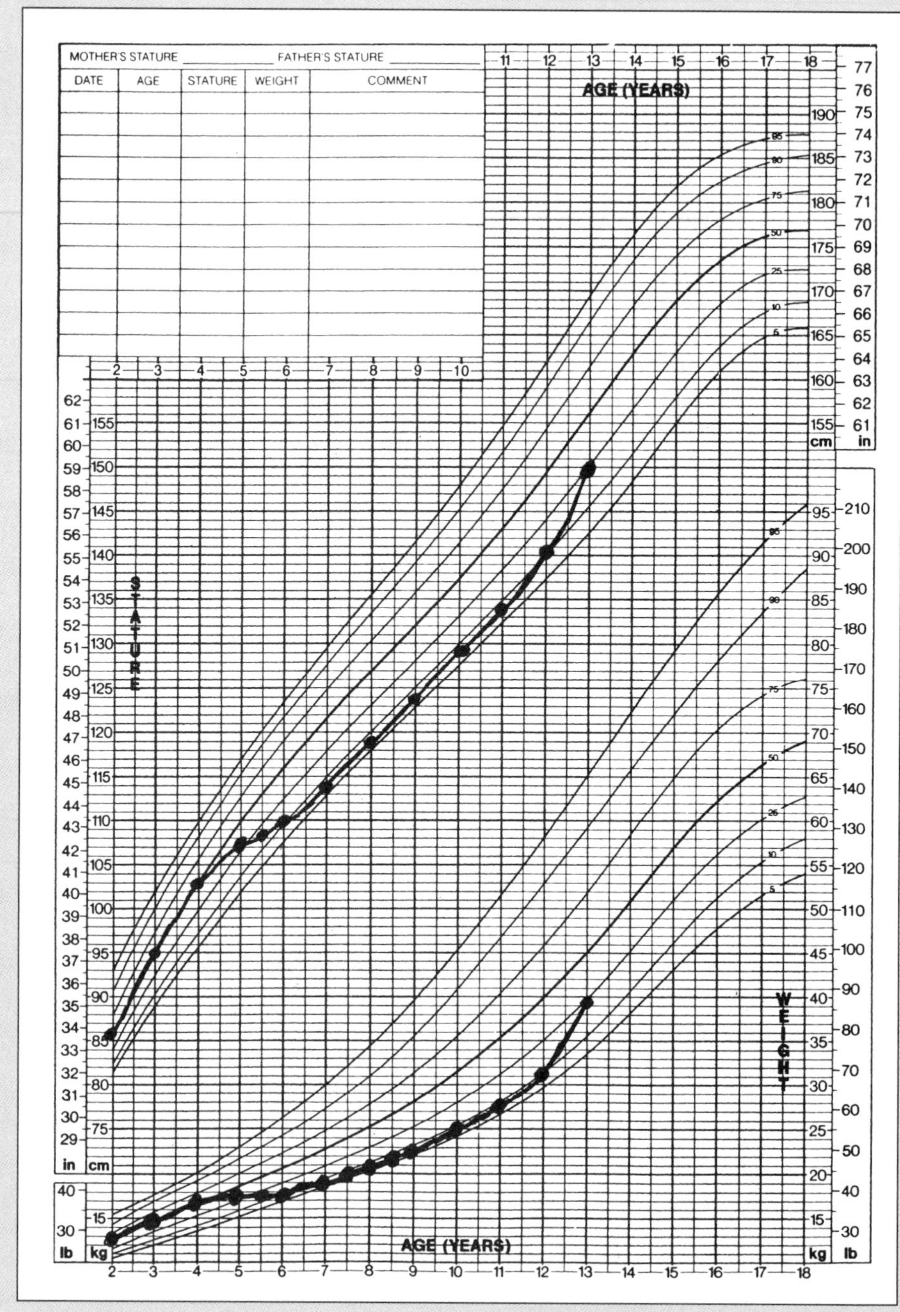

Constitutional delay pattern of growth. Note how the child has already started to catch up with peers at age 12 and 13. To make it more challenging, you could be shown the growth chart pattern only up to the age of 9 or 10 (before catch-up). In this case, the establishment of a stable pattern of steady but low-percentile growth is suggestive. (From Brochert A: Platinum Vignettes: Pediatrics. Philadelphia, Hanley & Belfus, 2002, p 50, with permission.)

4. **Hearing and vision.** Hearing should be measured objectively at birth and at least every two years starting at the age of 4 (until late adolescence). Vision should be measured objectively every few years starting at the age of 3 years (until late adolescence). Measure more often if history dictates.

Note: Check the red reflex at birth and routinely thereafter to detect congenital cataracts (classically due to congenital rubella/TORCH or galactosemia) or **retinoblastoma** (causes leukocoria, or a red reflex that becomes white).

➤ **CASE SCENARIO:** Until what age is a "lazy eye" normal? Consistent deviation of one eye is not normal at any age. Occasional misalignment of one eye may be normal until 3 months of age. After 3 months, refer to an ophthalmologist to prevent **amblyopia** (see ophthalmology section).

➤ **CASE SCENARIO:** What two classic infectious diseases are associated with acquired hearing loss in children? **Meningitis** and recurrent **otitis media.**

5. **Anemia.** Routine screening for anemia is now controversial and generally recommended only for those with risk factors for iron deficiency during infancy (e.g., prematurity, low birth weight, use of cow's milk before 12 months, poor dietary intake). All infants except full-term infants who are breastfed may be candidates for prophylactic iron supplements. Because baby formulas already contain iron supplements, preterm breastfed infants are the only ones for whom you have to worry about prescribing supplements. Menstruating adolescent females are also at risk for iron-deficiency anemia—consider screening if given the option.
6. **Lead.** Exposure to lead can cause neurologic damage ranging from mild learning disabilities or hyperactivity to mental retardation. Routine screening is now controversial and usually only recommended for high-risk children (e.g., the child lives in old building and is a paint-chip eater or lives near a battery recycling plant). If the level is $\geq$ 10 μg/dl, closer follow-up and intervention are needed. The best first course of action is to **stop the exposure.** Lead chelation therapy may be needed with **succimer** or dimercaptosuccinic acid (DMSA) if exposure stoppage fails.
7. **Fluoride.** Most children need no supplementation because fluoride is in most tap water. Supplementation is necessary in the first few years of life if water is inadequately fluoridated (primarily in rural areas). Too much fluoride can cause mottled bones and teeth. The first dentist appointment should be advised by the time the child is 3 years old.
8. **Vitamin D.** Most recommend supplementation only if the infant is at high risk (e.g., because of inadequate maternal vitamin D intake, little sunlight exposure and/or dark skin, or exclusive breastfeeding beyond 6 months of age). Start supplements by 6 months. Formula-fed infants are not at risk because formulas contains vitamin D supplements.
9. **Tuberculosis** (Tb). Do not screen for tuberculosis unless there are risk factors or symptoms. Screen annually at any age if risk factors are present (e.g., HIV infection, incarceration). If the only risk factor is that the child lives in a high-risk area or is the offspring of an immigrant, screen once at 4–6 years of age and once at 11–16 years of age.
10. **Urinalysis.** Controversial, but some recommend routinely in children at the age of 5. Screening urinalysis can help detect sexually transmitted diseases in sexually active adolescents.
11. **Immunizations**
    - A routine immunization schedule for healthy children with no specific risk factors follows:

VACCINE	WHEN TO GIVE IN ROUTINE CASES
Hepatitis B	0–1, 1–4, and 6–18 months (3 doses)
Diphtheria, tetanus, pertussis (DTP)	2, 4, 6, 15–18 months and 4–6 years (5 doses) plus tetanus booster (Td) every 10 years
Haemophilus influenzae, type b	2, 4, 6, 12–15 months (4 doses)
Polio, inactivated (IPV)	2, 4, 6 months and 4–6 years (4 doses)
Measles, mumps, rubella (MMR)	12–15 months and 4–6 years (2 doses)
Pneumococcus spp. (heptavalent)	2, 4, 6, 12–15 months (4 doses)
Varicella	12–18 months (1 dose)

- Information about contraindications and special patient populations

VACCINE	WHO SHOULD RECEIVE AND/OR CONTRAINDICATIONS
MMR	Avoid in children with anaphylactic reaction to eggs or neomycin; avoid in those with immunodeficiency other than HIV/AIDS
Hepatitis B	Give first dose at birth with hepatitis B immune globulin if mother has active hepatitis B
IPV	Avoid in children with anaphylaxis to neomycin or streptomycin
Varicella	Avoid in children with immunodeficiency or anaphylaxis to neomycin
Influenza	Give to children > 6 months old with immunodeficiency, severe heart/lung disease, or on chronic aspirin therapy (to prevent Reye syndrome)
Pneumococcus spp.	Give to children > 2 years old who have not been vaccinated if they have immunodeficiency of any kind, are asplenic, or lack splenic function (sickle cell disease)

➤ **CASE SCENARIO:** What routine screening tests should be performed in sexually active female pediatric patients? Annual Papanicolaou smear and gonorrhea/chlamydia culture. Culture in boys is more controversial because they do not get pelvic inflammatory disease and become sterile, but they can infect girls.

➤ **CASE SCENARIO:** What clinical scenario should prompt you to screen for urinary tract malformations? How should screening be done? Screen after a urinary tract infection (UTI) in boys < 6 years old and after a second UTI in girls < 6 years old. A **voiding cystourethrogram** and **renal ultrasound** are commonly performed for screening. Some recommend screening in girls < 6 years old after the first UTI.

INFANTS

Apgar score. The Apgar score is commonly done at 1 and 5 minutes. Do not wait until the 1-minute mark to evaluate the baby because you may have to suction or intubate the baby 5 seconds after delivery. The scale consists of five categories with a maximum score of 2 points per category, for a maximum total of 10 points. Resuscitation and close monitoring are usually performed until the child gets a score greater than 7 or goes to the intensive care unit (see table below).

Umbilical cord. Check the umbilical cord at birth for two arteries, one vein, and absence of the urachus. If only one umbilical artery is present, consider the possibility of **congenital renal malformations.**

Caput succedaneum is diffuse swelling/edema of the scalp at birth that **crosses the midline** and is benign. Cephalhematomas are subperiosteal hemorrhages that are sharply limited by sutures and **do not cross the midline.** Both result from birth trauma. Cephalhematomas are usually benign and self-resolving but in rare cases may indicate an underlying skull fracture. Consider ordering an x-ray or CT scan to rule out a fracture.

PARAMETER	NUMBER OF POINTS 0	1	2
Heart rate	Absent	< 100	>100
Respiratory effort	None	Slow, weak cry	Good, strong cry
Muscle tone	Limp	Some flexion of extremities	Active motion
Color	Pale, blue	Pink body, blue extremities	Completely pink
Reflex irritability*	None	Grimace	Grimace and strong cry/cough/sneeze

* Done by checking the response to stimulation of the sole of foot or a catheter put in the nose.

Cavernous hemangioma. First noticed a few days after birth, the tumor increases in size after birth and then gradually resolves within the first few years. The best initial treatment is to do nothing and observe at follow-up.

The anterior fontanelle usually closes by 18 months. A large anterior fontanelle or delayed closure may indicate **hypothyroidism, hydrocephalus,** rickets or intrauterine growth retardation (IUGR).

Moro and palmar grasp reflexes usually disappear by 6 months.

MILESTONES AND MISCELLANEOUS ISSUES

There are tons of milestones, but only the commonly tested ones are listed below. The exact age is not as important as the overall pattern when you are looking for dysfunctional development. When in doubt, use a formal developmental test. The following table gives rough *average* ages when milestones are achieved:

MILESTONE	AGE*	MILESTONE	AGE*
Social smile	1–2 months	Voluntary grasp with voluntary release	10 months
Cooing sounds	2–4 months	Waves "bye-bye"	10 months
While prone, lifts head up 90°	3–4 months	Separation anxiety	12–15 months
Rolls front to back	4–5 months	Walks without help	13 months
Voluntary grasp (no release)	5 months	Can build tower of 2 cubes	13–15 months
Stranger anxiety	6–9 months	Understands 1-step commands (no gesture)	15 months
Sits with no support	7 months	Good use of cup and spoon	15–18 months
Pulls to stand	9 months	Runs well	2 years
Plays pat-a-cake	9–10 months	Can build tower of 6 cubes	2 years
First words	9–12 months	Ties shoelaces	5 years
Imitates others' sounds	9–12 months		

* Remember that the age of a premature patient is reduced in the first 2 years in assessments of development (e.g., a premature child born after 6 months' gestation will have 3 months subtracted from his or her chronologic age; therefore, when 9 months old, the infant is expected to perform only at the 6-month-old level).

Tanner stages. Stage I is preadolescent; stage V is adult. Increasing stages are assigned for testicular and penile growth in males and for breast growth in females; both also use pubic hair development. Average age of puberty (when the patient first changes from stage I status) is 11.5 years in boys, usually with **testicular enlargement** as the first event, and 10.5 years in girls, usually with **breast development** as the first event.

Delayed puberty occurs when there is no testicular enlargement in boys by the age of 14 years and no breast development or pubic hair in girls by the age of 13 years. It is usually caused by a **constitutional delay,** which is a normal variant. Parents often have a similar history, and the growth curve lags behind peers of the same age but is consistent. Delayed puberty is rarely due to primary testicular failure (e.g., **Klinefelter syndrome,** cryptorchidism, history of chemotherapy, gonadal dysgenesis) or ovarian failure (e.g., **Turner syndrome,** gonadal dysgenesis); it also is rarely due to hypothalamic/pituitary defect such as a tumor.

Precocious puberty is usually idiopathic. Rare causes include **McCune-Albright syndrome** (café-au-lait spots, fibrous dysplasia and precocious puberty in girls), ovarian tumors (granulosa cell or theca-cell, which can secrete estrogen), testicular tumors (Leydig-cell, which can secrete testosterone), central nervous system (CNS) disease or trauma (e.g., pineal gland or hypothalamus affected), adrenal neoplasm, and **congenital adrenal hyperplasia** (in boys, usually 21-hydroxylase deficiency; in girls, causes ambiguous genitalia). Most patients with uncorrectable, idiopathic precocious puberty are given long-acting

gonadotropin-releasing hormone (GnRH) agonists to suppress progression of puberty and thus prevent premature epiphyseal closure.

The most common cause of nose-bleed in children is trauma (often nose-picking), but watch for a possible tumor (***nasopharyngeal angiofibroma***—adolescent boys with no trauma/blood dyscrasia and recurrent nose-bleeds and/or obstruction), ***leukemia*** (from pancytopenia, often associated with fever and anemia), and other causes of thrombocytopenia such as idiopathic thrombocytopenic purpura (ITP) and hemolytic uremic syndrome (HUS).

Sickle cell disease (SCD). A blood smear gives it away—look for a high percentage of reticulocytes also. SCD is seen almost always in blacks (8% are heterozygotes in U.S.). Watch for the classic manifestations of SCD: aplastic crises due to ***parvovirus B19*** infection; bone pain due to microinfarcts (often ***avascular necrosis*** of the femoral head); renal ***papillary necrosis;*** splenic sequestration crisis; ***autosplenectomy,*** often accompanied by increased infections with encapsulated organisms (give pneumococcal vaccine); ***acute chest syndrome,*** which mimics pneumonia; ***pigment*** cholelithiasis; priapism; and stroke. Diagnosis is made by hemoglobin electrophoresis. Screening is done at birth, but remember that symptoms usually do not begin until around 6 months of age because of the lack of adult hemoglobin production. Treat with prophylactic penicillin, which is started as soon as the diagnosis is made and continued until age 5 years; proper vaccination, including pneumococcal vaccine; folate supplementation; early treatment of infections; and proper hydration.

Note: Sickle "crisis" is severe pain in various sites due to acute red blood cell (RBC) sickling. Treat with oxygen, lots of intravenous fluid (IVF), and analgesics. Do not be afraid to use narcotics for pain. Consider transfusions if symptoms and/or findings are severe.

> ➤ ***CASE SCENARIO:*** A woman is watching her neighbor's 1-year-old, African-American child and brings her in for sudden, symmetric swelling and redness of the hands and feet that develop over a few hours. The child is very irritable. The woman thinks that there may be a family history of anemia. The child looks pale. What syndrome does the child probably have? "Hand-foot" syndrome, or ***dactylitis,*** a classic manifestation of sickle cell disease in young children.

Classic kidney/hematologic disorders:

	HUS	HSP	TTP	ITP
Most common age	Children	Children	Young adults	Children or adults
Previous infection	Diarrhea (*E. coli*)	URI	None	Viral (especially children)
RBC count	Low	Normal	Low	Normal
Platelet count	Low	Normal	Low	Low
Peripheral smear	Hemolysis	Normal	Hemolysis	Normal
Kidney manifestations	ARF, hematuria	Hematuria	ARF, proteinuria	None
Treatment	Supportive*	Supportive*	Plasmapheresis, NSAIDs Do not give platelets[†]	Steroids, splenectomy if medication fails[#]
Key differential points	Age, diarrhea	Rash, abdominal pain, arthritis, melena	CNS changes, age	Antiplatelet antibodies

HUS = hemolytic uremic syndrome, HSP = Henoch-Schönlein purpura, TTP = thrombotic thrombocytopenic purpura, ITP = idiopathic thrombocytopenic purpura, URI = upper respiratory infection, ARF = acute renal failure, NSAIDs = nonsteroidal anti-inflammatory drugs, CNS = central nervous system, RBC = red blood cell.

*In HUS and HSP, paients may need dialysis and transfusions.

[†]Do not give platelet transfusions to patients with TTP because they may form clots.

[#]Give steroids only if patient is symptomatic (bleeding) or counts fall to dangerous levels (< 20–40,000/µl).

PEDIATRIC CARDIOLOGY

Congenital heart defects. The following table provides a general description of several congenital heart defects:

DEFECT	SYMPTOM, TREATMENT, AND OTHER INFORMATION
PDA	Constant, machine-like murmur in upper left sternal border; dyspnea and possible CHF; close PDA with indomethacin (surgery is required if this approach fails); keep open with prostaglandin E_1; associated with congenital rubella and high altitudes.
VSD	Holosystolic murmur next to sternum; most VSDs resolve on their own; most common congenital heart defect.
ASD	Asymptomatic until adulthood; fixed, split S2 and palpitations; most ASDs do not require correction (unless they are very large)
TOF	Consists of four anomalies: (1) VSD, (2) right ventricular hypertrophy, (3) pulmonary stenosis, and (4) overriding aorta. Most common cyanotic congenital heart defect; loof for "tet" spells (squatting after exertion).
C of A	Upper extremity hypertension only, radiofemoral delay, systolic murmur heard over mid-upper back, rib notching on x-ray; associated with Turner syndrome.

PDA = patent ductus arteriosus, VSD = ventral septal defect, ASD = atrial septal defect, TOF = tetralogy of Fallot, C of A = coarctation of aorta, CHF = congestive heart failure.

Note: Endocarditis prophylaxis is required for all of the cardiac defects listed in the table except asymptomatic, secundum-type atrial septal defects (80% of ASDs).

Remember that a heart rate over 100 beats/min may be normal in pediatric patients (up to age 10).

In patients with a VSD, think about the possibility of **fetal alcohol syndrome, TORCH syndrome,** or **Down syndrome.**

> ➤ **CASE SCENARIO:** A 17-year-old male athlete with a family history of sudden death at an early age collapses suddenly during a basketball game. What condition should you consider? Hypertrophic obstructive cardiomyopathy. Treat with beta blockers to give the heart more time to fill, and consider a pacemaker. Positive inotropic agents (e.g., digoxin), diuretics, and vasodilators are contraindicated, because they make things worse.

Remember that in the fetal circulation oxygen content is highest in the umbilical vein and lowest in the umbilical arteries. In addition, oxygen content is higher in blood going to the upper extremities than in blood going to the lower extremities.

Circulation changes with the transition from intrauterine to extrauterine life. First breaths inflate the lungs and cause decreased pulmonary vascular resistance, which increases blood flow to the pulmonary arteries. This and the clamping of the cord increase left-sided heart pressures, which functionally closes the foramen ovale. Increased oxygen concentration shuts off prostaglandin production in the ductus arteriosus, causing gradual closure.

> ➤ **CASE SCENARIO:** A child has two episodes of dizziness, dyspnea, or passing out after playing, then is fine and has no other symptoms. You are shown an EKG taken while the child has no symptoms. What should you look for on the EKG to make the diagnosis? The **delta wave of Wolff-Parkinson-White syndrome.** The symptoms probably were caused by transient arrhythmias via accessory pathways.

PEDIATRIC GASTROENTEROLOGY

Gastrointestinal malformations in children. Each of the following gastrointestinal (GI) conditions (see table) must be treated with surgical repair.

NAME	PRESENTING AGE	VOMIT DESCRIPTION	FINDINGS/KEY WORDS
Pyloric stenosis	0–2 mo	Nonbilious, projectile	M >> F; palpable olive-shaped mass in epigastrium, low chloride, low potassium, metabolic alkalosis
Duodenal atresia	0–1 wk	Bilious	"Double-bubble" sign, Down syndrome
Tracheoesophageal fistula*	0–2 wk	Food regurgitation	Respiratory compromise with feeding, aspiration pneumonia; cannot thread nasogastric tube past esophagus; stomach distended by air
Hirschsprung disease	0–2 yr	Feculent	Abdominal distention, obstipation; no ganglia seen on rectal biopsy, M >> F
Anal atresia	0–1 wk	Late, feculent	Detected on initial exam in nursery; M >> F
Choanal atresia	0-1 wk	—	Cyanosis with feeding, relieved by crying; cannot pass nasogastric tube through nose

* Most common variant (85% of cases) has esophageal atresia with a fistula from bronchus to distal esophagus (which explains gastric distention, because each breath transmits air to GI tract). Be able to recognize a sketch of this most common variant (see figure). A classic chest x-ray shows the nasogastric tube coiled in the esophagus with a large, air-filled stomach.

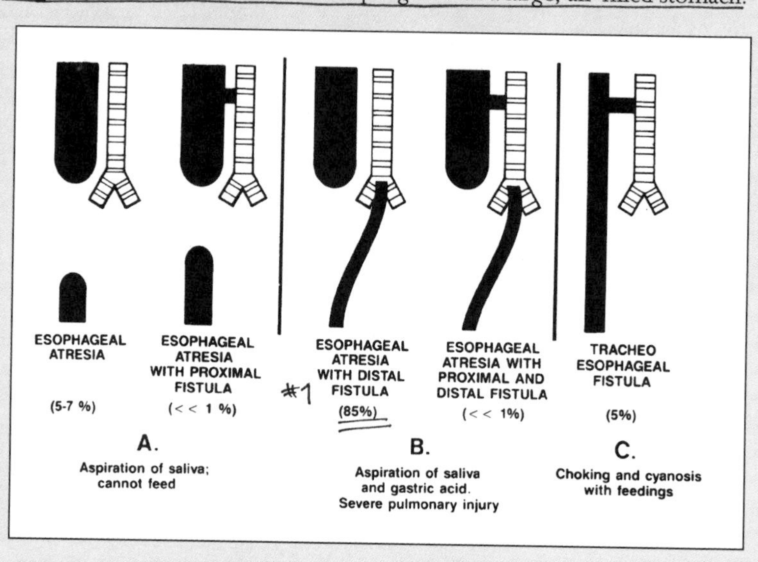

Types of tracheoesophageal anomalies and their presenting symptoms complexes. (From James EC, Corry RJ, Perry JF: Principles of Basic Surgical Practice. Philadelphia, Hanley & Belfus, 1987, with permission.)

Other pediatric GI conditions are listed in the table below.

NAME	PRESENTING AGE	VOMIT	FINDINGS/KEY WORDS
Intussusception	4 mo to 2 yr	Bilious	Currant-jelly stools (blood and mucus); palpable sausage-like mass; treat with air or barium enema (gives diagnosis and treats)
Necrotizing enterocolitis	0–2 mo	Bilious	Premature infants; fever, rectal bleeding, air in bowel wall; treat with NPO status, orogastric tube, intravenous fluids, antibiotics
Meconium ileus	0–2 wk	Feculent, late	Cystic fibrosis manifestation (as is rectal prolapse)
Midgut volvulus	0–2 yr	Bilious	Sudden onset of pain, distention, rectal bleeding, peritonitis, "bird's beak" in small bowel (not large bowel, as in adults) on contrast study; treat with surgery
Meckel diverticulum	0–2 yr	Varies	Rule of 2s*, GI ulceration/bleeding; use Meckel's scan to detect; treat with surgery
Strangulated hernia	Any age	Bilious	Physical exam detects bowel loops in the inguinal canal

NPO = nothing by mouth.

Rule of 2s: 2% of population affected (most common GI tract abnormality—remnant of the omphalomesenteric duct), 2 inches long, within 2 feet of ileocolic junction, presents in the first 2 years of life. Meckel diverticulum can cause GI bleeding, intussusception, obstruction, and/or volvulus.

Diaphragmatic hernia is more common on the left side (Bochdalek type) and affects boys more often than girls. Bowel herniates into the thorax, which compresses and impedes lung development (pulmonary hypoplasia results). Patients present with respiratory distress and have bowel sounds in the chest and bowel loops in the thorax on chest x-ray. Treat surgically. Prognosis related to lung development, not the hernia

Omphalocele vs. gastroschisis. Omphalocele is in the **midline,** the sac contains multiple abdominal organs, the umbilical ring is absent, and other anomalies are common. Gastroschisis is **to the right of the midline,** only small bowel is exposed (there is no true hernia sac), the umbilical ring is present, and other anomalies are rare.

Henoch-Schönlein purpura may present with GI bleeding and abdominal pain. Look for history of upper respiratory or GI infection, **characteristic rash on lower extremities and buttocks,** swelling in hands and feet, arthritis, and hematuria or proteinuria. Treat supportively.

Children develop nausea, vomiting, and/or diarrhea with **any systemic illness** more commonly than adults.

Children can develop inflammatory bowel disease (IBD) or irritable bowel syndrome (IBS) and often have GI complaints with **anxiety** or **psychiatric problems** (e.g., separation anxiety, dislike of school, depression, child abuse).

Neonatal jaundice may be physiologic or pathologic. The first step is to measure total, direct, and indirect bilirubin. The main concern is **kernicterus,** which is due to high levels of unconjugated bilirubin with subsequent deposit into the basal ganglia. Watch for poor feeding, seizures, flaccidity, opisthotonos (muscular spasm that results in spine beding, with body resting on heels and head), and/or apnea to accompany severe jaundice.

1. **Physiologic jaundice** is seen in 50% of normal infants and is even more common in premature infants. **Symptoms start 1–2 days after birth.** Bilirubin is mostly unconjugated. In full-term infants, bilirubin should be less than 12 mg/dl, peak at day 2–5, and return to normal by 2 weeks. In premature infants, the bilirubin should be less than 15 mg/dl and return to normal by 3 weeks.
2. **Pathologic jaundice.** Bilirubin levels are higher than normal and continue to rise or fail to decrease appropriately. **Any jaundice present at birth is pathologic.** The differential diagnosis includes the following:
   - Breast milk jaundice is seen in breastfed infants with peak bilirubin levels of 10–20 mg/dl at 2–3 weeks of age. Treat with temporary cessation of breastfeeding (switch to bottle) until jaundice resolves.
   - Illness. Infection or sepsis, hypothyroidism, liver insult, cystic fibrosis, and other illnesses may prolong neonatal jaundice and lower the threshold for kernicterus. The point to remember is that the youngest, sickest infants are at greatest risk for hyperbilirubinemia and kernicterus.
   - Hemolysis due to Rh incompatibility or congenital red cell diseases in the neonatal period. Look for anemia, peripheral smear abnormalities, family history, and higher levels of unconjugated bilirubin.
   - Metabolic. **Criggler-Najjar** disease causes severe unconjugated hyperbilirubinemia, and **Gilbert** disease causes mild unconjugated hyperbilirubinemia. **Rotor** and **Dubin-Johnson** diseases cause conjugated hyperbilirubinemia.
   - Biliary atresia may be seen in full-term infants with **clay or gray-colored stools** and high conjugated bilirubin. Treat with surgery.
   - Medications. **Avoid sulfa drugs in neonates;** they displace bilirubin from albumin and may precipitate kernicterus.

The **treatment for unconjugated hyperbilirubinemia** that persists, rises above 15 mg/dl, or rises rapidly is **phototherapy** (i.e., UV light exposure) to convert the unconjugated bilirubin to a water-soluble form that can be excreted. The last resort is exchange transfusion. Do *not* choose this option unless the level of unconjugated bilirubin is > 20 mg/dl and phototherapy has failed.

Any infant born to a mother with **active hepatitis B** should receive the first immunization shot and hepatitis B immune globulin at birth.

PEDIATRIC GYNECOLOGY

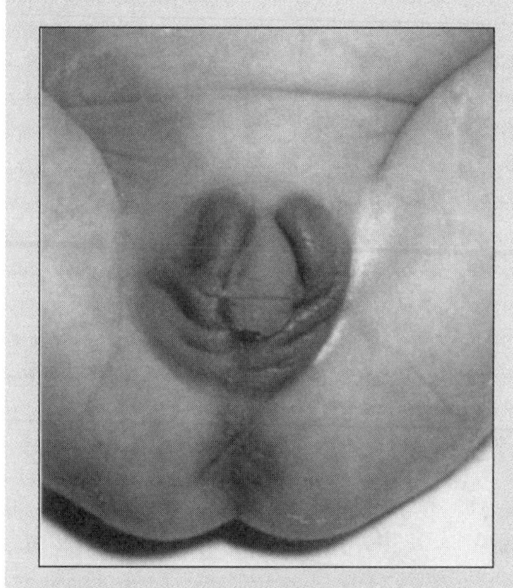

Ambiguous genitalia in a newborn infant with congential adrenal hyperplasia. (From Resnick MJ, Novick AC: Urology Secrets, 2nd ed. Philadelphia, Hanley & Belfus, 1999, with permission.).

Ambiguous genitalia. Look for adrenogenital syndrome/congenital adrenal hyperplasia (***21-hydroxylase deficiency*** in 90% of cases). Patients are usually female; boys with the disease experience precocious sexual development. Neonates with 21-hydroxylase deficiency rapidly develop salt-wasting (low sodium), ***hyperkalemia, hypotension,*** and elevated 17-hydroxyprogesterone. Treat with steroids and intravenous fluids immediately to prevent death. Any child with ambiguous genitalia (see figure) should not be assigned a sex until the work-up is complete and a karyotype is done.

➤ ***CASE SCENARIO:*** What does a female child with a "bunch of grapes" (vesicles) protruding from the vagina have? Sarcoma botryoides, a malignancy.

Premature/precocious puberty is usually idiopathic, but may be caused by a hormone-secreting tumor or CNS disorder, both of which must be ruled out. By definition, the patient must be younger than 8 years (9 years for boys). Treat the underlying cause, or, if the case is idiopathic, treat with a ***gonadotropin-releasing hormone (GnRH) analog*** to prevent premature epiphyseal closure and arrest or reverse puberty until an appropriate age.

➤ ***CASE SCENARIO:*** A mother brings in her 10-year-old daughter and is concerned because the child has just had her first period. What is the correct treatment? Reassurance only, because this is normal.

Vaginitis/discharge. Most cases of vaginitis or discharge are nonspecific or physiologic, but, on the boards, look for foreign body, ***sexual abuse*** (especially with sexually transmitted disease findings), or *Candida* as a presentation of diabetes (check serum and/or urine glucose in this case).

Vaginal bleeding in the neonate is usually physiologic from maternal estrogen withdrawal and resolves spontaneously within a few days.

PEDIATRIC IMMUNOLOGY

Primary immunodeficiencies are rare. Your job is simply to recognize the classic case presentations:

1. **IgA deficiency** is the most common primary immunodeficiency. Look for recurrent respiratory and GI infections. IgA levels are low.

   ➤ ***CASE SCENARIO:*** What therapy should be avoided in patients with IgA deficiency? ***Immunoglobulins,*** which may cause anaphylaxis due to anti-IgA antibodies. If a patient develops anaphylaxis after immunoglobulin exposure, think about a possible IgA deficiency.

2. **X-linked agammaglobulinemia (Bruton agammaglobulinemia)** is an X-linked recessive disorder that affects males. It is characterized by low or absent B cells and infections that begin after 6 months when maternal antibodies disappear. Look for recurrent lung or sinus infections with *Streptococcus* and *Hemophilus* spp.
3. **DiGeorge syndrome** is caused by hypoplasia of third and fourth pharyngeal pouches. Look for ***hypocalcemia*** or ***tetany*** (from absent parathyroids) in the first 24–48 hours of life, along with an absent or hypoplastic thymus. Congenital heart defects are common.
4. **Severe combined immunodeficiency** may be autosomal recessive or X-linked. Many cases are due to adenosine deaminase deficiency (autosomal recessive). Patients have B- and T-cell defects and

severe infections in the first few months of life. Cutaneous anergy usually is present. The thymus and lymph nodes may be absent or hypoplastic.

5. **Wiskott-Aldrich deficiency** is an X-linked recessive disorder that affects males. Look for the classic triad: **eczema, thrombocytopenia** (bleeding), and **recurrent infections** (usually respiratory).

6. **Chronic granulomatous disease** is usually an X-linked recessive disorder that affects males. Infections with catalase-positive organisms (e.g., *S. aureus*, *Pseudomonas* spp.) are common. The diagnosis is clinched when **deficient nitroblue tetrazolium dye reduction by granulocytes** is present (a test that measures the respiratory burst, which these patients lack).

7. **Chediak-Higashi syndrome** is usually autosomal recessive. Look for giant granules in neutrophils and associated **oculocutaneous albinism.** The syndrome is caused by a defect in microtubule polymerization.

8. **Complement deficiencies** (factors C5 through C9) cause **recurrent neisserial infections.** Specific complement components are low.

9. **Chronic mucocutaneous candidiasis** is a cellular immunodeficiency specific for *Candida* spp. Patients have thrush; candidal infections of the scalp, skin, and nails; and anergy to *Candida* spp. with skin testing. The condition often is associated with hypothyroidism; the rest of immune function is intact.

10. **Hyper-IgE syndrome (Job-Buckley syndrome)** is characterized by recurrent staphylococcal infections (especially of the skin). IgE levels are extremely high. Patients commonly have fair skin, red hair, and eczema.

PEDIATRIC INFECTIOUS DISEASE

Otitis media most commonly is due to *Streptococcus pneumoniae, Haemophilus influenzae,* and *Moraxella catarrhalis.* Manipulation of the auricle produces no pain, but the patient has earache, fever, nausea/vomiting, and erythematous and **bulging tympanic membrane** (light reflex and landmarks are difficult to see). Complications include tympanic membrane perforation (bloody or purulent discharge), mastoiditis (fluctuation and inflammation over mastoid process 2 weeks after otitis), labyrinthitis, palsies of cranial nerves VII and VIII, meningitis/cerebral abscess, venous thrombosis, and chronic otitis media. Chronic otitis media may lead to permanent perforation of eardrum, and patients may develop cholesteatomas with marginal perforations (treat with surgical excision). Treat otitis with antibiotics (amoxicillin, second-generation cephalosporin such as cefuroxime, or trimethoprim-sulfamethoxazole) to avoid these complications.

- **Recurrent otitis media** is a common pediatric clinical problem (as well as prolonged secretory otitis, a result of incompletely resolved otitis) and can cause **hearing loss with resultant developmental problems** (speech, cognitive functions). Treat with prophylactic antibiotics. Tympanostomy tubes are also used, but are now controversial. Adenoidectomy is thought to help in some cases by preventing blockage of the eustachian tubes, [illegible] screen girls < 6 after the first UTI.

Urinary tract infection (UTI). In children less than 5 years old, UTI is a cause for concern because it may be the presenting symptom of a **urinary tract malformation.** The most common examples are vesicoureteral reflux (males and females) and posterior urethral valves (males). Order a renal ultrasound and a voiding cystourethrogram to evaluate any boy under 6 years of age with a UTI and any girl under 6 with a second UTI or pyelonephritis.

Meningitis. The highest incidence of meningitis is seen in neonates; the majority of cases are seen in children younger than 2 years. Deciding when to do a lumbar puncture is difficult, because patients often do not have classic physical findings (Kernig and Brudzinski signs). Look for lethargy, fever or hypothermia, poor muscle tone, **bulging fontanelle,** vomiting, photophobia, **altered consciousness,** and signs of generalized sepsis (hypotension, jaundice, respiratory distress). Seizures also may be seen, but remember simple febrile seizures if the patient is between 5 months and 6 years old and has a fever > 102° F in the absence of other signs of meningitis. **Do not wait to start treatment** (i.e., antibiotics and IV fluids) if patients are doing poorly, even if you can't get an immediate lumbar puncture (treatment more important than precise diagnosis in this case, which is rare on the boards).

- Mumps and measles are now rare causes of aseptic (nonbacterial or culture-negative) meningitis. The best prevention is immunization.
- Watch for herpes encephalitis if the mother has herpes simplex virus (HSV) genital lesions at delivery. In older children and adults, herpes encephalitis is due to HSV-I (versus HSV-II in neonates) and those affected will have **temporal lobe abnormalities on a head CT scan or MRI.** Give acyclovir.

See neurology section for cerebrospinal fluid (CSF) findings in meningitis.

> ➤ **CASE SCENARIO:** A child has high fever, photophobia, vomiting, poor muscle tone, and altered level of consciousness. Vital signs include hypotension and tachycardia. Which should you do first—give antibiotics and IV fluids or perform lumbar puncture? Give antibiotics and IV fluids first. Empirical treatment may save the child's life, and delaying therapy is inappropriate, especially with new direct antigen tests that make CSF culture less important.

> ➤ **CASE SCENARIO:** A child recovers from a bout of meningitis after antibiotics. What does the child need as part of routine follow up? Formal hearing evaluation to check for hearing loss, the most common sequela of meningitis. Other sequelae include vision loss, mental retardation, motor deficits/paresis, epilepsy and learning/behavioral disorders.

> ➤ **CASE SCENARIO:** A child develops meningitis, and antibiotics are given. The direct antigen test is positive for *Neisseria meningitidis*. What do you need to do other than take care of the child? Give all the child's close contacts antibiotic prophylaxis (rifampin, ceftriaxone, or ciprofloxacin [in adults] usually given).

Infectious rashes are seen most often in children. Only supportive treatment is needed unless otherwise specified.

1. **Measles (rubeola).** Look for a reason for the patient not to be immunized. **Koplik spots** (tiny white spots on buccal mucosa) are seen 3 days after high fever, cough, runny nose, and conjunctivitis/photophobia. On the following day, a maculopapular rash begins on the head and neck and spreads downward to cover the trunk (head-to-toe progression). Complications include pneumonia ("giant-cell" pneumonia, especially in very young and immunocompromised patients), otitis media, and encephalitis (either an acute form or **subacute sclerosing panencephalitis,** which usually occurs years later).
2. **Rubella (German measles)** is most important because of infection in pregnant mothers. Screen and immunize any woman of reproductive age before she becomes pregnant. Rubella is milder than measles, with low fever, malaise, and tender swelling of the **suboccipital and postauricular nodes.** Arthralgias also may develop. After a 2- to 3-day prodrome, a faint maculopapular rash starts on the face and neck and spreads to the trunk (head-to-toe progression). Complications include encephalitis and otitis media.

   > ➤ **CASE SCENARIO:** A pregnant woman says that she was not vaccinated for rubella. She is 6 weeks pregnant. What should you do? Draw a baseline titer and observe. The vaccine is contraindicated during pregnancy. Then, if woman gets febrile illness during pregnancy, recheck titer to see if it has risen to make diagnosis.

3. **Roseola infantum (exanthem subitum).** Look for classic progression: high fever (may be > 40° C with febrile seizures) with no apparent cause for 4 days, then an abrupt return to normal temperature as a diffuse macular/maculopapular rash appears on the chest and abdomen. Roseola infantum is rare in children older than 3 years. It is caused by the **human herpesvirus type 6** (a DNA herpes family virus).

4. **Erythema infectiosum (fifth disease).** The classic **"slapped-cheek" rash** (confluent erythema over the cheeks) appears around the same time as mild constitutional symptoms (low fever, malaise). One day later, a maculopapular rash appears on the arms, legs, and trunk. Fifth disease is caused by **parvovirus B19** (the same virus that causes aplastic crisis in sickle cell disease).

5. **Chickenpox (varicella).** The description and progression of the rash should lead to the diagnosis. **Discrete macules (usually on the trunk) turn into papules, which turn into vesicles, which rupture and crust over.** These changes occur within 1 day. The lesions appear in successive crops; therefore, the rash is in different stages of progression in different areas. A **Tzanck smear** of tissue from the base of a vesicle shows multinucleated giant cells (rarely required for diagnosis). Varicella-zoster immune globulin is available for prophylaxis in patients with debilitating illness (e.g., leukemia, AIDS) if you see them within 4 days of exposure or for newborns whose mother has chickenpox. Acyclovir can be used in severe cases.

   Reactivation of the virus later in life can cause **shingles (zoster),** which are characterized by a dermatomal distribution of the rash. Pain and paresthesias often precede the rash. A person with active shingles can cause chickenpox in a person who has never been vaccinated or had chickenpox before.

   > ➤ ***CASE SCENARIO:*** A 14-year-old boy develops chickenpox, and the mother asks when he will no longer be contagious. What should you tell her? The child is contagious until the last lesion crusts over.

6. **Scarlet fever.** Look for a history of untreated streptococcal pharyngitis (only species that produce **erythrogenic toxin** can cause scarlet fever), followed by a sandpaper-like rash on the abdomen and trunk with classic **circumoral pallor** (i.e., area not affected by the rash) and a strawberry tongue. The rash tends to desquamate once the fever subsides. Treat with penicillin to prevent rheumatic fever from developing.

7. **Kawasaki syndrome** (mucocutaneous lymph node syndrome) is a rare disease that usually affects children younger than 5 years. Diagnostic criteria include **fever for longer than 5 days** (mandatory for diagnosis); bilateral **conjunctival injection;** changes in the lips, tongue, or oral mucosa (**strawberry tongue,** fissuring, injection); changes in the extremities (desquamation, edema, erythema); polymorphous **truncal rash** (which usually begins 1 day after the fever starts); and cervical lymphadenopathy. Also look for arthralgia/arthritis. The most feared complications involve the heart (**coronary artery aneurysms,** heart failure, arrhythmias, myocarditis, myocardial infarction). If Kawasaki syndrome is suspected, give **aspirin** and **IV immune globulin** (both reduce cardiac/coronary damage), and follow patient with echocardiography to detect heart involvement. This is one of the few times that aspirin is given to a pediatric patient.

8. **Infectious mononucleosis** (Epstein-Barr virus [EBV] infection). Look for fatigue, fever, pharyngitis, and lymphadenopathy (similar to streptococcal pharyngitis, but malaise tends to be prolonged and pronounced in EBV infection). To differentiate from streptococcal infection, look for **splenomegaly** (splenic rupture is rare, but patients should avoid contact sports and heavy lifting), hepatomegaly, **atypical lymphocytes** (bizarre forms that may resemble leukemia) with lymphocytosis, anemia/thrombocytopenia, and positive serology (**heterophile antibodies** [e.g., Monospot test] or specific EBV antibodies: viral capsid antigen, Ebstein-Barr nuclear antigen). Remember HIV in the differential diagnosis. EBV is associated with **nasopharyngeal carcinoma** and **African Burkitt lymphoma.**

   > ➤ ***CASE SCENARIO:*** A 22-year-old woman presents with a sore throat. She is given amoxicillin for presumed streptococcal infection and returns 3 days later with a diffuse maculopapular rash (see figure). Her sore throat has not improved. Does she have an allergy to amoxicillin? No—she has EBV infection. A rash occurs in roughly 90% of patients with EBV who are given ampicillin.

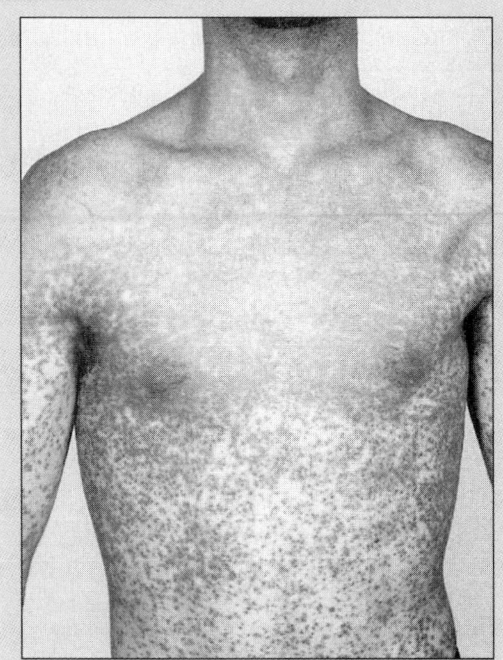

Toxic erythema. Nearly all patients who take amoxicillin or ampicillin for a sore throat that is due to the Epstein-Barr virus develop an erythematous rash, typically maculopapular. (From du Vivier A: Reactive disorders of the skin and adverse drug reactions. In du Vivier A (ed): Atlas of Clinical Dermatology, 3rd ed. New York, Churchill Livingstone, 2002, pp 367–416, with permission.)

9. **Rocky Mountain spotted fever** (*Rickettsia rickettsii* infection). Look for history of a **tick bite** (especially on the east coast) 1 week before the development of high fever or chills, severe headache, and prostration or severe malaise. The rash appears roughly 4 days after symptoms and **starts on the palms or wrists and soles or ankles, rapidly spreading to the trunk** and face (unique pattern of spread; see figure). Patients often are quite sick (disseminated intravascular coagulation, delirium) and need doxycycline (preferred) or chloramphenicol immediately.

10. **Impetigo.** Look for a history of skin break (e.g., previous chickenpox, insect bite, scabies, cut). Rash starts as thin walled vesicles that rupture and form yellowish crusts. The skin often is described as "weeping." Classically, lesions are seen on the face and tend to be localized. Impetigo is infectious; look for sick contacts. Treat with oral antistaphylococcal penicillin (to cover streptococci and staphylococci, the most common causative organisms).

Pediatric respiratory infections. The big three are croup, epiglottitis, and respiratory syncytial virus (RSV).

1. **Croup (acute laryngotracheitis).** Most patients are **1–2 years old.** Croup usually occurs in the fall or winter, and 50–75% of cases are due to **parainfluenza virus.** The other causative agent is influenza. Patients first develop symptoms of a viral upper respiratory infection (URI), such as rhinorrhea, cough, and fever. Roughly 1–2 days later, patients have a **"barking" cough,** hoarseness, and inspiratory stridor. The **"steeple sign"** (narrowing of the trachea just below the vocal cords due to subglottic edema) is classic on an AP x-ray of the neck, but is insensitive and nonspecific. Treat supportively with **humidified oxygen** (e.g., the "mist tent") and **racemic epinephrine.** Corticosteroids are controversial and take time to work.

2. **Epiglottitis.** Most patients are **2–7 years old.** The main cause is ***H. influenzae* type b,** thus widespread vaccination has decreased the incidence significantly. *S. pneumoniae* and *S. aureus* are are other potential causes. Look for little or no prodrome, with **rapid progression** to high fever, toxic appearance, **drooling,** and respiratory distress. No cough is present. The **"thumb sign"** (i.e., enlarged epiglottis looks like a thumb) is classic on lateral neck x-ray. Do not examine the throat or irritate the child in any way—you may precipitate airway obstruction! When a case of epiglottitis is presented, the first step is to **be prepared to establish an airway** (i.e., intubate, or perform a tracheostomy if needed). Treat with antibiotics (e.g., third-generation cephalosporin).

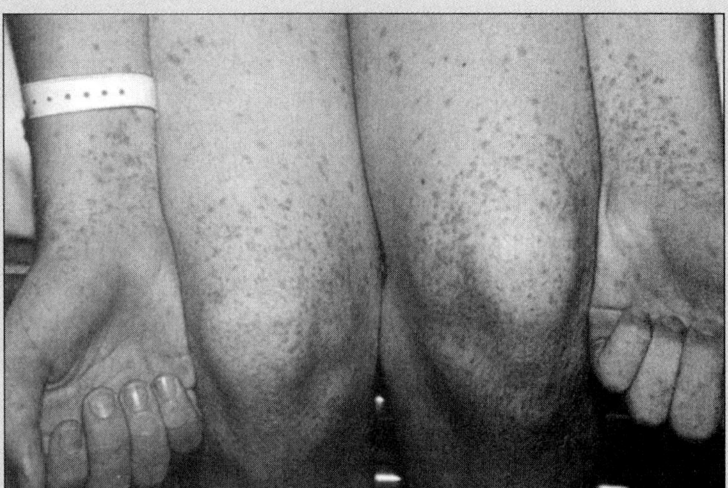

Rocky Mountain spotted fever. The petechial, macular rash characteristically starts on the palms, wrists, and lower extremities, then spreads toward the trunk. (From du Vivier A: Bacterial and spirochaetal infections. In du Viveier A (ed): Atlas of Dermatology, 3rd ed. New York, Churchill Livingstone, 2002, p 280, with permission.)

3. **RSV/bronchiolitis.** Most patients are **≤ 18 months.** Bronchiolitis usually occurs in the fall or winter, and > 75% of cases are caused by **respiratory syncytial virus (RSV).** Other causes are parainfluenza and influenza. Initial symptoms of viral URI are followed 1–2 days later by rapid respirations, intercostal retractions, and **expiratory wheezing.** Crackles may be heard on auscultation of the chest. Diffuse hyperinflation of the lungs is classic on x-rays; look for flattened diaphragms. Treat supportively (humidified oxygen, saline nasal drops, bronchodilators, IV fluids). Use **ribavarin** treatment only in patients with severe symptoms and high risk (cyanosis, other health problems). **Palivizumab** prophylaxis (a monoclonal antibody against RSV) can be used in very premature children and those with chronic lung disease during RSV season.

4. **Diphtheria** (*Corynebacterium diphtheriae*) and **pertussis** (*Bordetella pertussis*). Consider both if the patient has not been immunized. Diphtheria is associated with **grayish pseudomembranes** (necrotic epithelium and inflammatory exudate) on the pharynx, tonsils, and uvula, and myocarditis. Pertussis is associated with severe paroxysmal coughing and a high-pitched, whooping inspiratory noise (classically called "**whooping cough**"). Treat both with antibiotics; for diphtheria, add an antitoxin.

Streptococcus pyogenes (group A streptococcus) causes multiple important infections. The most common is **pharyngitis.** Look for sore throat with fever, tonsillar exudate, enlarged tender cervical nodes, and leukocytosis. Streptococcal throat culture confirms the diagnosis. The "rapid strep test" is more commonly used, as results are available within minutes. Do *not* treat empirically without a positive test. Elevated titers of antistreptolysin O and anti-DNase can be used retrospectively, as needed (e.g., to diagnose rheumatic fever or poststreptococcal glomerulonephritis). Treat with **penicillin** to avoid rheumatic fever and scarlet fever.

1. **Rheumatic fever.** The diagnosis is based on a history of streptococcal pharyngitis and the Jones criteria: major (**migratory polyarthritis, carditis, chorea, erythema marginatum** [see figure], **subcutaneous nodules**) and minor (elevated sedimentation rate, elevated levels of C-reactive protein, increased WBC count, elevated streptococcal antibody titer, prolonged PR interval on EKG, arthralgia). Treat with anti-inflammatories and corticosteroids (if needed) for carditis.

2. **Scarlet fever.** Some untreated pharyngitis cases progress to scarlet fever if the streptococcal species produces erythrogenic toxin. Symptoms include a red flush to the skin (which blanches with pressure and classically is associated with **circumoral pallor**), truncal rash, strawberry tongue, and late skin desquamation. Remember **Kawasaki syndrome** as another cause of this set of symptoms.

3. **Poststreptococcal glomerulonephritis** occurs most commonly after a skin infection but may occur after pharyngitis. The patient presents with a history of infection by a nephritogenic streptococcal strain 1–3 weeks earlier and abrupt onset of **hematuria,** proteinuria (mild—not in the nephrotic range), **RBC casts ("smoke-colored urine"** is the classic symptom), **hypertension,** edema (especially periorbital), and elevated BUN/creatinine. Treat supportively. Control blood pressure, and use diuretics for severe edema.

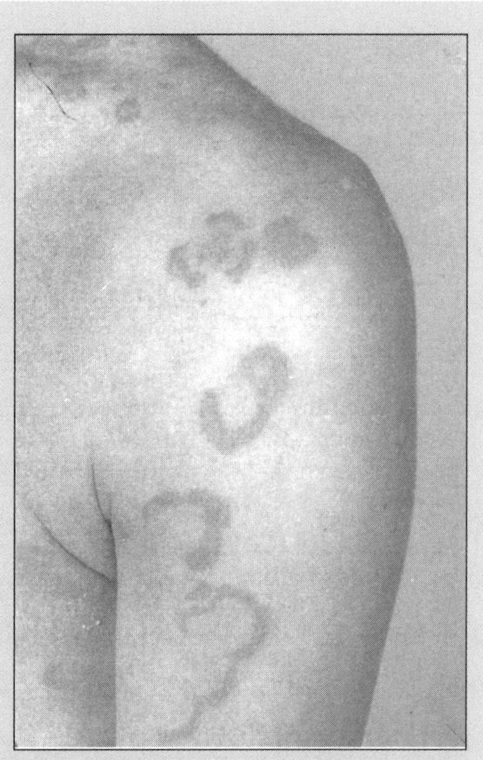

Erythema marginatum. The rash is classically flat to slightly elevated, erythematous and annular (ring-like) in appearance. (From Forbes CD, Jackson WF: Cardiovascular disorders. In Forbes CD, Jackson WF: Atlas and Text of Clinical Medicine. London, Mosby-Wolfe, 1993, pp 209–264, with permission.)

> ➤ *CASE SCENARIO:* Of the three above conditions, which can be prevented by giving antibiotics for strep throat? Rheumatic fever and scarlet fever. Glomerulonephritis cannot be prevented by treating strep throat.

Streptococcus agalactiae (streptococcus B) is the most common cause of neonatal meningitis and sepsis. The organism is acquired from the maternal birth canal, where it is part of the normal flora. Pregnant mothers are tested and treated (with amoxicillin) near term to prevent neonatal infection, a measure that has reduced the incidence significantly.

TORCH syndromes. Most TORCH intrauterine fetal infections can cause mental retardation, microcephaly, hydrocephalus, hepatosplenomegaly, jaundice, anemia, low birth weight, and/or IUGR:

1. ***Toxoplasma gondii.*** Look for ***maternal exposure to cats.*** Specific defects include intracranial calcifications and chorioretinitis.
2. **Other.** *Varicella-zoster* infection is associated with limb hypoplasia and ***scarring of the skin,*** whereas ***syphilis*** is associated with rhinitis, saber shins, **Hutchinson teeth,** interstitial keratitis, and skin lesions.
3. **Rubella.** Some physicians recommend abortion if the mother contracts rubella in the first trimester, when the effects on the fetus are worst. Check maternal antibody status on the first prenatal visit if the immunization history is uncertain. Look for cardiovascular defects (patent ductus, ventricular septal defect), deafness, cataracts, and microphthalmia in the newborn.
4. **Cytomegalovirus (CMV)** is the most common TORCH infection. Look for deafness, cerebral calcifications, and microphthalmia.
5. **Herpes.** Look for ***vesicular skin lesions*** (with positive Tzanck smears) and history of maternal herpes lesions.

   Note: With all in utero infections that cause problems with the fetus, the mother may have a subclinical infection and be asymptomatic. The infant may also be asymptomatic at birth but develop symptoms at a later date.

PEDIATRIC NEUROLOGY

The "floppy" baby. Two specific concerns in infants with hypotonia/flaccidity are a genetic disorder and infant botulism:

1. **Werdnig-Hoffman disease** is an autosomal recessive degeneration of anterior horn cells in the spinal cord and brainstem (lower motor neurons). Most infants are hypotonic at birth, and all are affected by 6 months. Look for a positive family history. The disease onset and course are ***long and slowly progressive;*** treatment is supportive.
2. **Infant botulism.** Look for ***sudden onset*** in a previously normal child and a history of ***honey*** ingestion (or other ***home-canned foods***). Diagnosis can be made by finding *Clostridium botulinum* toxin or organisms in the feces. Treatment is given in the hospital, with close monitoring of respiratory status because the child may need intubation for respiratory muscle paralysis. Spontaneous recovery usually occurs within a week.

Muscular dystrophy (most commonly ***Duchenne*** muscular dystrophy) is an **X-linked** recessive disorder of ***dystrophin*** that usually presents in boys aged 3–7 years. Look for muscle weakness, ***markedly elevated creatine phosphokinase* (CPK),** and pseudohypertrophy of the calves (due to fatty and fibrous infiltration of the degenerating muscles). IQ often is less than normal. ***Gower sign*** is classic (when patients attempt to rise from a prone position, they "walk" their hands and feet towards each other). Muscle biopsy establishes the diagnosis. Treatment is supportive. Most patients die by age 20. Other muscular dystrophies:

1. **Becker muscular dystrophy:** also an X-linked recessive dystrophin problem but milder.
2. **Mitochondrial myopathies:** rare but interesting because they are inherited as mitochondrial defects (passed only from mother to offspring; males cannot transmit). Key phrase is "**ragged red fibers**" on biopsy specimen. **Ophthalmoplegia** is classically present.
3. **Myotonic dystrophy:** autosomal dominant disorder that presents between 20 and 30 years of age. Myotonia (inability of muscles to relax) classically presents as **inability to relax the grip** (e.g., the patient cannot release a handshake). Look for coexisting **mental retardation, baldness,** and testicular or ovarian atrophy. Treatment is supportive and includes genetic counseling. The diagnosis is made on clinical grounds.

Glycogen storage diseases (autosomal recessive) are a rare cause of muscular weakness. **McArdle** disease is characterized by a relatively mild deficiency in glycogen phosphorylase and presents in young patients with **weakness and cramping after exercise.**

Neural tube defects. A triangular patch of hair over the lumbar spine indicates spina bifida occulta, which is asymptomatic and common. More serious defects are usually obvious and occur most commonly in the lumbosacral region (**meningocele** is meninges outside the spinal canal; **myelomenigocele** is CNS tissue plus meninges outside the spinal canal). Most importantly, giving folate to potential mothers reduces the incidence of neural tube defects.

Hydrocephalus. In children, look for abnormally **increasing head circumference,** increased intracranial pressure, **bulging fontanelle,** scalp vein engorgement, and paralysis of upward gaze. Large ventricles are seen on CT scan or MRI, the confirmatory tests. The most common causes include congenital malformations, tumors, and inflammation (after hemorrhage or meningitis). Treat the underlying cause if possible; otherwise, a surgical shunt is created to decompress the ventricles.

PEDIATRIC ONCOLOGY

The most common malignancy in children is **acute lymphocytic leukemia** (ALL). Patients classically presents with pancytopenia. Watch for bleeding, signs of anemia, and infection. Patients with **Down syndrome** have a much higher risk than the general population.

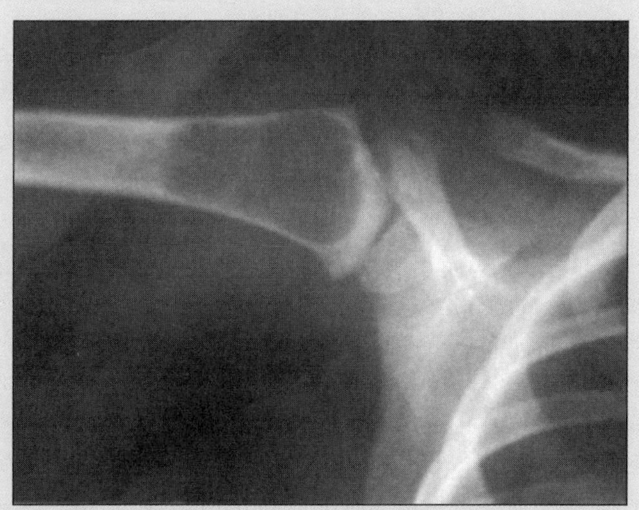

Unicameral (simple) bone cyst. (From West SG: Rheumatology Secrets. Phildelphia, Hanley & Belfus, 1997, with permission.)

Brain tumors in children usually are located in the posterior fossa (e.g., **cerebellum** or **brainstem**). Classic symptoms are due to increased intracranial pressure (vomiting, headaches) and tumor location (seizures, hydrocephalus, ataxia). The most common types are cerebellar **astrocytoma** and **medulloblastoma,** followed by ependymoma.

Wilms tumor vs. neuroblastoma. Both present as **flank masses** in young children. If the patient is younger than 6 months, neuroblastoma is more likely, but a tissue diagnosis is always obtained. Both have a peak incidence at around 2 years of age. Wilms tumor is much more common overall. Wilms tumor comes from kidney, neuroblastoma usually from the adrenal gland. Rarely, neuroblastomas may regress spontaneously (for unknown reasons). These tumors are the most common primary malignanacies of their respective organs in children. **Hepatoblastoma** is the classic and most common primary liver malignancy in young children.

Retinoblastoma is characterized by **leukocoria** in a young child (red reflex is white with a penlight) or unilateral exophthalmos. Tumor may be bilateral in the inherited form.

Unicameral bone cyst (i.e., simple bone cyst) is an expansile, lytic, well-demarcated lesion usually in the proximal portion of the humerus in children and adolescents (see figure). It is benign but may weaken bone enough to cause a pathologic fracture.

Osteosarcoma occurs in 10- to 20-year-olds, usually about the knee (distal femur, proximal tibia), and has a classic "**sunburst**" appearance of the associated periosteal reaction on x-ray. A mass may be palpable on exam.

PEDIATRIC OPHTHALMOLOGY

Neonatal conjunctivitis is classically due to one of three causes (though typical adult bacterial and viral etiologies are also possible during the neonatal period):

1. **Chemical reaction.** Silver nitrate, erythromycin or tetracycline drops are given prophylactically to newborns to prevent gonorrheal conjunctivitis. The drops may cause a chemical conjunctivitis (with no purulent discharge), which develops within 6–12 hours of instilling the drops and resolves within 48 hours. **Chemical reaction is "always" the answer if conjunctivitis appears in the first 24 hours of life.**
2. **Gonorrhea.** Look for symptoms of gonorrhea in the mother. The infant has an extremely purulent discharge that **starts 2–5 days after birth.** Treatment is topical (erythromycin ointment) plus IV or IM third-generation cephalosporin (e.g., ceftriaxone). Infants who are given prophylactic drops should not develop gonorrheal conjunctivitis.
3. **Chlamydial infection (inclusion conjunctivitis).** The mother often reports no symptoms. The infant has mild-to-severe conjunctivitis, which **begins 5–14 days after birth.** Patients must be treated with systemic antibiotics (oral erythromycin is the usual choice) to prevent chlamydial pneumonia, a common complication. Prophylactic eye drops do not effectively prevent chlamydial conjunctivitis.

> **CASE SCENARIO:** What is the most important point in the history for neonatal conjunctivitis? The age at presentation (≤ 1 day = chemical, 2–5 days = gonococcal; 5–14 days = chlamydial).

Cataracts in a neonate should make you think of **TORCH infections** or an inherited metabolic disorder (e.g., **galactosemia**).

Strabismus/amblyopia. Any child with a "lazy eye" (strabismus: the eye deviates, usually inward) that persists beyond 3 months of age needs ophthalmologic referral. This condition does not resolve and may cause blindness (amblyopia) in the affected eye. For this reason, visual screening must be done in all children. The visual system continues to develop until the age of 7 or 8 years. If one eye cannot see well or is turned outward, the brain cannot fuse the two different images and suppresses the bad eye. Thus the bad eye does not develop the proper neural connections and will never see well. Glasses will not correct the problem, which is neural rather than refractive.

Be able to differentiate **orbital cellulitis** from **preorbital cellulitis** (i.e., preseptal cellulitis). Both may be associated with swollen lids, fever, chemosis (swollen conjunctiva), and a history of facial laceration, trauma, or insect bite or sinusitis. **Ophthalmoplegia, proptosis, severe eye pain, or decreased visual acuity generally indicates orbital cellulitis** (an emergency). The most common causative agents in both are *Streptococcus pneumoniae*, *Hemophilus influenzae*, and staphylococci or streptococci (in patients with a history of trauma). Complications of orbital cellulitis include extension into the skull, dural sinus thrombosis, and blindness. Treat either condition with blood cultures and administration of broad-spectrum antibiotics until culture results are known. Inpatient IV antibiotics are needed for orbital cellulitis; surgery may be required for orbital abscess.

PEDIATRIC ORTHOPEDIC SURGERY

Pediatric hip problems:

NAME	AGE	EPIDEMIOLOGY	SYMPTOMS/SIGNS*	TREATMENT
CHD	At birth	Female, first-born, breech delivery	Barlow's and Ortolani's signs	Harness
LCP	4–10 yr	Male, short with delayed bone age	Knee, thigh, and groin pain, limp	Orthoses
SCFE	9–13 yr	Overweight, male, adolescent	Knee, thigh, and groin pain, limp	Surgical pinning

CHD = congenital hip dysplasia, LCP = Legg-Calvé-Perthes disease, SCFE = slipped capital femoral epiphysis (see figure).

*Pediatric hip problems are notorious for causing referred pain in the knee, but the knee is not tender, swollen, or otherwise abnormal.

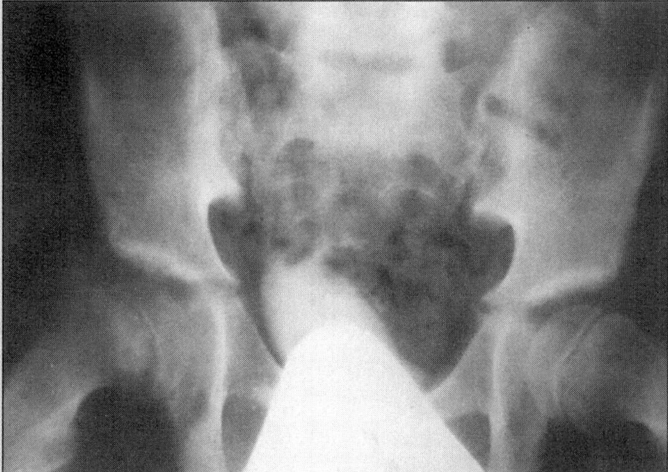

Slipped capital femoral epiphysis. The right femoral head is displaced medially and posteriorly relative to the right femoral shaft. (From Katz DS, Math KR, Groskin SA: Radiology Secrets. Philadelphia, Hanley & Belfus, 1998, with permission.)

➤ ***CASE SCENARIO:*** How do the above-mentioned hip disorders classically present in adults? As arthritis of the hip. Given the correct history (especially age at onset of symptoms), you may be able to tell which disorder the patient had. X-rays may be shown, but history can help you guess the answer if you are unsure.

Osgood-Schlatter disease is an osteochondritis of the tibial tubercle that is often bilateral and usually presents between 10 and 15 years of age in males with pain, swelling, and tenderness to palpation in the knee. Treat with rest, activity restriction, and NSAIDs. Most cases resolve spontaneously.

Scoliosis usually affects prepubertal girls and is idiopathic. Mild cases are observed. In more severe cases, treat with a brace. For deformities that are rapidly progressive or cause respiratory compromise, consider surgery. Check for scoliosis by having patient touch his or her toes while you look at the spine. An abnormal lateral curvature is seen in patients with scoliosis (see figure).

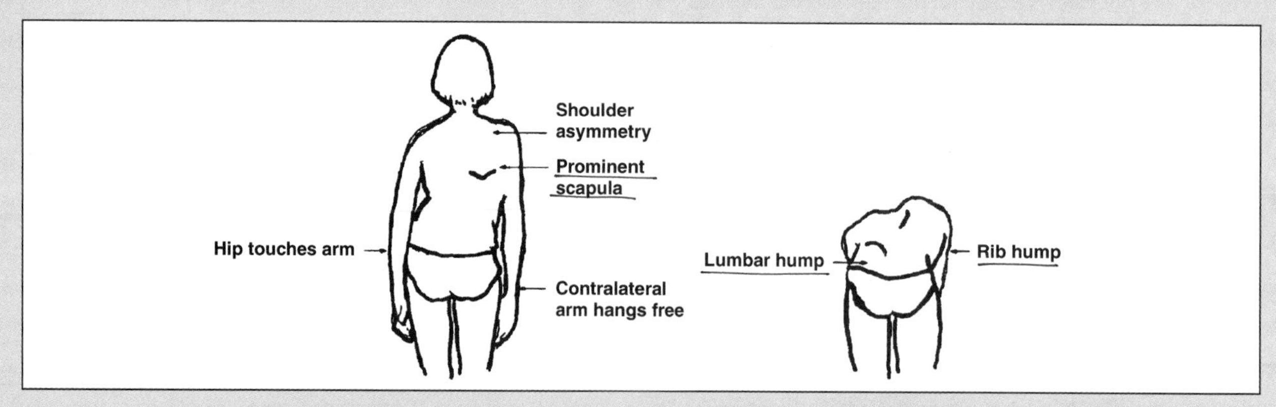

Scoliosis screening test showing the most important diagnostic features. (From Staheli LT: Pediatric Orthopedic Secrets. Philadelphia, Hanley & Belfus, 1998, with permisson.)

> ➤ **CASE SCENARIO:** A 4 year-old girl presents with irritated, red eyes. The mother also mentions that the child has been limping lately and has had a swollen, hot left knee for about 4 weeks. Rheumatoid factor is negative. Joint aspiration reveals inflammatory reaction in the joint fluid with no crystals or bacteria, and the culture is negative. What is the likely diagnosis and how should the eye symptoms be managed? The likely diagnosis is juvenile rheumatoid arthritis, which often has a negative rheumatoid factor. The child needs referral to an ophthalmologist for treatment of probable uveitis, which can be confirmed with a slit-lamp exam and requires treatment with steroid drops.

PEDIATRIC PSYCHIATRY

Eighty-five percent of cases of **mental retardation** (MR) are mild (IQ range = 55–70), and most are idiopathic. Patients can have a reasonable level of independence, with assistance or guidance during periods of stress. Look for **fetal alcohol syndrome,** which is the number-one preventable cause of MR. Down syndrome (number one overall cause of MR) and **fragile-X syndrome** (in boys) are other common causes.

Autism usually starts at a young age. Look for impaired social interaction (e.g., the child is isolated, unaware of surroundings), impaired verbal and nonverbal communication (e.g., strange words, babbling, repetition), and restricted activities and interests (e.g., head banging, strange movements). Autism is usually idiopathic, but look for congenital rubella as a potential cause. Occasionally, children have restricted, high-level abilities (i.e., "idiot savant"), as with Dustin Hoffman's character in the movie *The Rain Man*.

Learning disorder. Math, reading, writing, speech, language, or coordination is impaired, but everything else is normal. No mental retardation is present. ("Johnny just can't do math.")

Conduct disorder. Look for fire-setting, cruelty to animals, lying, stealing, and/or fighting.

> ➤ **CASE SCENARIO:** A 10-year-old boy repeatedly starts fires, lies, steals, and tortures animals. What disorder will the child likely have when he is an adult? Antisocial personality disorder (in fact, conduct disorder is required in order to make a diagnosis of antisocial personality disorder in adults).

Attention deficit-hyperactivity disorder (ADHD). As the name implies, affected children are hyperactive and have short attention spans. Boys develop the disorder more often than girls. Look for a fidgety child who is impulsive and cannot pay attention but is not cruel. Treat with stimulants (paradoxical calming effect) such as **modafinil** (Provigil), **methylphenidate** (Ritalin), and dextroamphetamine, all of which can cause **insomnia, abdominal pain, anorexia,** and **weight loss/growth suppression.** ADHD has become a hot topic because of concerns about overdiagnosis and overtreatment. Use "drug holidays" (stop drug for a brief period) to combat side effects.

Oppositional-defiant disorder. Affected children exhibit negative, hostile, and defiant behavior toward authority figures (e.g., parents or teachers). Such children may be a "pain in the butt," but only around adults; they are **normal around peers.** They are *not* cruel, lying, or criminally inclined.

Separation anxiety disorder. Look for a child who refuses to go to school. Basically, affected children think something will happen to them or their parents if they separate. Patients will do anything, from claiming to have **stomachache** or **headache** to throwing temper tantrums, to avoid separation.

Anorexia. Look for a female adolescent who is a good athlete, ballerina, and/or student with a perfectionist personality. With a body weight at least 15% below normal, the affected girl exhibits an intense fear of gaining weight, "feels fat" even though she is emaciated, and suffers from **amenorrhea.** All three are required for diagnosis. Death occurs in roughly 10–15% of patients from complications of starvation and/or bulimia (e.g., electrolyte imbalances, cardiac arrhythmias, infections). Patients are sometimes hospitalized against their will for IV nutrition. Roughly half of anorexics also have bulimia.

Bulimia. Look for a female adolescent who is of normal weight or overweight (unless suffering from coexisting anorexia). The patient has binge-eating episodes, during which she feels a lack of control, and then engages in purging behaviors such as **vomiting,** using **laxatives, exercising,** or **fasting.** Such patients also may require hospitalization for electrolyte disturbances. The classic physical findings in a patient with bulimia are **eroded tooth enamel** from frequent vomiting and/or **eroded skin over the knuckles** from putting fingers in the throat to induce vomiting.

Tourette disorder. Look for boys with **motor tics** (e.g., eye-blinking, grunting, throat clearing, grimacing, barking, or shoulder shrugging) and/or random bouts of swearing that are exacerbated by stress and remit during activity or sleep. Of interest, Tourette disorder can be caused and/or unmasked by the use of stimulants (e.g., for presumed ADHD). Antipsychotics such as haloperidol are used if symptoms are severe. Tourette syndrome tends to be a life-long disorder.

Encopresis/enuresis is not a disorder until after age 4 years (encopresis) or 5 years (enuresis). Rule out physical problems such as Hirschsprung disease and infection; then treat with **behavioral therapy** (e.g., "gold-star for being good" charts, alarms, biofeedback). **Imipramine,** which is not a first-line treatment, is used only for refractory cases of enuresis.

- *CASE SCENARIO:* A mother complains about her 2-year-old daughter who still wets her bed, although less often than a year ago. What is the preferred treatment? None, because bedwetting is normal for a 2 year old, and symptoms are already improving.
- *CASE SCENARIO:* List, in order, the top three causes of death in adolescents. **Accidents, homicide,** and **suicide.** Together, they cause about 75% of teen-age deaths. In black males, homicide is the number-one cause.

PEDIATRIC PULMONOLOGY

Respiratory distress syndrome: due to atelectasis from deficiency of surfactant; almost always in premature babies and/or babies of diabetic mothers. Look for rapid, labored respirations, **substernal retractions, cyanosis, grunting** and/or **nasal flaring** at birth. Blood gas shows hypoxemia and hypercarbia, X-ray shows diffuse atelectasis. Treat with O_2, intubate if needed, and give **surfactant.** Complications include intraventricular hemorrhage and pneumothorax/bronchopulmonary dysplasia (acute/chronic mechanical ventilation complications).

> ➤ ***CASE SCENARIO:*** What is the predominant presenting symptom of a newborn with a diaphragmatic hernia? Respiratory problems. Bowel herniated into the chest pushes on developing lung and causes lung hypoplasia on the affected side. Look for scaphoid abdomen and bowel sounds in the chest. Herniated bowel is seen on chest x-ray; 90% are left-sided.

Look for **meconium aspiration** if an infant is covered with meconium when delivered. Suction secretions first from the mouth (oropharynx) and then from the nose with a bulb syringe or suction catheter immediately after the head is delivered. If intubation is needed for depressed respiratory status, suctioning through the endotracheal tube is also commonly performed.

The most common type (85%) of **tracheoesophageal fistula** is an esophagus with a blind pouch proximally and a fistula between a bronchus/carina and the distal esophagus. Look for a neonate with ***excessive oral secretions, coughing and cyanosis with attempted feedings,*** abdominal distention, and aspiration pneumonia. The diagnosis should be suspected if a nasogastric tube cannot be passed into the stomach; the tube typically becomes ***coiled in the esophagus.*** An x-ray study using air injected through the NG tube (rarely needed) shows the proximal esophagus only. Treatment is early surgical correction.

Cystic fibrosis: autosomal recessive inheritance pattern; the most common lethal genetic disease in whites. Cystic fibrosis should be suspected in all children with ***rectal prolapse, meconium ileus,*** or ***esophageal varices;*** a "salty-tasting" infant; or any child with recurrent pulmonary infections and/or failure to thrive. The diagnosis can be made by an abnormal increase in the electrolytes of sweat (sodium and chloride) or a DNA probe test. Watch for ***pancreatic insufficiency,*** which should be treated with pancreatic enzyme replacements and fat-soluble vitamin supplements; ***infertility,*** which affects 98% of males and many females; and ***cor pulmonale*** (right heart failure from lung disease). Look for *Staphylococcus aureus* and *Pseudomonas* spp. to be the cause of the many respiratory infections. Treat with chest physical therapy, annual influenza vaccine, fat-soluble vitamin supplements, pancreatic enzyme replacement, and aggressive treatment of infections with antibiotics.

PEDIATRIC UROLOGY

Cryptorchidism is arrested descent of the testicle(s) somewhere between the renal area and the scrotum. The more premature the infant, the greater the likelihood of cryptorchidism. Many of the arrested testes eventually descend on their own within the first year of life. After 1 year, surgical intervention (orchiopexy) is warranted in an attempt to preserve fertility as well as facilitate future testicular exams (because of increased cancer risk). The higher the testicle is found (the further away from the scrotum), the higher the risk of developing testicular cancer and the lower the likelihood of retaining fertility.

> ➤ ***CASE SCENARIO:*** Does surgical correction of cryptorchidism alter the risk of testicular cancer in the affected testicle? No, but may preserve fertility and facilitates testicular exam.

Penile anomalies. In hypospadias, the urethra opens on the ventral side (undersurface when flaccid) of the penis; in epispadias, the urethra opens on the dorsal side (superior surface when flaccid) of the penis. Treat both surgically.

> ➤ ***CASE SCENARIO:*** Is epispadias or hypospadias associated with exstrophy of the bladder? Epispadias.

> ➤ ***CASE SCENARIO:*** Where do the left and right gonadal veins drain? The right testicular/ovarian vein drains into the inferior vena cava, whereas the left gonadal vein drains into the left renal vein.

Potter syndrome. Bilateral renal agenesis causes oligohydramnios in utero (the fetus swallows fluid but cannot excrete it), limb deformities, abnormal facies, and hypoplasia of the lungs. Potter syndrome is incompatible with life.

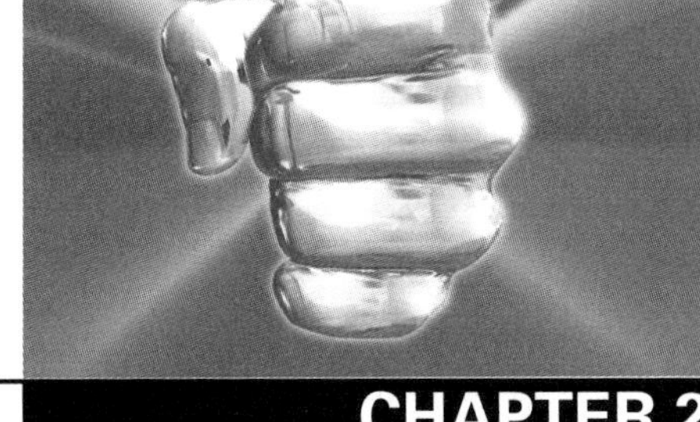

CHAPTER 2

Preventive Medicine, Epidemiology, and Biostatistics

VITAMINS AND MINERALS

VITAMIN	DEFICIENCY SIGNS AND SYMPTOMS	TOXICITY
A	Night blindness, scaly rash, xerophthalmia (dry eyes), Bitot spots (debris on conjunctiva); increased infections	Pseudotumor cerebri, bone thickening, **teratogenicity**
D	Rickets, osteomalacia, hypocalcemia	Hypercalcemia, nausea/vomiting, renal stones
E	Anemia, peripheral neuropathy, ataxia	Necrotizing enterocolitis in infants
K	Hemorrhage, prolonged prothrombin time	Hemolysis (kernicterus)
B_1 (thiamine)	Wet beriberi (high-output cardiac failure), dry beriberi (peripheral neuropathy), Wernicke/Korsakoff syndrome	
B_2 (riboflavin)	Cheilosis, angular stomatitis, dermatitis	
B_3 (niacin)	Pellagra (**d**ementia, **d**ermatitis, **d**iarrhea), stomatitis	
B_6 (pyridoxine)	Peripheral neuropathy, cheilosis, stomatitis, convulsions in infants, microcytic anemia, seborrheic dermatitis	Peripheral neuropathy (only B vitamin with known toxicity)
B_{12} (cobalamin)	Megaloblastic anemia *plus* neurologic symptoms	
Folic acid	Megaloblastic anemia *without* neurologic symptoms	
C	Scurvy (hemorrhages-skin petechiae, bone, gums; loose teeth; gingivitis), poor wound healing, hyperkeratotic hair follicles, bone pain (from periosteal hemorrhages)	

MINERAL	DEFICIENCY SIGNS AND SYMPTOMS	TOXICITY
Iodine	Goiter, cretinism, hypothyroidism	Myxedema
Fluorine	Dental caries (cavities)	Fluorosis with mottling of teeth/bone exostoses
Zinc	Hypogeusia (decreased taste), rash, slow wound healing	
Copper	Menke's disease (X-linked; kinky hair and mental retardation)	Wilson disease
Selenium	Cardiomyopathy and muscle pain	Loss of hair and nails
Manganese		"Manganese madness" in miners of ore
Chromium	Impaired glucose tolerance	

Deficiency of fat-soluble vitamins (A, D, E, K) is often due to **malabsorption** (e.g., cystic fibrosis, cirrhosis, celiac disease, sprue, pancreatic insufficiency). Parenteral supplements may be needed if high-dose oral supplements fail.

Rickets causes interesting physical and x-ray findings (see figure): craniotabes (skull is poorly mineralized and bones feel like the surface of a ping-pong ball), rachitic rosary (costochondral beading; small round masses on anterior rib cage), delayed fontanelle closure, bossing of the skull, kyphoscoliosis, bowlegs, knock-knees. Bone changes first appear at the lower ends of the radius and ulna.

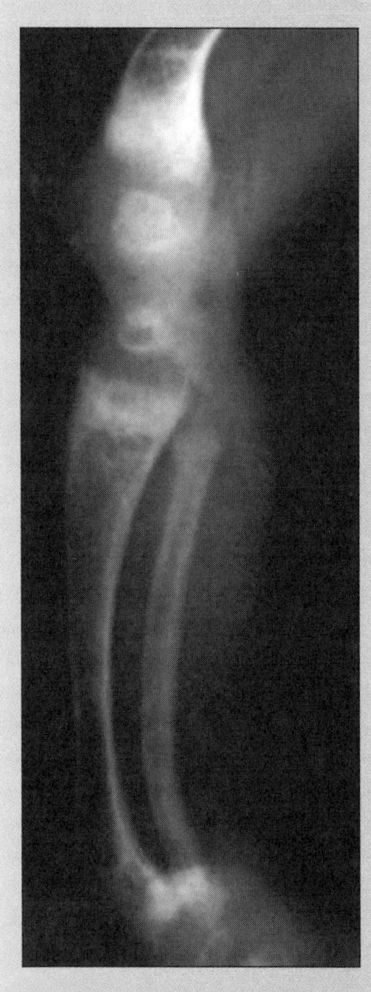

Radiologic findings in rickets. Lateral view of the lower leg. Note flared end of bones, bowing of long bones, and osteoporosis. (From West SG: Rheumatology Secrets. Philadelphia, Hanley & Belfus, 1997, with permission.)

- **CASE SCENARIO:** A 29-year-old woman with vitiligo develops numbness in her feet with decreased vibratory sense and megaloblastic anemia. She most likely has what condition? **Pernicious anemia,** the most common cause of vitamin B_{12} deficiency. This condition can be associated with other autoimmune disorders, such as vitiligo, hypothyroidism, and hypoadrenalism. Removal of the ileum and the tapeworm *Diphyllobothrium latum* are rare causes of B_{12} deficiency.
- **CASE SCENARIO:** What test is used to determine the cause of vitamin B_{12} deficiency? Schilling test.
- **CASE SCENARIO:** A 34-year-old man is put on a 6-month course of isoniazid for PPD skin test conversion. He develops tingling in his hands and feet. What vitamin deficiency might he have? Vitamin B_6 (pyridoxine).
- **CASE SCENARIO:** What test does a 22-year-old woman need before starting oral isotretinoin for acne? **Pregnancy test.** Vitamin A and its derivatives are teratogenic. She also should be offered some form of birth control and periodic pregnancy tests. Give counseling about the risks of teratogenicity.
- **CASE SCENARIO:** An infant born at home with no perinatal care develops bleeding problems shortly after birth. What is the likely nutritional cause? **Hemorrhagic disease of the newborn.** Vitamin K is given to all newborns as prophylaxis against this condition. Vitamin K is needed for the synthesis of factors II, VII, IX and X as well as proteins C and S.

➤ *CASE SCENARIO:* A patient with end-stage cirrhosis has a markedly prolonged prothrombin time. How should you treat it? With fresh frozen plasma. ***Vitamin K does not work in the setting of liver failure,*** because the liver cannot synthesize clotting proteins.

CANCER SCREENING

Guidelines for asymptomatic patients from the American Cancer Society:

CANCER	PROCEDURE	AGE (YR)	FREQUENCY
Colorectal	Sigmoidoscopy or double-contrast barium enema*	> 50	Every 5 years
	Stool occult blood test	> 50	Annually
Colon, prostate	Digital rectal exam	> 50	Annually
Prostate	Prostate-specific antigen test	> 50	Offer to patients annually, but still controversial
Cervical	Pap smear	18–65[t]	After 2 normal exams 1 year apart, every 3 years
Gynecologic	Pelvic examination	20–40 > 40	Every 3 years Annually
Endometrial	Endometrial biopsy	Menopause	Once at menopause
Breast	Breast self-examination	> 20	Monthly
	Physical exam	20–40 > 40	Every 3 years Annually
	Mammography	> 40	Annually
Cancer check-up[#]	Health counseling/exam	20–39	Every 3 years
		> 40	Annually

*Colonoscopy every 10 years is an alternative option.

[t]Start Pap smears at < 18 if patient sexually active.

[#]Includes examination for cancers of the thyroid, testis, ovary, lymph nodes, oral region, and skin.

Note: The preceding table is for screening of asymptomatic, healthy patients. Other committees have their own cancer screening recommendations, but this guide will prevent you from missing questions (controversial areas are not tested).

➤ *CASE SCENARIO:* What should you do to screen for lung cancer in a high-risk, asymptomatic patient? Nothing. No definite benefit has been shown so far.

No cancer screening: In general, urinalysis (screening for urinary tract cancer, which gives you hematuria), alpha fetoprotein (liver/gonadal cancer), and other serum markers are not appropriate for screening asymptomatic people with no physical findings, but look for these abnormal lab values as a clue to diagnosis. In high-risk individuals, screening with serum markers may be appropriate, but this is an evolving area. An example of such a screening program has been undertaken using alpha-fetoprotein (AFP) and liver ultrasound to screen for hepatocellular carcinoma in persons with cirrhosis and chronic viral hepatitis.

ADULT IMMUNIZATIONS

IMMUNIZATIONS IN ADULTS	
VACCINE	**WHICH ADULTS SHOULD RECEIVE AND OTHER INFORMATION**
Hepatitis B	Give to any adult who wants it and anyone at risk of hepatitis B (including health care workers).
Influenza	Advised for all adults over 50 and any high-risk patients (e.g., chronic respiratory, cardiovascular renal, or metabolic disease. Also give to women who will be pregnant during the influenza season (winter) and household contacts of high-risk patients (to protect the high-risk patient).
Pneumococcus	All adults over 65 and anyone with risks of higher morbidity/mortality from infection (e.g., patients with heart, lung, or kidney disease; diabetes; immunocompromise).
Rubella	All women of child-bearing age who lack immunity or history of immunization. Do not give to pregnant woman. Women should avoid pregnancy for 3 months after the vaccine. Also give to health care workers (to protect pregnant women's unborn children). Do not give to immunocompromised patients (except HIV-positive patients).
Tetanus (Td)	All people every 10 years. Give for any wound if vaccination history is unknown or patient has received < 3 total doses. Give booster in people with full vaccination history if more than 5 years have passed since last dose for all wounds other than clean, minor wounds (including burns). Give tetanus immunoglobulin with vaccine for patients with unknown/incomplete vaccination and nonclean/major wounds.

EPIDEMIOLOGY

Per-year rates that are commonly used to compare groups should be known:

- Birth rate: live births/1000 population
- Fertility rate: live births /1000 population of women aged 15–45
- Death rate: deaths/1000 population
- Neonatal mortality rate: neonatal deaths (in first 28 days)/1000 live births
- Perinatal mortality rate: neonatal deaths + stillbirths per 1000 total births. The major cause of perinatal mortality is prematurity. Rates are higher in nonwhites than in whites.

Note: A stillbirth (fetal death) is a prenatal or natal (during birth) death after 20 weeks' gestation.

- Infant mortality rate: deaths (from 0–1 year old)/1000 live births. The top three causes, in descending order, are congenital abnormalities, low birth weight/prematurity, and sudden infant death syndrome.
- Maternal mortality rate: maternal pregnancy-related deaths (deaths during pregnancy or in the first 42 days after delivery)/100,000 live births. The top three causes are pulmonary embolus, hypertension (e.g., pregnancy-induced hypertension, eclampsia), and hemorrhage. The rate increases with age and is higher in blacks.

Medicare is health insurance for people who are eligible for Social Security (primarily people > 65 years old as well as permanently/totally disabled people, and people with end-stage renal disease). Nursing home care is paid by Medicare only for a short term after a hospital admission; then it is paid by the patient (if the person has no money, the state usually pays).

Medicaid covers indigent persons who are deemed eligible by the individual states.

BIOSTATISTICS

Sensitivity: ability to detect disease; mathematically, the number of true positives divided by the number of people with the disease. Tests with high sensitivity are used for **screening;** they may have false-positive results but do not miss many people with the disease (low false-negative rate).

Specificity: ability to detect health (nondisease); mathematically, the number of true negatives divided by the number of people without the disease. Tests with high specificity are used for **disease confirmation;** they may have false-negative results but do not label as sick anyone who is actually healthy (low false-positive rate). The ideal confirmatory test must have high sensitivity *and* high specificity.Otherwise people with the disease may be called healthy.

- ***CASE SCENARIO:*** A researcher says that the cut-off fasting glucose value for the diagnosis of diabetes should be lowered from 126 mg/dl to 110 mg/dl. How would this change affect the test's number of false-negative and false-positive results? Fewer false negatives, more false positives. If the cut-off value is raised, fewer people will be called diabetic (more false negatives, fewer false positives).

Positive predictive value (PPV): when a test is positive for disease, the PPV measures how likely it is that the patient has the disease (probability of having a condition, given a positive test). Mathematically, the number of true positives is divided by the number of people with a positive test. **PPV depends on the prevalence of the disease and the sensitivity/specificity of the test** (e.g., an overly sensitive test that gives more false positives has a lower PPV).

- ***CASE SCENARIO:*** How does prevalence affect the PPV? The higher the prevalence, the greater the PPV.

Negative predictive value (NPV): when a test is negative for disease, the NPV measures how likely it is that the patient is healthy (probability of not having a condition, given a negative test). Mathematically, the number of true negatives is divided by the number of people with a negative test. Like PPV, **NPV depends on the prevalence of the disease and the sensitivity/specificity of the test** (the higher the prevalence, the lower the NPV).

- ***CASE SCENARIO:*** How does sensitivity affect NPV? The more sensitive the test, the fewer the number of false negatives and the higher the NPV.

Get in the habit of drawing a 2 × 2 table (see figure) to make calculations easier:

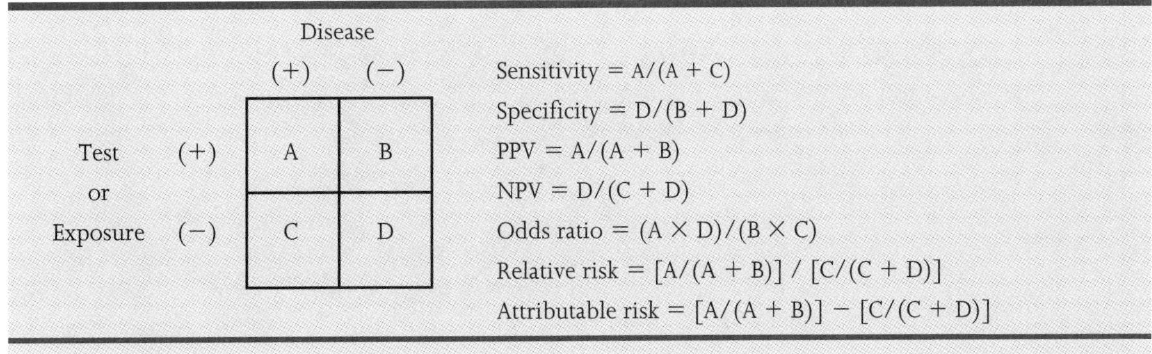

Attributable risk: number of cases attributable to one risk factor (put another way, the amount you would expect the incidence to decrease if a risk factor were removed). For example, if the incidence rate of lung cancer in the general population is 1/100 and in smokers it is 10/100, the attributable risk of smoking in causing lung cancer is 9/100, assuming a properly matched control (i.e., 10/100–1/100 = 9/100).

Relative risk: compares the disease risk in the exposed population to the disease risk in the unexposed population. **Relative risk can be calculated only after a prospective or experimental study.** A relative risk greater (or less) than one is clinically significant.

> ➤ **CASE SCENARIO:** After completing a chart and autopsy record review, a researcher finds that the incidence of pancreatic cancer is 5/1000 in smokers and 1/1000 in non-smokers. What is the relative risk of pancreatic cancer in smokers? The relative risk cannot be calculated because this is a retrospective study. Classic "fooled-you" type of question—choose "none of the above."

Odds ratio: used only for **retrospective studies** (e.g., case-control). The odds ratio compares disease in exposed and nondisease in unexposed populations with disease in unexposed and nondisease in exposed populations to determine whether there is a difference between the two. There should be more disease in exposed than unexposed populations and more nondisease in unexposed than exposed populations. The odds ratio is a less-than-perfect way to estimate relative risk from retrospective data.

> ➤ **CASE SCENARIO:** After a chart and autopsy record review, a researcher finds that the incidence of pancreatic cancer is 5/1000 in smokers and 1/1000 in nonsmokers. What is the relative risk of pancreatic cancer in smokers? Around 5 (See the 2 × 2 table for mathematical equation).

Standard deviation (SD): with a normal or bell-shaped distribution, 1 SD holds 68% of values, 2 SDs hold 95% of values, and 3 SDs hold 99.7% of values. In a normal distribution, the **mean = median = mode** (mean is the average value, median is the middle value, and mode is the most common value).

> ➤ **CASE SCENARIO:** A child scores 140 on an IQ test. A review of the literature reveals that the mean IQ in the child's community is 100, with an SD of 20. How does the child's score compare with that of other children? The child did better on the exam than 95% of children in the community.

Skewed distribution: a **positive skew** is asymmetry with an excess of high values (tail on right, mean > median > mode); a **negative skew** is asymmetry with an excess of low values (tail on left, mean < median < mode). Because positive and negative skews (see figure) are *not* normal distributions, standard deviation and mean are less meaningful values.

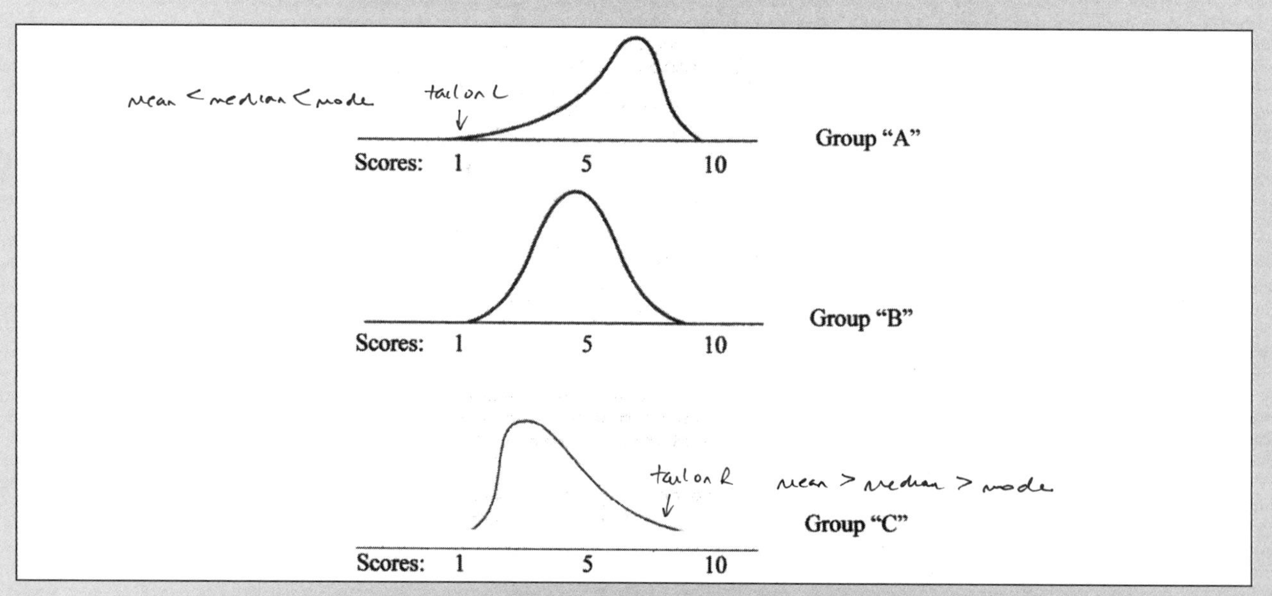

Group A demonstrates a negative skew (tail on the left), group B has a normal distribution, and group C has a positive skew (tail on the right).

Test reliability (synonymous with **precision**) measures the reproducibility and consistency of a test (e.g., the concept of interrater reliability: if two different people administer the same test, the examinee will get the same score if the test is reliable). **Random error reduces reliability/precision** (e.g., limitation in significant figures).

Test validity (synonymous with **accuracy**) measures the trueness of measurement—whether the test measures what it claims to measure (e.g., if you give a valid IQ test to a genius, the test should not indicate that he or she is retarded). **Systematic error reduces validity/accuracy** (e.g., miscalibrated equipment).

Correlation coefficient measures how related two values are (see figure). The range of the coefficient is −1 to +1. The important point in determining the strength of the relationship between two variables is how far the number is from zero (i.e. **absolute value**). Zero equals no association whatsoever, +1 equals a perfect positive correlation (when one goes up, so does the other), and −1 equals a perfect negative correlation.

➤ ***CASE SCENARIO:*** Which is a stronger correlation, + 0.3 or −0.3? They are equal.

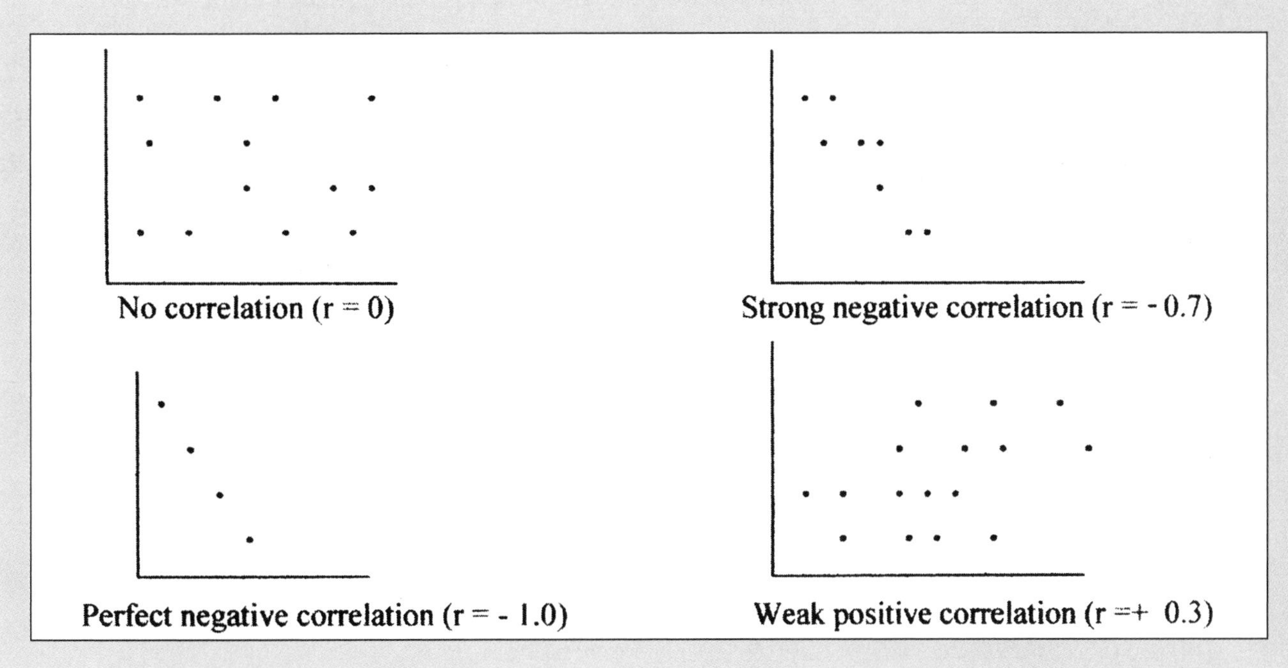

Confidence interval: when you take a set of data and calculate a mean, you want to say that the result is equivalent to the mean of the whole population, but usually the two values are not exactly equal. The confidence interval (usually set at 95%) says that you are 95% confident that the mean of the population is within a certain range (usually within 2 SD of your experimental or derived mean). For example, if you sample the heart rate of 100 people and calculate a mean of 80 beats/minute and a SD of 2, your confidence interval (confidence limits) would be written as $76 < X < 84 = 0.95$. This means that you are 95% certain that the mean heart rate of the whole population (X) is between 76 and 84, even though you sampled only a small percentage of the community.

Different types of studies (listed in decreasing order of quality and desirability):

1. **Experimental:** the gold standard type of study. Compares two equal groups in which one variable is manipulated and its effect is measured. Remember to check for double-blinding (or at least single-blinding) and well-matched controls.

2. **Prospective/longitudinal/cohort/incidence/follow-up:** choose a sample population, divide it into two groups based on presence or absence of a risk factor, and follow the groups over time to see what diseases they develop. This approach sometimes is called an **observational study** because all you do is observe. For example, you may follow people with and without asymptomatic hypercholesterolemia to determine whether people with hypercholesterolemia have a higher incidence of myocardial infarction later in life. You can calculate relative risk and incidence. This type of study is time-consuming, expensive, and good for common diseases, whereas retrospective studies are less expensive, less time-consuming, and good for rare diseases.
3. **Retrospective/case-control:** samples are chosen after the fact based on presence (cases) or absence (controls) of disease. Information then can be collected about risk factors. For example, you may look at people with lung cancer versus people without lung cancer to determine if the people with lung cancer smoke more.
4. **Case series:** good for extremely rare diseases. You simply describe the clinical presentation of people with a certain disease. Case series may suggest the need for a retrospective study.
5. **Prevalence survey/cross-sectional survey:** looks at the prevalence of a disease and prevalence of risk-factors. When two different cultures are compared, you may get an idea for the cause of a disease, which can be tested with a prospective study (e.g., more colon cancer and higher fat diet in U.S. versus less colon cancer and low fat diet in Japan).

Incidence: the number of new cases of disease in a unit of time (generally in 1 year, but any time frame can be used). The **incidence rate is equal to the absolute risk** (as opposed to relative or attributable risk). In an **epidemic,** the observed incidence greatly exceeds the expected incidence.

Prevalence: the total number of cases of disease (new or old).

> ➤ ***CASE SCENARIO:*** If a widely used new form of chemotherapy allows patients with lung cancer to survive an extra 2–3 years without curing the disease, what will happen to the incidence and prevalence of lung cancer? Nothing happens to the incidence, but the prevalence will increase because people live longer.

> ➤ ***CASE SCENARIO:*** For influenza, which is higher—incidence or prevalence? In short-term diseases (like the flu), the incidence is often higher than the prevalence (opposite of chronic diseases).

Comparison of data:

1. **Chi-squared test:** used to compare percentages or proportions (nonnumeric or nominal data).
2. **T-test:** used to compare two means.
3. **Analysis of variance (ANOVA):** used to compare three or more means.

P-value: If someone gives you data and tells you that $p < 0.05$ (commonly used as the cutoff for statistical significance), there is less than a 5% chance ($0.05 = 5\%$) that the data were obtained by random error or chance. If you read that the blood pressure (BP) in a control group is 180/100 mmHg, but the BP after use of drug X is 120/70 mmHg with $p < 0.10$, there is less than a 10% chance that the difference in BP is due to random error or chance (or up to a 9.99% chance that the result is due to chance). Three points: (1) the study still may have serious flaws; (2) a low p-value does *not* imply causation; and (3) a study that has statistical significance does not always have clinical significance (if drug X can lower the BP from 130/80 to 129/80 with $p < 0.001$, you still would not use drug X).

The p-value also ties into the **null hypothesis** (the hypothesis of no difference). For example, in a drug study of hypertension, the null hypothesis is that the drug does not work (any difference in BP is due to random error or chance). When the drug works beautifully and lowers the BP by 60 points, the null hypothesis must be rejected, because clearly the drug works. When $p < 0.05$, you can confidently *reject* the null hypothesis, because the p-value says that there is less than a 5% chance that the null hypothesis is correct. To reject the null hypothesis is to say that the difference in BP is not due to chance; it is due to the drug.

The p-value also represents the chance of making a **type I error** (concluding that there is an effect or difference when there is not or rejecting the null hypothesis when it is true).

A **type II error** is to accept the null hypothesis when it is false (the drug works but you say it does not).

Power: the probability of rejecting the null hypothesis when it is false (a good thing).

➤ **CASE SCENARIO:** What is the best way to increase the power of a study? Increase the sample size.

Experimental conclusions and errors

1. **Recall bias:** a risk for retrospective studies. When patients cannot remember things, they may inadvertently over- or underestimate risk factors. For example, John died of lung cancer, and his angry wife remembers him smoking "like a chimney," whereas Mike died of a non–smoking-related disease, and his loving wife denies that he smoked much. In realilty, both men smoked one pack per day.
2. **Interviewer bias:** occurs when there is no blinding. When a scientist receives big money to do a study and wants to find a difference between cases and controls, he or she may inadvertently interpret the same patient comment or outcome as "not significant" in the control group and "significant" in the treatment group.
3. **Unacceptability bias:** patients do not admit to embarrassing behavior or claim to exercise more than they do to please the interviewer—or they may claim to take experimental drugs when they spit them out.

➤ **CASE SCENARIO:** An experimenter measures the number of ashtrays owned and the incidence of lung cancer and finds that people with lung cancer have more ashtrays. He concludes that ashtrays cause lung cancer. What is the flaw in the study? **Confounding variable** (smoking tobacco is the confounding variable, because it causes the increase in both ashtrays and lung cancer).

➤ **CASE SCENARIO:** The mortality data of city A, a retirement community, and city B, a college town, are compared. A is much higher than B, and the researcher says that pollution or other toxic exposure must be the cause. What is the error? **Nonrandom or nonstratified sampling.** Of course city A will have higher a mortality rate (due to age differences) if the groups are not stratified into appropriate age-specific comparisons.

➤ **CASE SCENARIO:** A phone survey of 100 people finds 30 people who smoke and 20 who do not. The other 50 people did not answer the phone. The researcher concludes that the community has a smoking prevalence of 60%. What is the error? **Nonresponse bias.** In this case, the first step to try to salvage the results is repeated attempts to reach the nonresponders. If this approach is unsuccessful, list the nonresponders as unknown in the data analysis and see if any results can be salvaged. *Never* make up or assume responses.

➤ **CASE SCENARIO:** A prostate cancer screening test claims to prolong survival when compared with older survival data, using the same standard treatment as before. The researcher claims that earlier detection improves mortality from prostate cancer. What is the error? **Lead-time bias,** which is due to time differentials. The difference in survival is due only to earlier detection, not improved treatment or prolonged survival.

➤ **CASE SCENARIO:** In-hospital death rates for myocardial infarction (MI) are compared between hospital A and B. Hospital A has a higher in-hospital mortality rate. Hospital A also has a cardiac catheterization lab and dedicated coronary care unit; hospital B has neither and transfers patients to hospital A if they need a catheterization lab or coronary care unit. The researcher concludes that hospital B provides better care. What is the error? **Admission rate bias.** If you take on the tough cases (hospital B does not), you are sure to have higher mortality rates. The same error also can apply to surgeon's mortality/morbidity rates if the surgeon takes only tough cases.

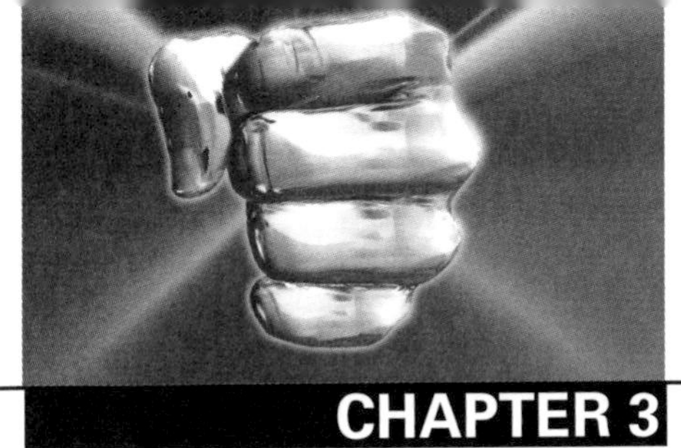

CHAPTER 3

Psychiatry and Ethics

SCHIZOPHRENIA

The diagnostic criteria are clues: **delusions, hallucinations, disorganized speech, grossly disorganized or catatonic behavior,** and **negative symptoms** (flat affect, alogia/refusal to talk, avolition/apathy). The typical age of onset is 15–25 years for men (look for a deteriorating college student) and 25–35 years for women. Roughly 1% of people in all cultures have schizophrenia. In the United States, most schizophrenic patients are born in the winter (reason unknown). Up to 10% of schizophrenics eventually commit suicide; a past attempt is the best predictor of eventual success. Treat with antipsychotic medications and psychosocial therapy and support, Medications are used first, but the best treatment (as in most psychiatric disorders) is medication plus therapy.

➤ **CASE SCENARIO:** What is the difference between brief/acute psychotic disorder, schizophreniform disorder, and schizophrenia? Only the **duration of symptoms**: < 1 month = brief psychotic disorder; 1–6 months = schizophreniform disorder; and > 6 months = schizophrenia.

Symptoms and prognosis:

POSITIVE SYMPTOMS	NEGATIVE SYMPTOMS	GOOD PROGNOSTIC FACTORS	POOR PROGNOSTIC FACTORS
Delusions	Flat affect	Good premorbid functioning	Poor premorbid functioning
Hallucinations	Alogia (no speech)	Late onset	Early onset
Bizarre behavior	Avolition (apathy)	Obvious precipitating factors	No precipitating factors
Thought disorder	Anhedonia	Married	Single, divorced, widowed
Poor attention		Family history of mood disorders	Family history of schizophrenia
		Positive symptoms	Negative symptoms
		Good support system	Poor support system

Antipsychotic medications:

	HIGH POTENCY	LOW POTENCY	ATYPICAL*
Example(s)	Haloperidol	Chlorpromazine	Risperidone, olanzapine
Extrapyramidal side effects	High incidence	Low incidence	Low incidence
Autonomic side effects[†]	Low incidence	High incidence	Medium incidence
Positive symptoms	Works well	Works well	Works well
Negative symptoms	Works poorly	Works poorly	Works somewhat

*Atypical, newer agents are the drugs of choice for maintenance therapy because of reduced extrapyramidal side effects and effect on negative symptoms.

[†]Autonomic side effects include anticholinergic (dry mouth, urinary retention, blurry vision, mydriasis), alpha-1 blockade (orthostatic hypotension), and antihistamine effects (sedation).

Extrapyramidal side effects are important and commonly tested:

1. **Acute dystonia** occurs in the **first few hours or days** of treatment. The patient has muscle spasms or stiffness (e.g., torticollis, trismus), tongue protrusions or twisting, opisthotonos, and oculogyric crisis (forced sustained deviation of the head and eyes). Most common in young men. Treat with **antihistamines** (e.g., diphenhydramine) or **anticholinergics** (e.g., benztropine, trihexyphenidyl).
2. **Akathisia** occurs in the first few days of treatment. The patient has a subjective feeling of restlessness and may pace constantly, alternate sitting and standing positions, or be unable to sit still. Beta blockers can be tried.
3. **Parkinsonism** occurs in the **first few months** of treatment. The patient has stiffness, cogwheel rigidity, shuffling gait, mask-like facies, and drooling. Most common in older women. Treat with **antihistamines** (e.g., diphenhydramine) or **anticholinergics** (e.g., benztropine, trihexyphenidyl).
4. **Tardive dyskinesia** occurs **after years** of treatment. Most patients have **perioral movements** (e.g., darting, protruding movements of the tongue, chewing, grimacing, puckering). Patients also may have involuntary, choreoathetoid movements of head, limbs, and trunk. There is no known treatment for tardive dyskinesia; if you have to make a choice, discontinue the antipsychotic and consider switching to an atypical antipsychotic (e.g., clozapine).
5. **Neuroleptic malignant syndrome** is a life-threatening condition that can occur at any time during treatment. The patient has **rigidity,** mutism, obtundation, agitation, **high fever** (up to 107°F), **high level of creatine phosphokinase** (often > 5000), sweating, and myoglobinuria. Treatment: (1) discontinue the antipsychotic; (2) give supportive care for fever and renal shutdown due to myoglobinuria; and (3) consider giving **dantrolene** (as in malignant hyperthermia).

Other facts about antipsychotic medication:

- Dopamine is a **prolactin-inhibiting factor** in the tuberoinfundibular tract of the brain. Thus, dopamine blockade causes an increase in prolactin, which may result in **high prolactin levels, galactorrhea** (typically bilateral), and impotence, **menstrual dysfunction,** or decreased libido.
- Individual antipsychotic side effects: thioridazine causes retinal pigment deposits, clozapine causes **agranulocytosis** (white blood cell counts must be monitored), and chlorpromazine causes jaundice and photosensitivity.

MOOD DISORDERS

Depression

Patients described on the boards usually do not come out and say, "I'm depressed." You have to watch for the clues: change in sleep habits (classically, **insomnia**), vague **somatic complaints,** anxiety, low energy level or **fatigue**, change in appetite (classically, **decreased appetite**), poor concentration, **psychomotor retardation,** and/or **anhedonia** (loss of pleasure; previously fun activities are no longer enjoyed). In children, depression often presents as an irritable mood instead of a depressed mood, and in the elderly, it may present as "**pseudodementia**."

Look for precipitating factors in the history, such as loss of a loved one, divorce or separation, unemployment or retirement, or chronic disease. Depression is more common in women. "Pencil-and-paper" tests (e.g., Beck's depression inventory) are sometimes used for screening. Treat with both antidepressants and psychotherapy; the combination works better than either modality alone.

- **Adjustment disorder with depressed mood:** the patient does not handle a stressful situation well and feels "bummed out" (for < 6 months) but does not meet criteria for full blown depression. A classic example is the teenage girl who breaks up with her boyfriend and seems to cry a lot, skips a few days of school, and does not want to talk to her friends for a week.

- **Dysthymia:** depressed mood on most days for more than 2 years, but no episodes of major depression, mania/hypomania, or psychosis.

Antidepressants

1. **Serotonin-specific reuptake inhibitors** (SSRIs; e.g., fluoxetine, paroxetine) prevent reuptake of serotonin only and have few serious side effects (**insomnia, anorexia, sexual dysfunction**). They are the first-line agents in all depressed patients.
2. **Tricyclic antidepressants** (TCAs; e.g., nortriptyline, amitriptyline) prevent reuptake of norepinephrine and serotonin. They also block alpha-adrenergic receptors (watch for orthostatic hypotension, dizziness, and falls) and muscarinic receptors as well as cause sedation and lower the seizure threshold (especially bupropion, which is not technically a TCA). TCAs are dangerous in overdose, primarily because of **cardiac arrhythmias,** which may respond to **bicarbonate.**
3. **Monoamine oxidase inhibitors** (MAOIs; e.g., phenelzine, tranylcypromine) are older medications and not first-line agents. They may be good for **atypical depression** (look for hypersomnia and hyperphagia—the opposite of classic depression). When patients eat **tyramine-containing foods** (especially wine and cheese), they may have a **hypertensive crisis.**

Bipolar Disorder

Mania is the only criterion required for a diagnosis. Depression commonly presents before or after mania. Look for classic symptoms such as **decreased need for sleep, pressured speech, sexual promiscuity, shopping sprees,** and **exaggerated self-importance** or delusions of grandeur. The initial onset classically is between 16 and 30 years of age. **Lithium** and **valproic acid** are first-line treatment agents. Carbamazepine is a second-line agent. Antipsychotics may be needed for patients with psychosis (used at the same time as the mood stabilizer). Antidepressants can trigger mania or hypomania, especially in bipolar patients.

- **Bipolar II** disorder is hypomania (mild mania without psychosis that does not cause occupational dysfunction) plus major depression.
- **Cyclothymia** is defined as at least 2 years of hypomania alternating with depressed mood (with no full-blown episodes of mania or depression).
- Lithium causes renal dysfunction (**diabetes insipidus**), thyroid dysfunction, **tremor,** and CNS effects at toxic levels. Valproic acid causes **liver dysfunction,** and carbamazepine may cause bone marrow depression.

Suicide

The major risk factors are **age > 45, alcohol or substance abuse, history of rage or violence, prior suicide attempts, male sex** (men *commit* suicide three times more often than women, but women *attempt* it four times more often than men), **prior psychiatric history, depression,** recent loss or separation, loss of health, unemployment or retirement, and single, widowed, or divorced status.

> ➤ ***CASE SCENARIO:*** What is the best predictor of future suicide? A past attempt.

Consider hospitalizing an acutely suicidal patient (against their will, if necessary) for treatment. Patients who are just coming out of a deep depression are at increased risk of suicide: the antidepressant may begin to work, and the person has more energy—just enough to commit suicide. Suicide rates are rising most rapidly among 15–24-year-olds, but the greatest risk is in people over age 65.

> ➤ ***CASE SCENARIO:*** True or false: Asking about suicide does not increase the risk of suicide.
> True. Always ask depressed patients about suicide to assess their risk.

Normal vs. pathologic grief, mourning, and bereavement: initial grief after a loss (e.g., death of a loved one) may include a state of shock, feeling of numbness or bewilderment, distress, crying, sleep disturbances, decreased appetite, difficulty in concentrating, weight loss, and survivor guilt for **up to 1 year**—in other words, the same symptoms as depression! Intense yearning (even years after the death) and even searching for the deceased are normal. **Feelings of worthlessness, psychomotor retardation,** and **suicidal ideation** are not signs of normal grief; they are signs of depression.

- *CASE SCENARIO:* A 68-year-old man comes to see you 2 weeks after his wife of 40 years died. He complains of poor appetite and crying spells and says that he keeps thinking he sees his wife, only to realize it is not her. He also feels guilty. He denies suicidal ideation. What does the patient have? Normal grief. It is normal to have an illusion or hallucination about the deceased. A normal grieving person knows that it was an illusion or hallucination, whereas a depressed person believes that the illusion or hallucination is real.

ANXIETY DISORDERS

Panic disorder: look for 20–40-year-old patient who thinks that he or she is dying or having a heart attack, even though the patient is healthy and has a negative work-up for organic disease. Patients often hyperventilate and are extremely anxious. Remember the association with **agoraphobia** (fear of leaving the house). Treat with SSRIs (e.g., fluoxetine), which are favored over benzodiazepines (because of the sedation and addiction potential with benzodiazepines).

Generalized anxiety disorder: patient **constantly worries about everything** (e.g., career, family, future, relationships, money) at the same time; not as dramatic as panic disorder. Treat with SSRIs, buspirone (nonaddictive, nonsedating) or benzodiazepines (addictive, sedating).

Simple phobias: fear of needles, blood products, animals, heights, other specific trigger. Treat with behavioral therapy, such as **flooding** (e.g., patient with fear of dogs locked in room with many dogs), **systematic desensitization** (e.g., patient with fear of dogs asked to think about dogs, then listen to a dog bark, then look at a live dog, etc.), biofeedback, and mental imagery. **Social phobia** is a specific subtype of simple phobia that is best treated with behavioral therapy. **Beta blockers** may be used before an unavoidable public appearance to reduce symptoms, and SSRIs may help.

Posttraumatic stress disorder: look for someone who has **been through a life-threatening event** (Vietnam veteran, survivor of severe accident or rape) who **recurrently experiences the event** (nightmares, flashbacks), **tries to avoid thinking about it,** and has **depression** or **poor concentration** as a result. Treat with (group) therapy with or without an antidepressant.

SOMATOFORM DISORDERS

Patients with somatoform disorders **do not intentionally create symptoms.** Treat with frequent return clinic visits and/or psychotherapy.

1. **Somatization disorder:** patients have multiple complaints in **multiple organ systems** over many years and have had extensive work-ups in the past.
2. **Conversion disorder:** after an obvious precipitating factor (e.g., fight with boyfriend), patients have **unexplainable neurologic symptoms** (blindness, stocking-and-glove numbness).
3. **Hypochondriasis:** patients continue to believe that they have a certain disease despite extensive negative work-up.
4. **Body dysmorphic disorder:** preoccupation with **imagined physical defect** (e.g., a teenager thinks that her nose is too big when its size is normal).

Somatoform disorder vs. factitious disorder vs. malingering

1. **Somatoform disorders:** patients do not intentionally create symptoms.
2. **Factitious disorders:** patients intentionally create their illness or symptoms (e.g., they inject insulin to induce hypoglycemia) and subject themselves to procedures to **assume the role of a patient** (unique type of secondary gain) with no financial or other secondary gain.
3. **Malingering:** patients intentionally create their illness for secondary gain (e.g., money, release from work or prison).

PERSONALITY DISORDERS

Personality disorders are lifelong disorders with no real treatment (although psychotherapy can be tried):

1. **Paranoid:** patients think that everyone (including friends) is out to get them; often start law-suits.
2. **Schizoid:** the classic loner; no friends and no interest in having friends.
3. **Schizotypal:** bizarre beliefs (e.g., extrasensory perception, cults, superstition, illusions) and bizarre manner of speaking but no psychosis.
4. **Avoidant:** patients have no friends but want them; fear of criticism or rejection causes them to avoid others (inferiority complex).
5. **Histrionic:** patients are overly dramatic and attention-seeking and may be inappropriately seductive; they must be the center of attention.
6. **Narcissistic:** patients are egocentric, lack empathy, use others for their own gain, and have a sense of entitlement.
7. **Antisocial:** patients may have a **long criminal record** (con men) and may have tortured animals or set fires as children (a history of childhood **conduct disorder** is required for this diagnosis). They are aggressive and do not pay bills or support children; they are also liars and **feel no remorse** (without conscience). The disorder has a strong association with alcoholism or drug abuse and **somatization disorder.** Most patients are male.
8. **Borderline:** instability of mood, behavior, relationships (many are bisexual), and self-image. Look for **splitting** (people and things are all good or all bad and may frequently change categories), suicide attempts, micropsychotic episodes (2 minutes of psychosis), impulsiveness and constant crisis (see Glenn Close in *Fatal Attraction*).
9. **Dependent:** patients cannot be (or do anything) alone; they are highly dependent on others. For example, a wife may stay with an abusive husband.
10. **Obsessive-compulsive:** patients are anal-retentive, stubborn, and cheap with restricted affect. Rules are more important than objectives. Different than obsessive-compulsive disorder (OCD)!

MISCELLANEOUS

Dissociative fugue/psychogenic fugue: patients have amnesia and travel, assuming a new identity.

Dissociative identity disorder/multiple personality disorder: most likely disorder to be associated with **childhood sexual abuse.**

Homosexuality and homosexual experimentation are not considered a disease at any age; they are normal variants.

- **CASE SCENARIO:** A woman complains that her husband has mentioned a few "kinky" fantasies and occasionally wears her underwear. What disorder does the man have? None. His behavior is within the realm of normal.

Obsessive-compulsive disorder: patients have recurrent **thoughts** or **impulses** (obsessions) and/or recurrent **behaviors** (compulsions) that cause marked dysfunction in their occupational or interpersonal lives. Look for washing (the patient may wash the hands 30 times a day) and checking rituals (the patient may check to see whether the door is locked 30 times a day). The onset usually is in adolescence or early adulthood. Treat with SSRIs (especially **fluvoxamine**) or clomipramine. Behavioral therapy (e.g., flooding) also may be effective.

Narcolepsy: daytime sleepiness; **decreased rapid eye movement (REM) latency** (patients enter the REM stage as soon as they fall asleep); **cataplexy** (loss of muscle tone, falls); and **hypnopompic** (as the patient wakes up) or **hypnagogic** (as the patient falls asleep) hallucinations. Treat with **modafinil** (an non-amphetamine stimulant) or amphetamines.

Note: Hospitalize patients (against their will, if necessary) who are a danger to themselves (suicidal or unable to take care of themselves) or others (homicidal).

DRUGS OF ABUSE

Marijuana is the most commonly abused illegal drug. Look for a teenager who listens to rock music, has **red eyes,** and acts "weird." Also look for "**amotivational syndrome**" (chronic use leads to laziness and lack of motivation), time distortion, and "munchies" (eating binge during intoxication). Patients have no physical withdrawal symptoms, although they may report psychological cravings. Overdoses are not dangerous, although patients may experience temporary dysphoria.

Cocaine is associated with sympathetic stimulation (**insomnia, tachycardia, mydriasis, hypertension, sweating**), hyperalertness, and possible paranoia, aggressiveness, delirium, psychosis, or **formications** (patients think that bugs are crawling on them). Overdoses can be fatal because of arrhythmia, heart attack, seizure, or stroke. On withdrawal, patients become sleepy, hungry (vs. anorexic with intoxication), and irritable with possible severe depression. Withdrawal is not dangerous, but psychological cravings usually are severe. Cocaine is **teratogenic** (vascular disruptions in fetus).

Amphetamines are more classically associated with psychotic symptoms (patients may appear to be full-blown schizophrenics) but otherwise similar to cocaine.

Opioids include heroin and related agents. They cause **euphoria, analgesia, drowsiness, miosis, constipation,** and CNS/respiratory depression. Overdose can be fatal because of respiratory depression; treat with **naloxone.** Because the drug is usually taken intravenously, there are associated morbidities and mortalities (e.g., endocarditis, HIV, cellulitis, talc damage to lung). Withdrawal is not life-threatening, but patients act as though they are going to die. Symptoms include **gooseflesh, diarrhea, insomnia,** and cramping or pain. **Methadone** treatment sometimes is given to opiate addicts. Methadone is a longer-acting opioid that allows patients to function by keeping them on a chronic, free, low dose. Its use is controversial.

Lysergic acid diethylamide (LSD)/mushrooms: symptoms of intoxication include **hallucinations** (usually visual vs. auditory in schizophrenia), **mydriasis,** tachycardia, diaphoresis, and perception and mood disturbances. Overdoses are not dangerous (unless the patient thinks that he can fly and jumps out a window), and there are no withdrawal symptoms. Patients may have "**flashbacks**" months to years later (brief feeling of being on the drug again, even though none was taken) or a "bad trip" (acute panic reaction or dysphoria). Treat bad trips with reassurance or a benzodiazepine/antipsychotic agent, if needed.

> **CASE SCENARIO:** What are the known teratogenic effects of LSD? None. Neither LSD nor marijuana has been definitely proved to be teratogenic, though smoke inhalation (marijuana) is thought to have ill effects on the fetus (a la cigarette smoking).

Phencyclidine (PCP):symptoms of LSD/mushroom intoxication plus confusion, agitation and aggressive behavior. Also look for **vertical and/or horizontal nystagmus,** plus possible schizophrenic-like symptoms (e.g., paranoia, auditory hallucinations, disorganized behavior and speech). Overdose can be *fatal* (convulsions, coma, respiratory arrest); treat with supportive care and **urine acidification** to hasten elimination. There are no withdrawal symptoms.

Inhalants (e.g., gasoline, glue, varnish remover): intoxication causes euphoria, dizziness, slurred speech, a feeling of floating, ataxia, and/or a sense of heightened power. Inhalant use usually is seen in **younger teenagers** (11–15 years). Overdoses can be fatal (respiratory depression, cardiac arrhythmias, asphyxiation) or cause severe permanent sequelae (nervous system, liver, or kidney toxicity, peripheral neuropathy). There is no known withdrawal syndrome.

Benzodiazepines/barbiturates: cause sedation and drowsiness as well as reduced anxiety and disinhibition. Overdoses can be fatal (respiratory depression); treat overdoses of benzodiazepines with **flumazenil.** In addition, *withdrawal can be fatal* (as with alcohol) because of seizures and/or cardiovascular collapse. Treat withdrawal on an inpatient basis with benzodiazepines, and gradually taper the dose over several days. Benzodiazepines and barbiturates are dangerous when mixed with alcohol (all three are CNS depressants).

Note: Caffeine can cause **headaches, irritability,** and **fatigue** in withdrawal.

ETHICS

Do *not* force **adult Jehovah's witness** patients to accept blood products.

If a child has a life-threatening condition and the parents refuse a simple, curative treatment (e.g., antibiotics for meningitis), first try to persuade the parents. Then get a court order to give the treatment; do not give the treatment until you talk to the courts, if you can avoid it.

Let competent people die if they want to do so; never force treatments on adults of sound mind. On the other hand, do not commit active euthanasia. Respect the patient's wishes for passive euthanasia.

Do not tell anyone how your patient is doing unless the person is directly involved with care and needs to know or is an authorized family member. If a colleague asks about a friend who happens to be your patient, ***refuse to answer.***

When it is permissible to break patient confidentiality:

1. At the patient's request
2. Suspected child abuse
3. Court mandate
4. Duty to warn and protect (if a patient says that he is going to kill Joe, you have to tell Joe, the proper authorities, or both)
5. Reportable disease
6. Danger to others. For example, if a driver is blind or has seizures, let the proper authorities know so that they can take away the patient's license to drive. If an airplane pilot is a paranoid, hallucinating schizophrenic, authorities need to know.

Informed consent involves giving the patient information about the diagnosis (his or her condition and what it means), the prognosis (the natural course of the condition without treatment), the proposed treatment (description of the procedure and what the patient will experience), the risk/benefits of the treatment, and alternative treatments. Patients then are allowed to make their own choice. The documents that patients are made to sign on wards are not required or sufficient for informed consent; they are used for documentation and medicolegal purposes (i.e., lawsuit paranoia).

When a patient is incompetent, a court-appointed guardian should be arranged (surrogate decision-maker or health care power of attorney).

Living wills and do-not-resuscitate (DNR) orders should be respected and followed if done correctly. For example, if a patient says in his living will that he does not want to be put on a ventilator, do not put the patient on a ventilator, even if a spouse, child, or significant other tells you to do so. Of course, be nice about it, and discuss it with those concerned in a caring, professional manner.

Depression should always be evaluated as a reason for "incompetence." A patient who is suicidal may refuse all treatment. This refusal should not be respected until the depression is treated.

Psychiatric patients can be hospitalized against their will if they are a danger to self or others for a limited time. After 1–3 days, most states require a formal hearing to determine whether the patient has to remain in custody. This practice is based on the principle of beneficence (doing good and avoiding harm).

Restraints can be used on an incompetent or violent (delirious, psychotic) patient if needed, but their use should be brief and reevaluated frequently.

> ➤ **CASE SCENARIO:** How effective are restraints in preventing falls in demented or delirious patients? Restraints generally do not reduce the risk of falls and can cause serious injury.

Patients under 18 do not require parental consent if they are emancipated (married, living on their own and financially independent, raising children, serving in the armed forces), have a sexually transmitted disease, want contraception, are pregnant, want drug treatment or counseling, or have psychiatric illness. Some states have exceptions to these statements, but for the boards, let minors make their own decisions in such settings.

If a patient is comatose and no surrogate decision-maker has been appointed, the wishes of the family should generally be respected. If there is a family disagreement or ulterior motives are suspected, talk to the hospital ethics committee. Use courts as a last resort.

> ➤ **CASE SCENARIO:** What should you do in a pediatric emergency when parents, caretakers, or family members are not available to give consent? Treat the child as you see fit.

Do not hide a diagnosis from patients (including children) if they want to know the diagnosis (even if the family asks you to do so). Do not lie to any patient because the family asks you to do so. Conversely, do not force patients to receive information against their will; if they do not want to know the diagnosis, do not tell them.

> ➤ **CASE SCENARIO:** A family asks you not to tell grandma the diagnosis. What should you do first? Ask the family about their concerns. If this approach does not resolve the issue, ask the patient whether she wants to know the diagnosis. If she does, tell the family that you are obligated to give her the information.

> ➤ **CASE SCENARIO:** What should you do if a patient who needs treatment cannot communicate (e.g., comatose or unconscious patients)? Give all required care unless you know that the patient does not want it.

Withdrawing and withholding care are legal equivalents. The fact that a patient is on a ventilator does not mean that you can never turn it off.

In **terminally ill patients,** give enough pain medication to relieve pain. Do not be afraid to use narcotics, and do not worry about addiction in this setting.

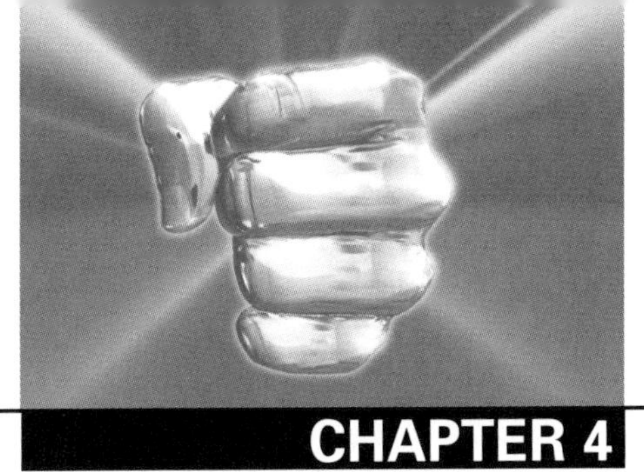

CHAPTER 4

Obstetrics and Gynecology

OBSTETRICS

Preventive Care/Normal Pregnancy

if pregnant or can be pregnant
No CT/XR
No teratogenic meds

Consider pregnancy in all women of reproductive age before treating any condition. Do not give a teratogenic drug or order an x-ray/CT scan without knowing whether the woman is pregnant. A patient who says that she is on birth control may still be pregnant; no contraception is 100% effective, especially when compliance is taken into account. The standard human chorionic gonadotropin (HCG) pregnancy test becomes positive roughly 2 weeks after conception.

Give **folate** to all women of reproductive age to prevent neural tube defects. This prevention is most effective in the first trimester, when many women do not even know that they are pregnant.

Signs of pregnancy: amenorrhea, morning sickness with nausea or vomiting, ***Hegar sign*** (softening and compressibility of the lower uterine segment), ***Chadwick sign*** (dark discoloration of the vulva and vaginal walls), linea nigra (see figure), ***melasma*** and weight gain.

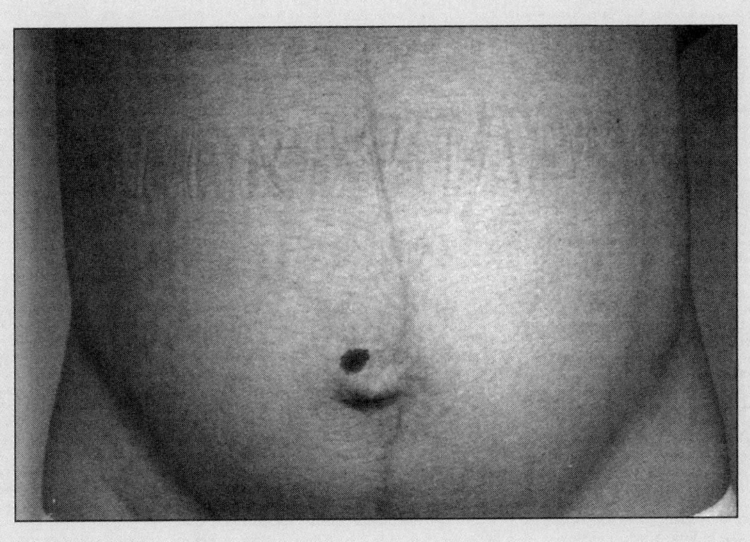

The midline vertically-oriented thin hyperpigmented line over the abdomen is consistent with linea nigra, a normal, benign finding in pregnancy. (From du Vivier A: Pregnancy and female disorders. In du Vivier A (ed): Atlas of Clinical Dermatology, 3rd ed. New York, Churchill Livingstone, 2002, pp 683–691, with permission.)

Changes and complaints associated with normal pregnancy: nausea and vomiting (morning sickness), heavy (possibly even painful) feeling of the breasts, increased pigmentation of the nipples and areolae, backache, striae gravidarum, and mild ankle edema. Heartburn and increased frequency of urination are also frequent problems in pregnancy. **Quickening** (the mother's first perception of fetal movements) usually occurs at 18–20 weeks in a primigravida and at 16–18 weeks in a multigravida.

Routine lab tests in a pregnant patient:

1. **Pap smear.** Every woman should have a Pap smear at the first visit, unless she has had a normal smear in the past 6 months.
2. **Urinalysis** should be done at every visit to screen for pre-eclampsia, bacteriuria, and diabetes. **Treat asymptomatic bacteriuria in pregnancy;** 20% of pregnant women develop cystitis or pyelonephritis if untreated at least in part because progesterone decreases the tone of the ureters and the uterus compresses the ureters.
3. **Complete blood count** should be done at the first visit to see whether the patient is anemic (pregnancy aggravates anemia). Give iron supplements (in prenatal vitamin formulations) to prevent anemia.
4. **Blood type, Rh type, and antibody screen** should be done at the first visit to identify possible isoimmunization/Rh incompatibility.
5. **Syphilis test** should be done at the first visit (mandated in most states) and at subsequent visits in high-risk patients.
6. **Rubella antibody screen** should be done at the first visit if the patient's vaccination history is unknown; otherwise, it is not needed.
7. **Diabetes screening** should be performed in all women at 24–28 weeks. Screen with fasting serum glucose and serum glucose 1 or 2 hours after an oral glucose load. Consider screen at the first visit if the patient has risk factors for diabetes (obese, family history, age over 30).

    ➤ **CASE SCENARIO:** What is the most likely cause of macrosomia in a term infant? Maternal diabetes.

8. **Serum alpha-fetoprotein (AFP) or "triple screen"** should be done between 15 and 20 weeks for older or other high-risk women. **Low AFP = Down syndrome, fetal demise or inaccurate dates. High AFP = neural tube defects (e.g., anencephaly, spina bifida), ventral wall defects (e.g., omphalocele, gastroschisis), multiple gestation, or inaccurate dates.** If AFP or triple screen is positive at 16–20 weeks, first order an ultrasound to rule out inaccurate dates or obvious fetal abnormality. If the results are inconclusive, the patient should undergo amniocentesis for a diagnosis of chromosomal disorders (cell culture) or neural tube defects (amniotic fluid AFP level).
9. **Group B streptococcal culture** should be done at 35–37 weeks. If the patient is positive, treat during labor with ampicillin to prevent neonatal meningitis.
10. **Others:** hepatitis B serology, tuberculosis skin test, HIV test, and ultrasound are done only when the patient has a suggestive history or risk factors. If asked, you should do routine chlamydial and gonorrhea cultures for any sexually active woman younger than 25, especially if she has multiple partners or is indigent, even if she is asymptomatic.

At every prenatal visit, listen for fetal heart tones and evaluate uterine size for any size/dates discrepancy. Fetal heart tones can be heard with Doppler at 10–12 weeks and with a stethoscope at 16–20 weeks. Uterine size is evaluated by measuring the distance from the symphysis pubis to the top of the fundus in centimeters. At 12 weeks' gestation, the uterus enters the abdomen, and at 20 weeks it reaches the umbilicus. Between roughly 20 and 35 weeks, the measurement in cm should equal the number of weeks' gestation. A discrepancy greater than 2–3 cm is called a **size/dates discrepancy,** and ultrasound should be done. A size/dates discrepancy may indicate problems such as intrauterine growth retardation, multiple gestation, or inaccurate dates.

HCG levels roughly double every two days in the first trimester of pregnancy, and an HCG that stays the same or increases only slowly with serial testing indicates a fetus in trouble, ectopic pregnancy or fetal demise. A rapidly increasing HCG or one that does not decrease after delivery may indicate a hydatiform mole or choriocarcinoma.

Transvaginal ultrasound can detect intrauterine pregnancy at roughly ***5 weeks*** or when the HCG level > 2000 mIU. Use this information when trying to determine the possibility of an ectopic pregnancy. If patient's last menstrual period was 3 weeks ago and the pregnancy test is positive, you cannot rule out an ectopic pregnancy. If, however, the patient's last menstrual period was 8 weeks ago and an ultrasound of the uterus does not show a gestational sac, be highly suspicious of ectopic pregnancy.

Pregnant women can have the same surgical conditions as nonpregnant woman. In general, treat the disease, regardless of the pregnancy. This rule of thumb applies to all acute surgical conditions (e.g., appendicitis, cholecystitis). With semiurgent conditions (e.g., ovarian neoplasm), it is best to wait until the second trimester, when the patient and fetus are most stable. Purely elective cases are avoided. Appendicitis may present with right upper quadrant pain or tenderness due to the uterine displacement of the appendix. Do a laparoscopy if you are unsure and the patient has peritoneal signs.

The **average weight gain** in pregnancy is 28 lbs (12.5 kg). With larger gains, think of diabetes. With smaller gains, think of hyperemesis gravidarum, psychiatric disorder, or major systemic disease.

Normal physiologic changes in pregnancy

1. Lab tests

- Sedimentation rate is markedly elevated (worthless test in pregnancy).
- Overall levels of thyroxine (T_4) and thyroid-binding globulin increase, but the level of free T_4 remains normal.
- Hemoglobin increases, but plasma volume increases more; the net result is a decrease in hematocrit and hemoglobin.
- Blood urea nitrogen (BUN) and creatinine decrease as the glomerular filtration rate increases. Levels of BUN and creatinine at the high end of normal indicate renal disease in pregnancy.
- Alkaline phosphatase increases markedly.
- Mild proteinuria and glycosuria are normal in pregnancy.
- Electrolytes and liver function tests remain normal.

2. Cardiovascular changes

- Blood pressure decreases slightly.
- Heart rate increases by 10–20 beats/minute.
- Stroke volume and cardiac output increase (up to 50%).

3. Pulmonary changes

- Minute ventilation increases because of increased tidal volume with same or only slightly increased respiratory rate.
- Residual volume decreases.
- Carbon dioxide decreases (***physiologic hyperventilation/respiratory alkalosis***).

Prenatal Fetal Monitoring

Consider ultrasound for all women with a size/dates discrepancy > 2–3 cm and all women who have risk factors for pregnancy problems (e.g., hypertension; diabetes; renal disease; lupus erythematosus; cigarette, alcohol, or drug use; history of previous problems). There are fewer and fewer women who do not have an indication (or desire) for an ultrasound exam.

Intrauterine growth retardation (IUGR) is defined as size below the tenth percentile for age. The causes are many and are best understood in broad terms as due to one of three types of factors: **maternal** (e.g., smoking, alcohol or drugs, lupus), **fetal** (e.g., TORCH infections, congenital anomalies), or **placental** (e.g., hypertension, pre-eclampsia). The ultrasound parameters measured for determination of IUGR determination are biparietal diameter, head circumference, abdominal circumference, and femur length.

The **biophysical profile** (BPP) is used to evaluate fetal well-being. It consists of a heart tracing and ultrasound to measure four parameters:

1. **Nonstress test:** fetal heart rate tracing is obtained for 20 minutes to look for normal variability.
2. **Amniotic fluid index:** measures the amount of amniotic fluid to screen for oligo- or polyhydramnios.
3. **Fetal breathing movements**
4. **Fetal body movements**

Use the BPP if there is any concern about fetal well-being and in high-risk pregnancies near term. If the fetus scores low on the BPP, the next test is the **contraction stress test** for uteroplacental dysfunction. The mother is given oxytocin, and the fetal heart strip is monitored. If late decelerations are seen on the fetal heart strip with each contraction, the test is positive; usually a cesarean section is done.

Oligohydramnios: decreased amniotic fluid (≤ 300–500 ml). Causes include **IUGR, premature rupture of membranes** (PROM), postmaturity, and renal agenesis (Potter disease). Oligohydramnios may cause fetal problems such as **pulmonary hypoplasia,** cutaneous or skeletal abnormalities due to compression, or hypoxia due to cord compression.

Polyhydramnios: too much amniotic fluid (≥ 1700–2000 ml). Causes include **maternal diabetes, multiple gestation, neural tube defects** (anencephaly, spina bifida), **GI anomalies** (omphalocele, esophageal atresia), and **hydrops fetalis** (Rh incompatibility, fetal heart failure, etc.). Polyhydramnios can cause postpartum **uterine atony** (with resultant postpartum hemorrhage) and maternal dyspnea (the overdistended uterus compromises pulmonary function).

Monitoring of fetal heart and uterine contraction patterns during labor is routinely done, but the benefit is controversial. At term, the normal fetal heart rate is 110–160 beats/minute. Any value outside this range is worrisome. The following abnormalities are fair game, and you may be shown a fetal heart strip:

1. **Early deceleration,** in which the nadir (low-point) of fetal heart deceleration and the peak of uterine contraction coincide, signifies **head compression** (probable vagal response) and is **normal.**
2. **Variable deceleration** (variable with relation to uterine contractions) is the most commonly encountered abnormality and signifies **cord compression.** Place the mother in the lateral decubitus position, administer oxygen by face mask, and stop any oxytocin infusion. If bradycardia is severe (< 80–90 beats/min) or the variable pattern fails to resolve, measure fetal oxygen saturation and/or fetal scalp pH.
3. **Late deceleration,** in which fetal heart deceleration occurs after uterine contraction, signifies **uteroplacental insufficiency** and is the most worrisome pattern. First, place the mother in lateral decubitus position, give oxygen by face mask, and stop oxytocin. Next, give a tocolytic agent (beta$_2$ agonist such as ritodrine or magnesium sulfate) and IV fluids if the mother is hypotensive (especially with epidural anesthesia!). If late decelerations persist, measure fetal oxygen saturation and/or scalp pH.
4. **Loss of variability in heart rate:** if the fetal heart rate stays constant, consider checking fetal scalp pH. Any loss of variability associated with significant late or variable decelerations is a very worrsiome pattern and typically indicates the need for delivery.

5. **Fetal tachycardia or bradycardia** is worrisome if it is prolonged or if the heart rate is well outside the normal range
6. **Any recurrent or prolonged (> 2 minutes) decelerations** are worrisome.

   Note: Any fetal scalp pH < 7.2 or abnormally decreased fetal oxygen saturation is an indication for delivery. If the pH > 7.2 or fetal oxygen saturation is normal, you may consider continuing to observe or deliver.

Labor and Delivery

In **true labor,** normal contractions occur at least every 3 minutes, are fairly regular, and are associated with cervical changes (effacement and dilation). In **false labor** (Braxton-Hicks contractions), contractions are irregular and associated with no cervical changes.

Normal labor:

STAGE	CHARACTERISTICS	NULLIGRAVIDA	MULTIGRAVIDA
First	Onset of true labor to full cervical dilation	< 20 hr	< 14 hr
Latent phase	From 0 to 3–4 cm dilation (slow, irregular)	Highly variable	Highly variable
Active phase	From 3 to 4 cm to full dilation (rapid, regular)	> 1 cm/hr dilation	> 1.2 cm/hr dilation
Second	From full dilation to birth of baby	30 min to 3 hr	5–30 min
Third	Delivery of baby to delivery of placenta	0–30 min	0–30 min
Fourth	Placental delivery to maternal stabilization	Up to 48 hr	Up to 48 hr

Protraction disorder occurs once true labor has begun if the mother takes longer than the above chart indicates (see figure). **Arrest disorder** occurs once true labor has begun if no change in dilation occurs over 2 hours (as opposed to slow change in protraction disorder) or no change occurs in descent over 1 hour. First, rule out ***abnormal lie*** and ***cephalopelvic disproportion.*** If neither is present, treat with labor augmentation (oxytocin, prostaglandin gel, amniotomy). If this approach fails, observe and do a cesarean section at the first sign of trouble.

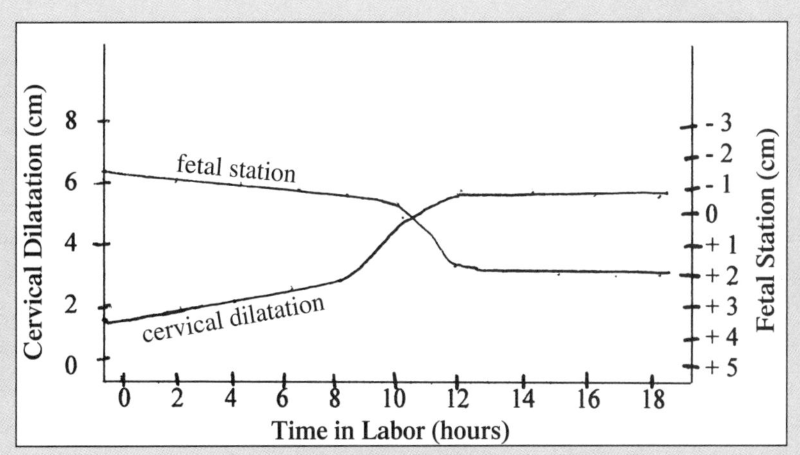

Arrested labor. A normal course of cervical dilatation and fetal station is present until 12–13 hours, when complete arrest is evident because of a "flattening out" of parameter lines. (From Brochert A: Platinum Vignettes: Obstetrics and Gynecology. Philadelphia, Hanley & Belfus, 2002, p 75, with permission.)

The most common cause of "failure to progress" (protraction or arrest disorder), also known as dystocia ("difficult birth"), is **cephalopelvic disproportion** (CPD), defined as disparity between the size of the baby's head and the mother's pelvis. Labor augmentation is contraindicated in this setting.

When **oxytocin** is given to augment ineffective uterine contractions, watch out for **uterine hyperstimulation** (painful, overly frequent, and poorly coordinated uterine contractions), **uterine rupture,** fetal heart rate decelerations, and ***water intoxication*** (**hyponatremia** from antidiuretic hormone-like effect of oxytocin). Treat all of these problems by first discontinuing oxytocin infusion (half-life = < 10 minutes).

Prostaglandin E_2 (PGE_2 or dinoprostone) also may be used locally to induce the cervix ("ripening") and is highly effective in combination with oxytocin. PGE_2 also may cause uterine hyperstimulation. ***Amniotomy*** hastens labor but exposes the fetus and uterus to possible infection if labor does not occur.

Contraindications to labor induction/augmentation are placenta previa, vasa previa, umbilical cord prolapse or presentation, prior classic uterine cesarean section incision, transverse fetal lie, active genital herpes, known cervical cancer, and known CPD (similar to contraindications for vaginal delivery).

When the mother has **genital herpes simplex virus (HSV) infection,** delay the decision about whether to do a cesarean section until the mother goes into labor. If, at the time of true labor, the mother has lesions of HSV, do a cesarean section. If, at the time of true labor, she has no HSV lesions, allow vaginal delivery. **Acyclovir** given to the mother during the last month of pregnancy can reduce the risk of having active lesions at the time of labor.

After a cesarean section with a classic (vertical) uterine incision, the mother must have cesarean sections for all future deliveries because of increased rate of uterine rupture. After a cesarean section with a lower (horizontal) uterine incision, a woman may attempt to deliver future pregnancies vaginally.

Epidural anesthesia is preferred in obstetric patients. General anesthesia involves a higher risk of aspiration and resulting pneumonia, because the gastroesophageal sphincter is relaxed in pregnancy and most patients have not been put on NPO (nothing-by-mouth) status for very long. There are also concerns that general anesthetic agents may cross the placenta and affect the fetus. Spinal anesthesia can interfere with the mother's ability to push and is associated with a higher incidence of hypotension than epidural anesthesia.

Signs of placental separation: fresh blood appears from the vagina, the umbilical cord lengthens, and the fundus rises and becomes firm and globular.

- **CASE SCENARIO:** What is the first maneuver to try if shoulder dystocia occurs during delivery? The **McRobert maneuver.** Have the mother sharply flex her thighs against her abdomen, which may free the impacted shoulder. If this maneuver does not work, your options are limited. An extended episiotomy or other more complex maneuvers are generally needed.

- **CASE SCENARIO:** What is the correct order of labor positions? Descent, flexion, internal rotation, extension, external rotation, and expulsion.

Fetal malpresentations. Although under specific guidelines some frank and complete breeches may be delivered vaginally, it is acceptable to do a cesarean section for any breech presentation. With shoulder presentation or incomplete/footling breech, cesarean section is mandatory. For face and brow presentations, watchful waiting is best, because most convert to vertex presentations. If they do not convert, do a cesarean section.

Postpartum Period

For the first several days postpartum, it is normal to have some discharge (lochia), which is red the first few days and gradually turns to a white/yellowish-white color by day ten.

➤ ***CASE SCENARIO:*** If lochia becomes foul smelling, what condition should you suspect? Endometritis.

The **major causes of maternal mortality** are pulmonary embolism, pregnancy-induced hypertension (PIH), and hemorrhage.

➤ ***CASE SCENARIO:*** When a newly postpartum mother develops dyspnea, tachypnea, chest pain, and hypotension, what condition does she probably have? Amniotic fluid pulmonary embolism.

Postpartum hemorrhage: > 500 ml blood loss during a vaginal delivery or > 1000 ml during a cesarean section. The most common cause is **uterine atony** (75–80% of cases). Other causes include lacerations, retained placental tissue (**placenta accreta,** increta, or percreta), coagulation disorders (e.g., disseminated intravascular coagulation, von Willebrand disease), low placental implantation, and uterine inversion. Patients with severe hemorrhage may develop hypopituitarism (**Sheehan syndrome**). The major risk factors for retained placental tissue are previous uterine surgery and previous cesarean section.

Uterine atony is often caused by **overdistention of the uterus** (multiple gestation, polyhydramnios, macrosomia), **prolonged labor, oxytocin usage,** grandmultiparity (history of 5 or more deliveries), and precipitous labor (< 3 hr). Treat with bimanual compression and massage of the uterus while giving a dilute oxytocin infusion. If this approach fails, you can try ergonovine or another ergot drug (contraindicated with maternal hypertension) or prostaglandin F_2-alpha. If these also fail to stop bleeding, a hysterectomy may be needed.

In patients with **retained products of conception** (which is probably the most common cause of *delayed* postpartum hemorrhage), remove the placenta manually to stop bleeding; then do curettage in the operating room under anesthesia. If the patient has placenta accreta, increta, or percreta (placental tissue grows into or through the myometrium), a hysterectomy is usually necessary to stop the bleeding.

With **uterine inversion** (the uterus inverts and can be seen outside the vagina), put the uterus back in place manually (anesthesia may be required) and give IV fluids and oxytocin. Uterine inversion is usually iatrogenic (due to **pulling too hard on the cord**).

Postpartum fever, defined as a fever for at least two consecutive days, is usually due to breast engorgement; urinary tract infection; or endometritis, endomyometritis, or puerperal sepsis. Important predisposing factors for endometritis are cesarean section, PROM or preterm PROM, prolonged labor, frequent vaginal exams during labor, and manual removal of the placenta or retained placental fragments. Look for **tender uterus** and/or **foul-smelling lochia.** Treat with broad-spectrum antibiotics after performing cultures of the endometrium, vagina, blood, and urine.

- If a postpartum fever from endometritis fails to resolve with broad-spectrum antibiotics, there are two main possibilities: progression to pelvic abscess or pelvic thrombophlebitis. Order a CT scan, which will show an abscess (which needs to be drained). If there is no abscess on CT, think of pelvic thrombophlebitis, which presents with persistent spiking fevers and lack of response to antibiotics. Give **heparin** for an easy cure (and diagnosis in retrospect).

If a postpartum patient goes into shock and no bleeding is seen, think of amniotic fluid embolism, uterine inversion, or concealed hemorrhage (e.g., uterine rupture with bleeding into the peritoneal cavity).

Breastfeeding

If a woman does not want to breastfeed, prescribe tight-fitting bras, ice packs, and analgesia. Bromocriptine and estrogens or birth control pills also can be used to suppress lactation. Breastfeeding is generally encouraged, because it is good for mother-child bonding and may protect the baby from infections.

If a woman breast-feeds, watch for **mastitis,** which usually develops in the first 2 months postpartum. Breasts are red, indurated, and painful and nipple cracks or fissuring may be seen. **Staphylococcus aureus** is the usual cause. Treat with analgesics (e.g., acetaminophen, ibuprofen), warm and/or cold compresses, and continued breast-feeding with the affected breast(s) even though it is painful (use breast pump to empty breast if needed) to prevent further milk duct blockage and abscess formation. Antistaphylococcal antibiotic (e.g., cephalexin, dicloxacillin) is usually given for more than mild symptoms. If a **fluctuant** mass develops or there is no response to antibiotics within a few days, an abscess is likely present and must be drained.

Breastfeeding is contraindicated with maternal HIV and when the mother uses illicit drugs, prescription sedatives or stimulants, lithium, or chemotherapy.

Abortion

Abortion is defined as termination of a pregnancy at < 20 weeks (fetus < 500 gm). Most abortions occur in the first trimester and are spontaneous (i.e. a miscarriage). Treat all patients with IV fluids and/or blood, if needed, and give Rh immune globulin (Rhogam) in the proper setting.

1. **Threatened abortion:** uterine bleeding without cervical dilation and no expulsion of tissue. Treat with pelvic rest (no sex/tampons/douching). Half of women go on to have a normal pregnancy.
2. **Inevitable abortion:** uterine bleeding with cervical dilation, crampy abdominal pain, and no tissue expulsion. Treat with observation, often followed by dilatation and curettage (D&C) of the uterine cavity.
3. **Incomplete abortion:** passage of some products of conception through the cervix. Treat with observation, often followed by D&C.
4. **Complete abortion:** expulsion of all products of conception from the uterus. Treat with serial HCG testing to make sure it goes down to zero. Consider D&C with pain or open cervical os.
5. **Missed abortion:** fetal death without expulsion of fetus. Most women will go on to have spontaneous miscarriage, but D&C commonly performed.
6. **Induced abortion:** intentional termination of pregnancy < 20 weeks (may be elective, which is requested by patient, or therapeutic if done to maintain the health of the mother).
7. **Recurrent abortion:** two or three successive, unplanned abortions. Causes include:
   - Infectious (syphilis, *Listeria, Mycoplasma, Toxoplasma* spp.)
   - Environmental (alcohol, tobacco, drugs)
   - Metabolic (diabetes, hypothyroidism)
   - Autoimmune (lupus and/or **antiphospholipid antibodies/lupus anticoagulant**)
   - Anatomic abnormalities (**cervical incompetence,** congenital female tract abnormalities, fibroids)
   - Chromosomal abnormalities (e.g., maternal/paternal translocations)
     - **CASE SCENARIO:** What condition classically causes painless, recurrent abortions in the second trimester? **Cervical incompetence.** Future pregnancies can be treated with cervical cerclage (suture to keep cervical os closed) at 14–16 weeks. Other anatomic abnormalities also should be considered.

Classic symptoms of ectopic pregnancy (which usually presents between 4 and 10 weeks and ends in spontaneous or therapeutic abortion, sometimes with catastrophic tubal rupture) are **amenorrhea, vaginal bleeding,** and **abdominal pain** with a **positive HCG** test. Palpation of an adnexal mass may indicate an ectopic pregnancy or a corpus luteum cyst. Ultrasound is generally done to help exclude this condition. When you are in doubt and the patient is crashing (e.g., hypovolemia, shock, severe abdominal pain/rebound tenderness), consider laparoscopy for a definitive diagnosis and treatment. In stable cases, the tube may be salvaged (salpingostomy). Medical abortion (e.g., with methotrexate) is gaining acceptance in compliant patients who desire it.

> ➤ **CASE SCENARIO:** What is the major risk factor for ectopic pregnancy? A previous history of **pelvic inflammatory disease** (10-fold increased risk). Other risk factors include previous ectopic pregnancy, history of tubal sterilization or tuboplasty, and pregnancy that occurs with an intrauterine device in place.

Third-trimester Bleeding

Always do an ultrasound before a pelvic exam. The differential diagnosis includes:

1. **Placenta previa.** Predisposing factors include multiparity, increasing age, multiple gestation, and prior previa. This condition is why you do an ultrasound before a pelvic exam. **Bleeding is painless** and may be profuse. Ultrasound is 95–100% accurate in diagnosis. Cesarean section is mandatory for delivery, but you may try to admit with bed/pelvic rest and tocolysis if the patient is preterm and stable and the bleeding stops.
2. **Abruptio placentae.** Predisposing factors include hypertension (with or without pre-eclampsia), trauma, polyhydramnios with rapid decompression after membrane rupture, **cocaine** or tobacco use, and preterm PROM.

   Note: The patient can have this condition *without visible bleeding* because the blood may be contained behind the placenta. Watch for **uterine pain and tenderness** and increased uterine tone with **hyperactive contraction pattern.** Fetal distress is apparent. Abruptio placentae also may cause disseminated intravascular coagulation if fetal products enter the maternal circulation. Ultrasound may be falsely normal. Treat with rapid delivery (vaginal preferred).
3. **Uterine rupture.** Predisposing factors include previous uterine surgery, trauma, **oxytocin,** grand multiparity (several previous deliveries), excessive uterine distention (e.g., multiple gestation, polyhydramnios), abnormal fetal lie, CPD, and shoulder dystocia. Look for sudden onset of severe pain, often accompanied by maternal hypotension or shock. Fetal parts may be palpated in the abdomen, or the **abdominal contour may change.** Treat with immediate laparotomy and usually hysterectomy after delivery.
4. **Fetal bleeding** usually results from **vasa previa** or velamentous insertion of the cord. The major risk factor is **multiple gestation** (the higher the number of fetuses, the higher the risk). **Bleeding is painless,** and the mother is completely stable, whereas the fetus shows worsening distress (tachycardia initially, then bradycardia as fetus decompensates). The **Apt test** is positive on uterine blood (differentiates fetal from maternal blood cells). Treat with immediate cesarean section.
5. **Cervical or vaginal lesions:** herpes, gonorrhea, *Chlamydia, Candida* spp.
6. **Cervical or vaginal trauma:** usually from intercourse.
7. **Bleeding disorder:** antepartum presentation is rare (more common postpartum).
8. **Cervical cancer:** can occur in pregnant patients, too!
9. **"Bloody show":** with cervical effacement, a blood-tinged mucus plug may be released from the cervical canal and heralds the onset of labor (this is a normal occurrence and a diagnosis of exclusion).

In all patients with third-trimester bleeding:

- Start IV fluids, and give blood if needed.
- Give oxygen.
- Order a complete blood count, coagulation profiles, and ultrasound.
- Set up fetal and maternal monitoring.

- Do an illicit drug screen if drug abuse is suspected (cocaine causes placental abruption).
- Give Rh immune globulin if the mother is Rh-negative.
- The **Kleihauer-Betke** test can be used to quantify the amount of fetal blood in the maternal circulation and calculate the dose of Rhogam.

Preterm and Postterm Labor

Preterm labor: labor occurring between 20–37 weeks. Treat with lateral decubitus position, bed/pelvic rest, oral or IV fluids, and oxygen administration (all may stop the contractions). Then give a tocolytic agent (**beta$_2$ agonist** or **magnesium sulfate**) if no contraindications are present. The patient can be discharged on oral tocolytics. The many contraindications to tocolysis include heart disease, hypertension, diabetes, hemorrhage, pre-eclampsia, chorioamnionitis, IUGR, ruptured membranes, cervical dilation $\geq$ 4 cm, fetal demise, and fetal anomalies incompatible with survival.

Fetal fibronectin can be detected in vaginal secretions of women presenting with signs and symptoms of preterm labor and if negative between 22–34 weeks, there is a very low likelihood of delivery in the next 2 weeks. Thus, a more conservative, observational approach can be used. When fetal fibronectin is positive in this setting, the woman remains at a higher risk for delivery in the next 2 weeks and a more aggressive approach to tocolysis and fetal lung maturity hastening is employed.

If fetal lungs are immature (amniocentesis reveals **lecithin:sphingomyelin [L:S] ratio < 2:1** or is negative for **phosphatidylglycerol**) and the fetus is between 26–34 weeks of age, corticosteroid administration may hasten lung maturity and thus reduce the risk of respiratory distress syndrome.

Premature rupture of the membranes (PROM) is rupture of the amniotic sac before the onset of labor. Diagnosis of rupture of the membranes (whether premature or not) is based on history and sterile speculum exam, which shows (1) **pooling of amniotic fluid,** (2) **ferning pattern** when the fluid is placed on a microscopic slide and allowed to dry, and/or (3) **positive nitrazine test** (nitrazine paper turns blue in the presence of amniotic fluid). Ultrasound should be done to assess amniotic fluid volume (as well as gestational age and any anomalies that may be present). Spontaneous labor often follows membrane rupture. If labor does not occur within 6–8 hours and the mother is at term, consider inducing labor.

Chorioamnionitis is a prenatal/natal infection that presents with **fever** and **tender, irritable uterus.** The classic cause is PROM or preterm PROM. Do a culture and Gram stain of the amniotic fluid, and treat with ampicillin while awaiting culture results. Chorioamnionitis may result in neonatal sepsis and/or maternal sepsis or endomyometritis.

Preterm PROM is premature rupture of the membranes before 36–37 weeks. Risk of infection increases with the duration of ruptured membranes. Do a culture and Gram stain of the amniotic fluid. If the results are negative, treat with pelvic/bed rest and frequent follow-up. If the results are positive for group B streptococci, treat the mother with amoxicillin even if she is asymptomatic.

Multiple gestations usually result in premature labor and delivery due to limitations of uterine size. If the sex or blood type is different, twins are **dizygotic.** If the placentas are monochorionic, the twins are **monozygotic.** These three simple factors differentiate monozygotic from dizygotic twins in 80% of cases. In the remaining 20%, HLA typing studies may be needed.

Other complications of multiple gestations (the higher the number of fetuses, the higher the risk of most of these conditions)

1. **Maternal:** anemia, hypertension/pre-eclampsia, postpartum uterine atony, postpartum hemorrhage.

2. **Fetal:** polyhydramnios, malpresentation, placenta previa, abruptio placentae, velamentous cord insertion/vasa previa, umbilical cord prolapse, IUGR, congenital anomalies, increased perinatal morbidity and mortality.

   Note: With vertex-vertex twin presentations, you can try vaginal delivery for both infants; with any other combination of presentations or more than two fetuses, do a cesarean section.

Postterm pregnancy is defined as **> 42 weeks'** gestation. Generally, if the gestational age is known to be accurate, such patients are induced into labor (e.g., with oxytocin). If dates are uncertain, do twice-weekly biophysical profile. At 43 weeks, most physicians induce labor or do a cesarean section. Remember that both prematurity and postmaturity increase perinatal morbidity and mortality.

> ***CASE SCENARIO:*** Prolonged gestation is classically associated with what congenital anomaly? Anencephaly (see figure).

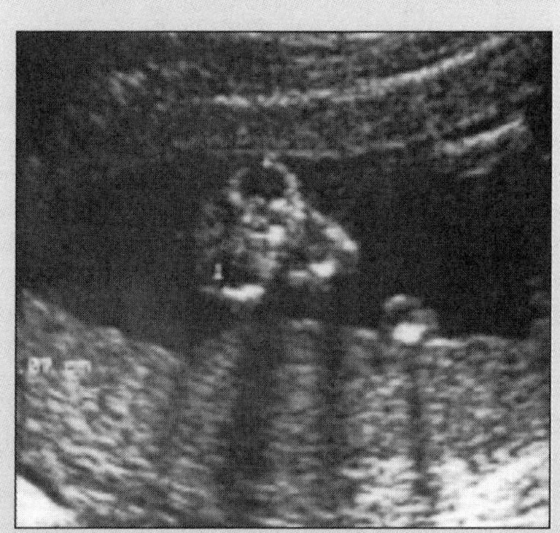

Anencephalic fetus with frog-like appearance. (From Katz DS, Math KR, Groskni SA: Radiology Secrets. Philadelphia, Hanley & Belfus, 1998, p. 229, with permission.)

High-risk Obstetrics/Problem Pregnancies

Hyperemesis gravidarum: intractable nausea and vomiting leading to dehydration and possible electrolyte disturbances. The condition presents in the first trimester, usually in **younger women with their first pregnancy** and some **underlying social stressors** or psychiatric problems. Treat with supportive care, including small, frequent meals and antiemetics (fairly safe in pregnancy). With severe dehydration and/or electrolyte disturbances, admit to the hospital for treatment with IV fluids and observation.

Note: With all high-risk pregnancies, consider BPP once or even twice a week in the third trimester until delivery.

> ***CASE SCENARIO:*** A pregnant woman's last child had spina bifida, and she wants to know if her fetus has it. Should you do chorionic villi sampling? No, because chorionic villi sampling cannot detect neural tube defects. It is generally reserved for women with previously affected offspring with a known genetic disease, because it can be done at 9–12 weeks (earlier than amniocentesis), which gives women the advantage of a first-trimester abortion if a fetus is affected. Chorionic villi sampling causes a slightly higher miscarriage rate than amniocentesis.

Pre-eclampsia: look for **hypertension** (if the woman has preexisting hypertension, look for >30/15-mmHg increase in blood pressure over baseline), urinalysis with 2+ or more **proteinuria,** oliguria, **swelling or edema of the hands and/or face,** headache, visual disturbances, and HELLP syndrome (**h**emolysis, **e**levated **l**iver enzymes, **l**ow **p**latelets, often with right upper quadrant or epigastric pain). Pre-eclampsia usually occurs in the **third trimester.** The main risk factors are chronic renal disease, chronic hypertension, family history, multiple gestation, nulliparity, extremes of reproductive age (the classic case is a **young female with her first child**), diabetes, and black race. Treatment includes stabilization and delivery if the patient is at term. If the patient is premature and has mild disease, give **hydralazine** or **labetalol** for hypertension, **magnesium sulfate** for seizure prophylaxis, prescribe bed rest, and observe in the hospital. If the patient has severe disease (oliguria, mental status changes, headache, blurred vision, pulmonary edema, cyanosis, HELLP, blood pressure > 160/110 mmHg, progression to eclampsia [seizures]), deliver regardless of gestational age because both mother and infant may die. **Pre-eclampsia plus seizures =** eclampsia.

Mild ankle edema is normal in pregnancy, but severe ankle edema or hand edema should make you suspect pre-eclampsia.

Hypertension plus proteinuria in a pregnant patient is pre-eclampsia until proved otherwise.

- Do not wait to remeasure very high blood pressure in a pregnant patient. Err on the safe side: assume that it represents pre-eclampsia, and start treatment.
- Do not try to deliver the infant until the mother is stable (e.g., do not perform a cesarean section while the mother has seizures).
- Pre-eclampsia and eclampsia cause uteroplacental insufficiency, IUGR, fetal demise, and increased maternal morbidity and mortality rates.
- Pre-eclampsia and eclampsia generally are not considered risk factors for future development of hypertension or end-organ effects of hypertension.

  ➤ ***CASE SCENARIO:*** Pre-eclampsia symptoms that develop before the third trimester should make you consider what disorder? Molar pregnancy.

  ➤ ***CASE SCENARIO:*** What is the best way to prevent eclampsia? Regular prenatal care, which allows you to detect the disorder in the pre-eclampsia stage and treat appropriately.

  ➤ ***CASE SCENARIO:*** What is the initial treatment of choice for eclamptic seizures? Magnesium sulfate, which also lowers blood pressure. Toxic effects include **hyporeflexia (first sign of toxicity), respiratory depression, CNS depression,** coma, and death. If toxicity occurs, the first step is to stop the magnesium infusion.

Maternal complications of gestational diabetes: polyhydramnios, pre-eclampsia, and complications of diabetes. Problems in infants born to diabetic mothers include **macrosomia** (gestational diabetes) or IUGR (pre-existing diabetes); **respiratory distress syndrome; cardiovascular, colon, craniofacial,** and **neural tube defects;** and **caudal regression syndrome** (the lower half of the body is incompletely formed).

- Treat with diet, exercise, and/or insulin. Do not use oral hypoglycemics, which can cross the placenta. Tighter control results in better outcomes for mother and baby. Check HbA1c to determine compliance and glucose fluctuations.

  ➤ ***CASE SCENARIO:*** What is the classic glucose problem after birth in an infant born to a diabetic mother? Postdelivery **hypoglycemia.** In utero, fetal islet-cell hypertrophy results from maternal and thus fetal hyperglycemia. After birth, when the infant is cut off from the mother's glucose supply, hyperglycemia resolves, but islet cells continue to overproduce insulin and cause hypoglycemia. Treat with IV glucose.

Maternal hypertension causes IUGR and is a risk factor for pre-eclampsia.

IgG is the only maternal antibody that crosses the placenta. An elevated neonatal IgM concentration is *never* normal, whereas an elevated neonatal IgG often represents maternal antibodies.

Rh incompatibility/hemolytic disease of the newborn occurs when the mother is Rh-negative and the infant is Rh-positive. If both mother and father are Rh-negative, there is nothing to worry about;

the infant will be Rh-negative. If the mother is Rh-negative and the father is Rh-positive, the infant has a 50/50 chance of being Rh-positive. If there is a potential for hemolytic disease, check maternal Rh antibody titers.

Give Rh immune globulin automatically at 28 weeks and within 72 hours after delivery as well as after any procedures that may cause transplacental hemorrhage (e.g., amniocentesis). There **must be previous sensitization** for disease to occur. In other words, if a nulliparous mother has never received blood products, her first Rh-positive infant most likely will not be affected by hemolytic disease. The second Rh-positive infant, however, will be affected (unless Rh immune globulin is administered at the right times during the first pregnancy). If you check maternal Rh antibodies and they are strongly positive, Rh immune globulin does not help, because sensitization has already occurred. Rh immune globulin administration is a good example of **primary prevention.**

- If not detected or prevented, Rh incompatibility can lead to fetal hydrops (edema, ascites, pleural/pericardial effusions) and demise.
- Amniotic fluid spectrophotometry can gauge the severity of fetal hemolysis.
- Treatment of hemolytic disease involves delivery if the fetus is mature (check lung maturity with L:S ratio), **intrauterine blood transfusion,** and **phenobarbital,** which helps the fetal liver break down bilirubin by inducing enzymes.
- ABO blood group incompatibility (and other minor antigens) also can cause hemolytic disease of the newborn when the mother is type O and the infant is is type A, B, or AB. Previous sensitization is not required, because IgG antibodies (which can cross the placenta) occur naturally in people with blood type O. The disease usually is less severe than Rh incompatibility, but treatment is the same.

> ➤ **CASE SCENARIO:** The mother is Rh-negative and has a high titer of Rh antibodies. The father is Rh-positive. Should you give Rh immune globulin? No—you are too late. Antibodies have already formed. Instead, monitor fetus closely.

Hydatiform mole: essentially, the products of conception become a tumor. Look for **pre-eclampsia before the third trimester;** an **HCG level** that does not return to zero after a delivery/abortion or rapidly rises during pregnancy; first- or second-trimester bleeding with possible expulsion of "**grape-like vesicles;**" uterine size/date discrepancy; and/or a "**snow storm**" pattern on ultrasound. **Complete moles** are 46 XX (all chromosomes from the father) and contain **no fetal tissue; incomplete moles** are usually 69 XXY and **contain fetal tissue.** The gross appearance suggests a "bunch of grapes." Treat with uterine dilatation and curettage, then follow HCG levels until they fall to zero. If HCG does not fall to zero or rises, the patient has either an invasive mole or choriocarcinoma (choriocarcinoma can only arise de novo or from a complete mole, not from an incomplete mole). In either case, the patient needs chemotherapy (usually **methotrexate** or actinomycin D).

In women with **antiphospholipid antibodies** and previous problem pregnancies (e.g., recurrent abortions), low-dose **aspirin** with low-dose subcutaneous **heparin** may help in subsequent pregnancies (normally, aspirin and other NSAIDs should be avoided in pregnancy).

If a woman develops **tuberculosis** (Tb) during pregnancy (positive purified protein derivative [PPD] skin test and suspicious chest x-ray and/or positive sputum culture), treat as you would any other patient. If the woman is a known recent PPD converter or has additional risk factors (e.g., HIV infection or living with an active case of Tb), treat with isoniazid prophylaxis just like a regular patient. Be sure to give the mother vitamin B_6 with isoniazid to prevent deficiency in her and the fetus. Avoid **streptomycin,** which may cause deafness and/or nephrotoxicity in the fetus.

Obstetric Pharmacology and Teratogenesis

Teratogenic agents:

AGENT	DEFECT(S) CAUSED
Thalidomide	Phocomelia
Antineoplastics	Many
Tetracycline	Yellow or brown teeth
Aminoglycoside	Deafness
Valproic acid	Spina bifida, hypospadias
Progesterone	Masculinization of females
Cigarettes	Intrauterine growth retardation, low birth weight, prematurity
Birth control pills	VACTERL syndrome (**v**ertebral, **a**nal, **c**ardiac, **t**rachoe**e**sophageal, **r**enal, and **l**imb malformations)
Lithium	Cardiac (Ebstein) anomalies
Aminopterin	Intrauterine growth retardation, central nervous system defects, cleft lip/palate
Radiation	Intrauterine growth retardation, central nervous system/face defects, leukemia
Alcohol	Fetal alcohol syndrome
Phenytoin*	Craniofacial and limb defects, mental retardation, cardiovascular defects
Trimethadione	Craniofacial and cardiovascular defects, mental retardation
Warfarin	Craniofacial and central nervous system defects, intrauterine growth retardation, stillbirth
Carbamazepine	Fingernail hypoplasia, craniofacial defects
Isotretinoin[t]	Central nervous system, craniofacial/ear, and cardiovascular defects
Iodine	Goiter, cretinism
Cocaine	Cerebral infarcts, mental retardation
Diazepam	Cleft lip/palate
Diethylstilbestrol	Clear cell vaginal cancer, adenosis, cervical incompetence

*Diphenylhydantoin.

[t]Vitamin A in general is considered teratogenic when recommended intake levels are exceeded.

Drugs that are generally safe in pregnancy: acetaminophen, penicillin, cephalosporins, erythromycin, nitrofurantoin, H_2 blockers, antacids, heparin, hydralazine, methyldopa, labetalol, insulin, and docusate.

GYNECOLOGY

Infections

Pelvic inflammatory disease (PID): look for a female patient aged 13–35 years with **abdominal pain, adnexal tenderness,** and **cervical motion tenderness** (all three should be present). Patients also have at least one of the following: elevated sedimentation rate, leukocytosis, fever, or **purulent cervical discharge.** Treat with more than one antibiotic (e.g., cefoxitin/ceftriaxone and doxycycline on an outpatient basis; clindamycin and gentamicin on an inpatient basis) to cover multiple organisms (e.g., *Neisseria gonorrhoeae, Chlamydia* spp., *Escherichia coli*). In patients with a history of intrauterine device use, think of ***Actinomyces israeli.***

- PID is the most common cause of preventable infertility (causes scarring of tubes) and the most likely cause of infertility in a woman under age 30 with normal menstrual cycles.

- Watch for progression to tubo-ovarian abscess (palpable on exam) and abscess rupture. Rupture is treated with emergent laparotomy and excision of affected tube (unilateral disease) or hysterectomy and bilateral salpingo-oophorectomy (severe bilateral disease). An unruptured abscess may respond to antibiotics (unlike many abscesses) alone.

Vaginal infections*:

ORGANISM	FINDINGS	TREATMENT
Candida spp.	Cottage-cheese discharge, pseudohyphae on KOH prep, history of diabetes/antibiotic treatment/pregnancy	Oral or topical antifungal
Trichomonas spp.	Organisms are seen swimming under microscope; pale green, frothy, watery discharge, "strawberry" cervix	Metronidazole
Gardnerella spp.	Malodorous discharge; fishy smell on KOH prep, clue cells	Metronidazole
Human papillomavirus	Venereal warts, koilocytosis on Pap smear	Many (acid, cryotherapy, laser, podophyllin)
Herpes	Multiple shallow, painful ulcers; recurrence and resolution	Acyclovir, valacyclovir
Chlamydia spp.	Most common sexually transmitted disease; dysuria; positive culture and antibody tests	Doxycycline or azithromycin†
Neisseria gonorrhoeae	Mucopurulent cervicitis; gram-negative	Ceftriaxone or ciprofloxacin
Molluscum	Characteristic appearance of lesions, intracellular inclusions	Many (curette, cryotherapy, coagulation)
Pediculosis	"Crabs," itching, see lice on pubic hairs	Permethrin cream

KOH = potassium hydroxide.

*Findings are similar in men and treatment is the same.

†Chlamydial infection is treated with erythromycin or amoxicillin if the patient is pregnant. When compliance is an inssue (e.g., alcoholic/drug abuser, homeless or unreliable partner), give 1 gm of azithromycin orally as a one-time dose. It may be wise to watch the person take it.

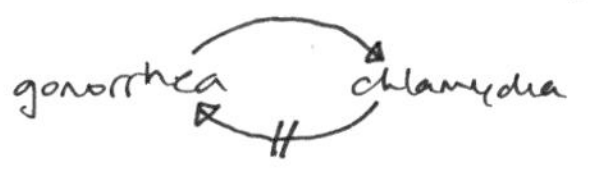

➤ ***CASE SCENARIO:*** A 19-year-old woman presents with a purulent cervical discharge. Culture reveals gonorrhea. What should the treatment be? Ceftriaxone and doxycycline (the doxycycline is given to treat presumed chlamydial coinfection). The reverse is not true, however; do not treat patients with chlamydial infection for gonorrhea unless you know they have both.

➤ ***CASE SCENARIO:*** A woman presents with a malodorous discharge, and a fishy odor is detected when you perform a potassium hydroxide preparation of a swab sample. How should you handle treatment of the woman's sexual partner? The patient is infected with *Gardnerella* spp. You do not need to treat the patient's sexual partners. The same is true for candidal infection. Remember to treat partners and give counseling (e.g., condoms) for the other infections in the chart above.

Amenorrhea

Primary amenorrhea: any female who has not menstruated by age 16 has primary amenorrhea. In the absence of secondary sexual characteristics by age 14 or absence of menstruation within 2 years of developing secondary sex characteristics, patients should be evaluated. **First get a pregnancy test** (pregnancy can cause primary amenorrhea!). If it is negative and no abnormalities are seen on physical exam (e.g., absent uterus, Turner syndrome phenotype), **administer progesterone.** If bleeding occurs, estrogen and a normal uterus are present. If bleeding does not occur, the patient probably has either an absence of estrogen or an anatomic abnormality. See below for specifics.

- If a patient is older than 14 and has no secondary sexual characteristics, there is most likely a congenital problem.
- In a phenotypically normal female (normal breast development) with an absence of both axillary and pubic hair, think of **androgen insensitivity syndrome.** The uterus is absent, and the patient is XY or a genotypic male but should be treated as a female.
- **Imperforate hymen** presents in a menarche-aged patient with blood in the vagina that cannot escape. On exam, the hymen bulges outward. Treatment is surgical opening of the hymen.

Secondary amenorrhea in a previously menstruating, sexually active woman of reproductive age is **pregnancy until proved otherwise** with a negative HCG assay. If the pregnancy test is negative and no obvious abnormality is apparent in the history or physical exam, administer progesterone, which will tell you the patient's estrogen status:

- If the patient has vaginal bleeding within 2 weeks, she has sufficient estrogen. Next, check the luteinizing hormone (LH) level. If it is high, think of **polycystic ovary syndrome.** If it is low or normal, think of three possibilities: (1) pituitary adenoma (check **prolactin**); (2) **hypothyroidism** (check thyroid-stimulating hormone [TSH]); or (3) low gonadotropin hormone levels due to drugs, stress, **exercise,** or **anorexia nervosa** (normal prolactin and TSH). Any of these patients can try **clomiphene** to become pregnant.
- If the patient has no bleeding, estrogen is insufficient. Check follicle-stimulating hormone (FSH) next. If it is elevated, the patient has **premature ovarian failure/menopause;** check for an autoimmune disorder, karyotype abnormalities, and history of chemotherapy. If FSH is low or normal, the patient may have a neoplasm affecting the hypothalamus; consider an MRI of the brain.
  - ➤ ***CASE SCENARIO:*** What is the first test to order in any woman of reproductive age who has amenorrhea, whether primary or secondary? A pregnancy test.

Other Menstrual Disorders

Endometriosis: ectopic endometrial glands that are outside the uterus. Patients are classically **nulliparous** and **over age 30,** with the following symptoms: **dysmenorrhea, dyspareunia** (painful intercourse), **dyschezia** (painful defecation), and/or perimenstrual spotting. The most common site of occurrence is the **ovaries;** look for tender adnexae in a patient without other evidence of PID. Other exam findings include nodularities of the broad/uterosacral ligaments and retroverted uterus. The gold standard of diagnosis is laparoscopy with visualization of endometriosis (described as raised blue-colored "**mulberry spots;**" flat, brown-colored "**powder burns;**" or blood-filled "**chocolate cysts**").

- Most likely cause of infertility in a menstruating woman over age of 30.
- Treat first with **birth control pills** (danazol and gonadotropin-releasing hormone ([GnRH] agonists are second-line agents).
- Surgery/cautery can be used to destroy endometriomas and often **improves fertility**. In an older patient, consider hysterectomy with bilateral salpingo-oopherectomy for severe symptoms.

Adenomyosis: ectopic endometrial glands that are within the uterine musculature. Patients usually are **over age 40** with **dysmenorrhea** and menorrhagia. Physical exam reveals a **large, boggy uterus.** Do dilatation and curettage to rule out endometrial cancer, and consider hysterectomy to relieve severe symptoms. GnRH agonists also may relieve symptoms.

Dysfunctional uterine bleeding (DUB): defined as abnormal uterine bleeding not associated with tumor, inflammation, or pregnancy. DUB is the most common cause of abnormal uterine bleeding and is a diagnosis of exclusion. Over 70% of cases are associated with anovulatory cycles (unopposed estrogen). The age of the patient is very important. After menarche and just before menopause, DUB is common and, in fact, physiologic. Most other women have **polycystic ovary syndrome.** Perform a dilatation and curettage to rule out endometrial cancer in women over 35. Also get a complete blood count to make sure that the patient is not anemic from excessive blood loss. Uncommon causes of DUB are infections, endocrine disorders (thyroid, adrenal, pituitary/prolactin), coagulation defects, and estrogen-producing neoplasms.

- In the absence of pathology, treat first with nonsteroidal anti-inflammatory drugs (NSAIDs), which are first-line agents for DUB and dysmenorrhea.
- Birth control pills are also a first-line agent for menorrhagia/DUB if patient does not desire pregnancy and her menstrual cycles are irregular.
- Progesterone is sometimes given for severe bleeding.

Polycystic ovarian syndrome (PCOS): look for an **overweight** woman who has **hirsutism, amenorrhea,** and/or **infertility** (i.e. "heavy, hirsuit, and [h]amenorrheic"). PCOS is the most likely cause for infertility in a woman under 30 with abnormal menstruation. Multiple ovarian cysts often are seen on ultrasound. The primary event is thought to be **androgen excess;** the **LH:FSH ratio is greater than 2:1.** Unopposed estrogen increases risk for **endometrial hyperplasia** and **carcinoma.** Treat with birth control pills or cyclic progesterone. If the woman desires pregnancy, clomiphene may be used.

Premenstrual dysphoric disorder (aka PMS): occurs every month just before menstruation. The patient is symptom-free at other times. Classic symptoms include bloating, breast swelling/tenderness, headaches, irritability, and depression. Treat with NSAIDs; consider antidepressants for depression symptoms.

Menopause: average age of menopause is around 50. Patients have irregular cycles or **amenorrhea, hot flashes, mood swings,** and an **elevated FSH level.** See pharmacology section for information about hormone replacement therapy (HRT). Bone density test may show osteoporosis. Patients also may complain of **dysuria, dyspareunia, incontinence,** and/or **vaginal itching, burning, or soreness**—symptoms that often are due to atrophic vaginitis in this age group. Look for vaginal mucosa to be thin, dry, and atrophic with increased parabasal cells on cytology. Estrogen, either topical or systemic, improves these symptoms.

Leiomyoma (fibroid): benign tumors (see figure) that are the most common indication for hysterectomy (when they grow too large or cause symptoms). Malignant transformation is rare (< 1%), and some believe it is nonexistent. Look for **rapid growth during pregnancy or use of estrogen** (e.g., birth control pills) or regression after menopause (estrogen-dependent). Fibroids may cause infertility (which may be restored by myomectomy), pain, or menorrhagia/metrorrhagia; anemia due to fibroids is an indication for hysterectomy. Perform dilatation and curettage to rule out endometrial cancer and malignant transformation in women older than 40. Patients may present with a polyp protruding through cervix.

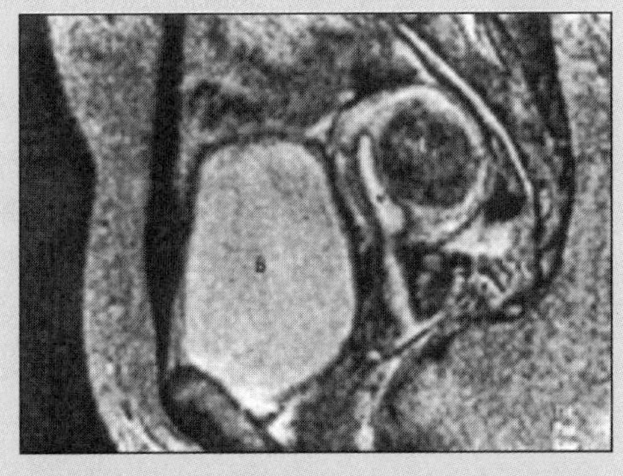

Leiomyoma on a T2-weighted sagittal image. A round, low signal intensity intraumural leiomyoma (L) is seen in the posterior aspect of the uterus. E = endometrium, B = bladder. (From Katz DS, Math KR, Groskin SA (eds): Radiology Secrets. Philadelphia, Hanley & Belfus, 1998, p 252, with permission.)

Breast Disorders

Breast discharge: watch for history of birth control pills, hormone therapies, antipsychotic medications, or hypothyroidism symptoms, all of which can cause discharge. When the discharge is **bilat-**

lateral and nonbloody, the cause is not breast cancer. The patient may have a prolactinoma (check prolactin level) or endocrine disorder. When the discharge is unilateral, whether bloody or not, and/or associated with a mass, it should raise concern about possible breast cancer. Biopsy any mass in this setting.

Breast mass in a woman under 35 (unlikely to be cancer)

1. **Fibrocystic disease:** **bilateral,** multiple, tender (especially premenstrually), cystic lesions. Most common breast disorder. Generally, no further work-up needed—just routine follow-up. Progesterone for a week at the end of each month or danazol may help relieve symptoms.
2. **Fibroadenoma:** painless, discrete, **sharply circumscribed, rubbery, mobile mass.** Fibroadenoma is the most common benign tumor of the female breast. It may be observed for one or more menstrual cycles in the absence of symptoms. **Pregnancy and estrogen-containing medicines** (e.g., oral contraceptives) **may stimulate growth** (tumors are estrogen-dependent). Excision is curative but not often required unless the patient desires or there is clinical concern for cancer.
3. **Mastitis/abscess:** Lactating woman in the first few months postpartum with reddish, painful breast that develops into a fluctuant mass (abscess). See page 48 for treatment.
4. **Fat necrosis:** look for history of trauma.

   Note: Mammography in women under 35 is rarely useful, because the breast tissue is too dense to allow characterization of masses. If cancer (rare in this age group) is suspected, proceed directly to biopsy or consider ultrasound of the breast.

Breast mass in a woman 35 or over (always consider cancer in the differential)

1. **Fibrocystic disease:** as above, but aspiration of cyst fluid and baseline mammography are recommended. If cyst fluid is nonbloody and the mass resolves after aspiration, the patient needs only reassurance and follow-up. If the fluid is bloody or the cyst recurs quickly, do a biopsy to rule out cancer.
2. **Fibroadenoma:** get a baseline mammogram. You can observe briefly if the mass is small *and* seems benign clinically *and* the woman is premenopausal *and* has no risk factors for breast cancer. Otherwise, do a biopsy! Watch out for phylloides tumor, a potentially malignant tumor that can masquerade as a rapidly growing fibroadenoma.
3. **Breast cancer:** classic presentation of **nipple retraction** and/or **peau d'orange** may or may not be seen in a **nulliparous** woman with a **strong family history.** In a woman 35 or older, you will almost never be faulted for doing a biopsy of any mass. In the absence of a classic benign case presentation (such as trauma to the breast with fat necrosis or bilateral masses with premenstrual breast pain every month), always consider biopsy. In addition, get a baseline mammogram. See oncology section for more information on breast cancer.

   ➤ **CASE SCENARIO:** What is a new breast mass in a postmenopausal female? Cancer until proved otherwise. Get a biopsy.

In patients with a clinically evident breast mass, mammography and ultrasound are secondary tools. The decision to perform a biopsy is a **clinical decision** based on risk factors, physical exam, history, and imaging characteristics. Mammography is best used to detect nonpalpable breast masses (as a screening tool) and is only one of many tools used to evaluate a palpable mass. On the other hand, if a suspicious lesion is found on mammogram, it should be biopsied *even if it seems benign on physical exam.*

Miscellaneous

Pelvic relaxation/vaginal prolapse: due to weakening of pelvic ligaments. Look for history of several vaginal deliveries, feeling of heaviness or fullness in the pelvis, backache, worsening of symptoms with standing, and resolution with lying down.

1. **Cystocele:** bladder bulges into the **upper anterior vaginal wall.** Symptoms include urinary urgency, frequency, and incontinence.
2. **Rectocele:** rectum bulges into **lower posterior vaginal wall.** The major symptom is difficulty in defecating.
3. **Enterocele:** loops of bowel bulge into the **upper posterior vaginal wall.**
4. **Urethrocele:** urethra bulges into the **lower anterior vaginal wall.** Symptoms include urinary urgency, frequency, and incontinence.

   Note: Conservative treatment involves pelvic strengthening exercises and/or a **pessary** (artificial, removable device that provides support). Surgery is used for refractory or severe cases.

Infertility: two-thirds of cases are due to a female problem, one-third to a male problem. If nothing is apparent after the history and physical exam, the first step is a **semen analysis** (cheap, noninvasive test that may lead to an easy diagnosis).

- Consider ovluation disorders in women with irregular menstrual cycles.
- Consider a tubal problem in patients with a history of PID or previous ectopic pregnancy.
- Consider a uterine problem in patients with a history of dilatation and curettage (which may cause intrauterine synechiae), fibroids, or signs or symptoms of endometriosis or adenomyosis.
- Consider cervical factors in patients with a history of cervicitis, birth trauma, or previous cone biopsy of the cervix.
- Laparoscopy is a last result or is done in patients with a history suggestive of endometriosis. Lysis of adhesions and destruction of endometriosis lesions may restore fertility.
  - ➤ ***CASE SCENARIO:*** What test can be used to look for structural abnormalities of the uterus and tubes? A hysterosalpingogram.
  - ➤ ***CASE SCENARIO:*** In which women can clomiphene be used to induce ovulation? Women who produce adequate estrogen. If the woman is hypoestrogenic, use human menopausal gonadotropin (hMG), which is a combination of FSH/LH. If these approaches fail, consider in vitro fertilization.

If a patient does not desire sterilization, the most effective form of birth control is hormones: birth control pills (see pharmacology section), long-acting progesterone depot injections, or long-acting subcutaneous implants. Only condoms (male or female) protect from sexually transmitted diseases. An intrauterine device (IUD) should be used only in older women, preferably those who are monogamous, because IUDs increase the risk of ectopic pregnancy and PID. A recent hot topic is postcoital contraception, which is essentially a high-dose of birth control pills taken within 48–72 hours after intercourse.

♀ makes estrogen – give clomiphene

♀ does not make estrogen – give hMG

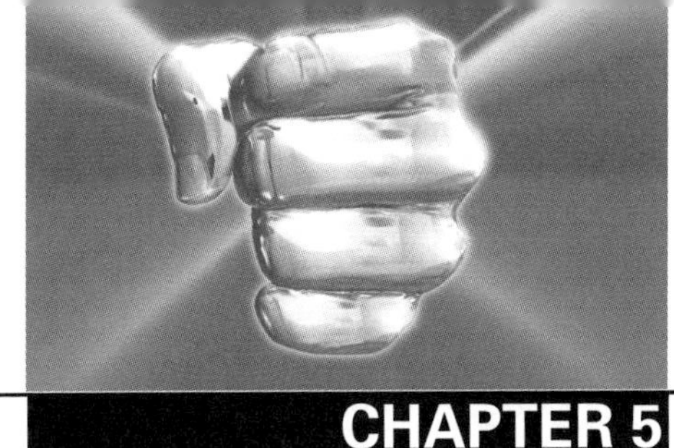

CHAPTER 5

Surgery, Surgical Subspecalties, and Trauma

TRAUMA

The ABCDEs are the key to the initial management of patients with trauma. Always do them in order. For example, if the patient is bleeding to death and has a blocked airway, you may have to choose which issue to address first. The first priority is airway management.

A = **Airway maintenance and cervical spine care.** Provide, protect, and maintain an adequate airway at all times and assume a cervical injury is present while doing so (i.e., place cervical collar, and do not hyperextend neck) until it is excluded. If the patient can answer questions, the airway is fine. You can use an oropharyngeal or nasopharyngeal airway in uncomplicated cases and give supplemental oxygen. When you are in doubt or when the airway is blocked, intubate. If intubation fails, do a cricothyroidotomy.

B = **Breathing and ventilation.** Similar to airway, but even when the airway is patent, the patient may not be spontaneously breathing. The end result is the same. When you are in doubt or the patient is not breathing, intubate. If intubation fails, do a cricothyroidotomy.

C = **Circulation and control of hemorrhage.** If the patient seems hypovolemic (tachycardia, bleeding, weak pulse, paleness, diaphoresis, capillary refill > 2 seconds), give IV fluids and/or blood products. The initial procedure is to start 2 large-bore catheters and give a bolus of 10–20 ml/kg (roughly 1 liter) of lactated Ringer's solution (IV fluid of choice in trauma) and blood. Then reassess the patient for improvement. Repeat the bolus if needed.

D = **Disability and neurologic status.** Check neurologic function (Glasgow coma scale).

E = **Exposure by undressing the patient.** Remove the patient's clothing and "put a finger in every orifice" so that you do not miss any occult injuries.

In general, **all trauma patients** should have cervical spine, chest, and pelvic x-rays with CT exams used as needed for further evaluation or persistent symptoms despite negative x-rays.

Evaluate **head trauma** with a **noncontrast CT** (better than MRI for trauma).

Blunt abdominal trauma. Initial findings determine a course of action:

- If the patient is awake and stable and your exam is benign, observe and repeat the abdominal exam later.
- If the patient is hemodynamically unstable (hypotension and/or shock that does not respond to a fluid challenge), proceed directly to laparotomy.
- If the patient has altered mental status, the abdomen is unexaminable or tender, or there is no obvious source of blood loss to explain a hemodynamically unstable status, order a **CT scan** of the abdomen and pelvis with oral and IV contrast (CT scan is preferred; diagnostic peritoneal lavage is no longer widely used).

Penetrating abdominal trauma. Type of injury and initial findings determine the course of action:

- With a gunshot wound, proceed directly to laparotomy.
- With a wound from a sharp instrument, management is more controversial. Either proceed directly to laparotomy (better choice if the patient is unstable) or do a CT scan. If the results are positive, consider laparotomy based on the injury; if the results are negative, observe and repeat the exam later.

Six thoracic injuries can be rapidly fatal and must be recognized immediately:

1. **Airway obstruction.** The patient has no audible breath sounds and cannot answer questions even though they may be awake and gurgling. Clear the airway if possible and treat with **endotracheal intubation.** If intubation fails, do a **cricothyroidotomy** (or tracheostomy in the operating room if there is time).
2. **Open pneumothorax.** An open defect in the chest wall causes poor ventilation and oxygenation. Treat with **endotracheal intubation, positive-pressure ventilation,** and **closure of the defect in the chest wall.** Gauze should be used and taped *on three sides only* to allow excessive pressure to escape so that you do not convert an open pneumothorax into a tension pneumothorax.
3. **Tension pneumothorax.** Usually seen after blunt trauma, tension pneumothorax occurs when air is forced into pleural space and cannot escape. It collapses the affected lung, then **shifts the mediastinum and trachea to the opposite side** of the chest. The patient has **absent breath sounds** and a **hypertympanic or hyperresonant percussion sound** on the affected side. Impaired cardiac filling may result in hypotension and/or **distended neck veins.** Treat with **needle thoracentesis** (anterior second intercostal space usually preferred), followed by insertion of a chest/thoracostomy tube.
4. **Cardiac tamponade.** The classic history is penetrating trauma to the left chest. Patients have hypotension (due to impaired cardiac filling), **distended neck veins, muffled heart sounds, pulsus paradoxus** (exaggerated fall in blood pressure on inspiration), and **normal breath sounds.** Treat with **pericardiocentesis** if the patient is unstable: put a catheter in the pericardial sac (via a subxiphoid approach) and aspirate the blood or fluid. If the patient is stable, you can do an echocardiogram to confirm the diagnosis.
5. **Massive hemothorax.** With loss of more than 1 liter of blood into thoracic cavity, patients have **decreased breath sounds** on the affected side, **dull note on percussion,** hypotension and/or **collapsed neck veins** (from blood leaving the vascular tree), and tachycardia. Placement of a chest tube causes the blood to come out. Give intravenous fluids and/or blood before you place the chest tube. If bleeding stops after the initial outflow, order an x-ray and/or CT scan to check for remaining blood or pathology and treat supportively. Emergent thoracotomy is required if the bleeding does not stop or is massive.
6. **Flail chest.** When several adjacent ribs are broken in multiple places, the affected part of the chest wall can move paradoxically (inward during inspiration, outward during expiration) during respiration (see figure). There is almost always an associated **pulmonary contusion,** which, combined with pain, may make respiration inadequate. When you are in doubt or the patient is not doing well, **intubate** and give **positive-pressure ventilation.**

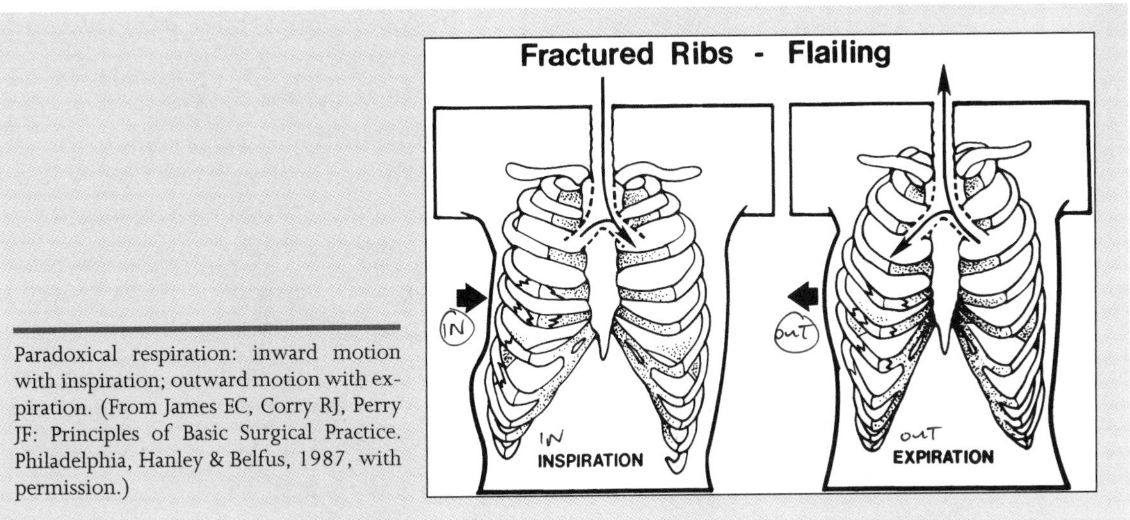

Paradoxical respiration: inward motion with inspiration; outward motion with expiration. (From James EC, Corry RJ, Perry JF: Principles of Basic Surgical Practice. Philadelphia, Hanley & Belfus, 1987, with permission.)

Other injuries

Thoracic aortic rupture: the most common cause of immediate death after an automobile accident or fall from great height. Usually occurs just beyond the take-off of the subclavian artery (aortic isthmus). Thoracic aortic laceration with a contained rupture (i.e., intact adventitia) can allow survival, but many (up to 50%) rupture and die within 24 hours of reaching the hospital, thus treat with immediate surgical management. Untreated survival beyond 4 months is less than 5%.

- **CASE SCENARIO:** What is the classic chest x-ray finding with aortic dissection? **Widened mediastinum.** Order a CT scan or angiogram if you are suspicious (because of x-ray or trauma degree, location, or type). Treat with immediate surgical repair for aortic involvement proximal to the take-off of the subclavian artery (a Stanford A-type dissection).
- **CASE SCENARIO:** On which side does a traumatic diaphragm rupture usually occur? The left. The liver is believed to protect the right side. The classic findings are hearing bowel sounds in the chest or seeing bowel loops in the thorax on chest x-ray. Fix surgically.

Head trauma. See Neurosurgery section.

Neck trauma. The neck is divided into three zones for trauma:

Zone I: base of the neck (from 2 cm above the clavicles to the level of the clavicles).

Zone II: midcervical region (2 cm above the clavicle to the angle of the mandible).

Zone III: the angle of the mandible to the base of the skull.

- With symptomatic zone I and III injuries, do an arteriogram (or CT angiogram) before going to the operating room in a stable patient.
- With zone II injuries, proceed to the operating room for surgical exploration in symptomatic patients; do *not* do an arteriogram first.
- In patients with obvious bleeding or a rapidly expanding hematoma, proceed directly to operating room no matter where injury is.

Choking victim: leave choking patients alone if they are speaking, coughing, or breathing. If they stop doing all of these things, perform the Heimlich maneuver.

If a tooth is knocked out, put it back in place with no cleaning (or rinse it only with saline) and stabilize as soon as possible. The sooner this is done, the better the prognosis for salvage of the tooth.

Burns may be thermal, chemical, or electrical. Initial management of all burns includes *lots* of intravenous fluids (use lactated Ringer's [LR] solution or normal saline if LR is not a choice), removal of all clothes and other smoldering items on the body, copious irrigation of chemical burns, and, of course, the ABCs. You should have a very low threshold for intubation; use 100% oxygen until significant carboxyhemoglobin from carbon monoxide inhalation is ruled out.

- **Electrical burns.** Because most of the destruction is internal, patients may have myoglobinuria, acidosis, and renal failure. Use aggressive IV fluids to prevent renal failure. The immediate, life-threatening risk with electricity exposure and burns (including lightning and putting a finger in an electrical outlet) is cardiac arrhythmias. Order an electrocardiogram.
- **Chemical burns.** Alkali burns are worse than acidic burns, because alkali penetrates more deeply. Treat all chemical burns with copious irrigation from the nearest source (e.g., tap water).
- **Thermal burns.** Burned skin is much more prone to infection, usually by *Staphylococcus aureus* or *Pseudomonas* spp. Pseudomonal infection causes a **fruity smell** and/or **blue-green color.** Prophylactic antibiotics are given topically, *not* systemically. Severity is classified as follows:

  1. **First-degree burns** involve epidermis only (painful, dry, red areas with no blisters). Keep clean.
  2. **Second-degree burns** involve epidermis and some dermis (swollen, with blisters and open weeping surfaces). Remove blisters, then apply antibiotic ointment (e.g., silver nitrate, silver sulfadiazine, neomycin) and dressing.
  3. **Third-degree burns** involve all layers of the skin, including nerve endings. The skin is dry and charred. Surgical excision of eschar and skin grafting are required. Watch for compartment syndrome, which is treated with escharotomy.

     ➤ *CASE SCENARIO:* What is the major difference in symptoms between second- and third-degree burns? Second-degree burns are very painful, whereas third-degree burns are classically **painless** initially because of nerve damage.

     ➤ *CASE SCENARIO:* What vaccine should burn victims receive? Tetanus.

Hypothermia: body temperature < 95°F (35°C), usually accompanied by mental status changes and generalized neurologic deficits. If the patient is conscious, use slow rewarming with blankets. If the patient is unconscious, consider immersion in a tub of warm water. The most important point is to monitor the EKG for arrhythmias, which are common with hypothermia. The rare but classic finding is the ***J wave,*** a small, positive deflection following the QRS complex. Also monitor electrolytes, renal function, and acid-base status.

- With frostnip (cold, painful areas of skin; mild injury) and frostbite (cold, anesthetic areas of skin; more severe injury), treat by rewarming affected areas with warm water (not scalding hot) and generalized warming (e.g., blankets).

  ➤ *CASE SCENARIO:* In the setting of hypothermia, finish the following phrase: "A patient is not considered dead until [.........]." A patient is not considered dead until he or she is "warm and dead." In other words, do not give up resuscitation efforts until the patient has been warmed.

Hyperthermia may be due to heat stroke. Look for a history of heat exposure and high temperature (> 104°F), without other possible culprits. Treat with immediate cooling (wet blankets, ice, cold water). The immediate threats to life are convulsions (treat with diazepam) and cardiovascular collapse. Rule out infection and other classic culprits:

1. **Malignant hyperthermia:** look for succinylcholine or halothane exposure. Treat with supportive care and **dantrolene.**
2. **Neuroleptic malignant syndrome:** patient is taking an antipsychotic. First, stop the medication. Second, treat with support (especially lots of intravenous fluids to prevent renal shutdown from rhabdomyolysis) and possibly dantrolene.

- **CASE SCENARIO:** What lab value is markedly elevated in patients with neuroleptic malignant syndrome? The **creatine phosphokinase (CPK)** level, because of muscle breakdown.

3. **Drug fever:** idiosyncratic reaction to a medication that usually was started within the past few weeks.

Near drowning. Fresh water is said by some to be worse than salt water, because fresh water, if aspirated, can cause hypervolemia, electrolyte disturbances, and hemolysis. Others think this is nonsense. Intubate patients if they are unconscious, and monitor arterial blood gases if they are conscious. Patients who almost drown in cold water often do better than those who almost drown in warm water (due to decreased metabolic needs). Death usually results from hypoxia and/or cardiac arrest.

GENERAL SURGERY

Acute abdomen. An inflamed peritoneum often buys the patient a laparotomy because it signifies a potentially life-threatening condition; important exceptions are **pancreatitis,** some cases of **diverticulitis,** and **spontaneous bacterial peritonitis.** The best physical confirmation of peritonitis is **rebound tenderness** and **involuntary guarding**/abdominal muscular rigidity. Voluntary guarding is a softer sign, as is tenderness to palpation; both are often present in benign diseases. When you are in doubt and the patient is stable, withhold narcotics, which mask symptoms, until you have a diagnosis. Do serial abdominal exams. Consider CT scan with oral and IV contrast. If the patient is unstable or worsening, proceed to laparoscopy/laparotomy.

Acute abdomen localization

1. **Right upper quadrant** (RUQ): think of gallbladder (cholecystitis), bile ducts (cholangitis), or liver (abscess).
2. **Left upper quadrant** (LUQ): think of spleen (rupture with blunt trauma or rarely, abscess).
3. **Right lower quadrant** (RLQ): think of appendix (appendicitis) or obstetric/gynecologic problem.
4. **Left lower quadrant** (LLQ): think of sigmoid colon (diverticulitis) or obstetric/gynecologic problem.
5. **Epigastric:** think of stomach (penetrating ulcer) or pancreas (pancreatitis).

Cholecystitis. The five Fs summarize the classic patient with **cholesterol** stones: fat, forty, fertile, female, and now febrile, especially if gallstones are seen on ultrasound or the patient has a history of gallstones and/or gallstone-type symptoms (e.g., postprandial RUQ colicky pain with bloating and/or nausea and vomiting). Look for **Murphy's sign.** Do a cholecystectomy. Remember that **pigment gallstones** are seen in patients with hemolytic anemias, not "5-F" patients.

- **CASE SCENARIO:** What triad of findings is associated with cholangitis? **RUQ pain, fever** or shaking chills, and **jaundice.** Patients often have a history of gallstones. Start antibiotics after getting blood cultures, and do a cholecystectomy once the patient is stable.
- **CASE SCENARIO:** What is the best first imaging test for suspected gallbladder disease? Ultrasound. For cholecystitis, a nuclear hepatobiliary/scintigraphy study (e.g., HIDA scan) clinches a difficult diagnosis (positive scan = nonvisualization of the gallbladder).

Splenic rupture. Patients have a history of blunt abdominal trauma, hypotension or tachycardia, shock, and **Kerr sign** (referred left shoulder pain). Do not let patients with Epstein-Barr virus (EBV) infection play contact sports. Do not forget to immunize postsplenectomy patients (see immunization section).

Appendicitis. The incidence peaks in 10–30-year-olds. The classic history is **crampy, poorly localized periumbilical pain followed by nausea and vomiting, then localization of pain to the RLQ and peritoneal signs** with worsening of nausea and vomiting. Patients who are hungry and asking for food do not have appendicitis. Remember the positive **Rovsing sign** and **McBurney point tenderness.** Use CT scan of the abdomen (see figure) or ultrasound to help make the diagnosis in uncertain cases. Do an appendectomy.

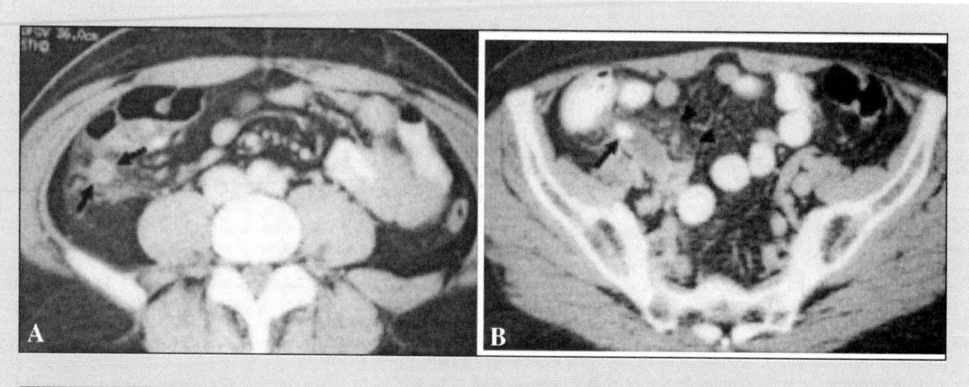

Two cases of acute appendicitis on CT. **A,** Contrast-enhanced CT. The appendix (seen in cross-section) is distended, its wall enhances (*arrows*), and there is periappendiceal inflammation. **B,** Contrast-enhanced CT of a different patient. The appendix (seen as a tubular structure) is dilated and contains an appendicolith (*arrow*); there is inflammation of the surrounding fat (*arrowheads*). (From Katz DS, Math KR, Groskin SA (eds): Radiology Secrets. Philadelphia, Hanley & Belfus, 1998, p 111, with permission.)

Diverticulitis. Localized LLQ pain in a patient over 50 is diverticulitis unless you have a good reason to think otherwise. Treat medically with broad-spectrum antibiotics and place the patient on NPO (nothing-by-mouth) status. **CT scan** with oral and IV contrast is the best test to confirm disease and rule out a complicating abscess. If disease is recurrent or refractory to medical therapy, consider colon (usually sigmoid) resection.

Pancreatitis, acute. Look for epigastric pain in an alcohol abuser or a patient with a known history of gallstones. Pain may radiate to the back, and serum **amylase** or **lipase** is elevated (if these values are not given, order them). Other common symptoms include decreased bowel sounds, local ileus (sentinel loop of bowel on x-ray), nausea, vomiting, and anorexia. Treat with pain medications, NPO status, nasogastric tube, intravenous fluids, and supportive care. Watch for complications of **pseudocyst** and **pancreatic abscess,** which can be diagnosed by CT scan and may require surgical intervention.

> **CASE SCENARIO:** Which narcotic should be avoided in patients with pancreatitis? **Morphine,** which causes sphincter of Oddi spasm and can worsen symptoms. Use other opiates instead (typically, meperidine is used).

> **CASE SCENARIO:** A patient has history of ulcers, epigastric pain, peritoneal signs, mildly elevated amylase, and normal lipase. A small amount of free air is noted under the diaphragm on abdominal x-ray. What is the likely diagnosis? Perforated peptic ulcer, which can cause elevated amylase (but lipase typically normal).

Small bowel obstruction (SBO). Symptoms include **bilious vomiting** (early symptom), **abdominal distention,** constipation, hyperactive bowel sounds (high-pitched, rushing sounds), and pain that usually is poorly localized. X-ray shows multiple air-fluid levels in small bowel loops (see figure). Patients often have a **history of previous surgery;** the most common cause of SBO in adults is **adhesions,** which usually develop from prior surgery. In children, think of **incarcerated inguinal hernia** or **Meckel diverticulum.** Start treatment with NPO status, nasogastric tube, and intravenous fluids. If symptoms do not resolve or if the patient develops peritoneal signs, laparotomy is needed to relieve the obstruction.

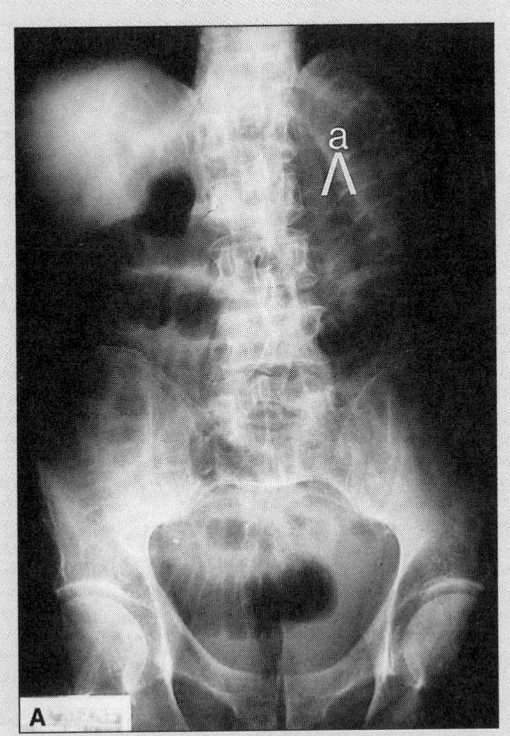

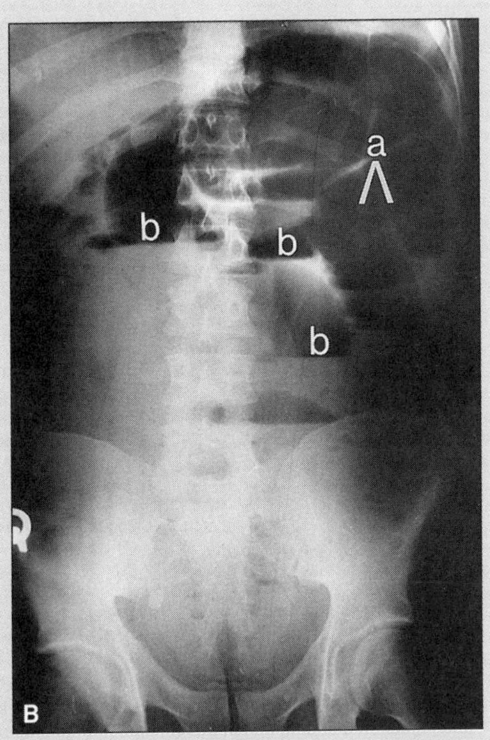

Small intestinal obstruction. A, Supine flatplate showing dilated loops of small intestine (a). B, Upright flatplate showing dilated loops of small intestine (a) and multiple air-fluid levels (b). (From James EC, Corry RJ, Perry FJ: Principles of Basic Surgery. Philadelphia, Hanley & Belfus, 1987, p 276, with permission.)

Large bowel obstruction. Symptoms include gradually increasing abdominal pain, **abdominal distention,** constipation, and **feculent vomiting** (late symptom). This condition is seen more often in older patients as a result of **diverticulitis, colon cancer,** or **volvulus.** Treat early with NPO status and nasogastric tube. Sigmoid volvulus often can be decompressed with an endoscope. Other causes or refractory cases require surgery to relieve the obstruction. In children, watch for **Hirschsprung disease.**

Hernia. The four common types (there are others) are treated with surgical repair if they are symptomatic:

1. **Indirect:** most common in both sexes and all age groups. The hernia sac travels through the inner and outer inguinal rings (protrusion begins **lateral to the inferior epigastric vessels**) and **into the scrotum (or labia)** due to a patent processus vaginalis (congenital defect).
2. **Direct:** the hernia (no sac) protrudes **medial to the inferior epigastric** vessels (and not into the scrotum or labia) due to weakness in the abdominal musculature (of Hesselbach's triangle).
3. **Femoral:** more common in women. The hernia (no sac) goes through the femoral ring onto the **anterior thigh (located below the inguinal ring).** Femoral hernias are the most susceptible to incarceration and strangulation.
4. **Incisional:** after any wound (especially surgical), a hernia can occur through the site of the incision.
   - **Incarceration** is when herniated organs are trapped and become swollen or edematous.
   - **Strangulation** is when the entrapment/incarceration becomes so severe that the blood supply is cut off. **Strangulation can lead to necrosis and is a surgical emergency.** Patients may present with SBO symptoms and shock.

➤ **CASE SCENARIO:** What is the most common cause of small bowel obstruction in a person who has never had surgery before? Incarcerated hernia (second most common in patients with prior abdominal surgery).

Preoperative and postoperative points

1. Preoperatively, keep the patient on NPO status for at least 8 hours (when possible) to reduce chance of aspiration
2. Spirometry (and, of course, a good history) is the best preoperative test to order for assessment of pulmonary function. It measures forced vital capacity (FVC), forced expiratory volume in 1 second (FEV_1), FEV_1/FVC ratio (%), and maximum voluntary ventilation.
3. Use compressive/elastic stockings, early ambulation, and/or low-dose heparin or prophylactic dose low-molecular weight heparin to help prevent deep venous thrombosis and pulmonary embolism. Warfarin often is used for orthopedic procedures.
4. The most common cause of postoperative fever in the first 24 hours is **atelectasis** (usually low-grade fever). Prevent or treat with early ambulation, chest physiotherapy/percussion, incentive spirometry, and proper pain control. Both too much pain and too many narcotics increase the risk of atelectasis.
5. The mnemonic "**water, wind, walk, wound, and weird drugs**" helps to recall the causes of postoperative fever: wound = surgical wound infection, water = urinary tract infection, walk = deep venous thrombosis, wind = atelectasis/pneumonia, weird drugs = drug fever. If daily fever spikes occur, think about an intra-abdominal abscess; consider a CT scan to locate the abscess. Abscesses often need surgical or CT-guided catheter drainage.
6. Fascial/wound dehiscence typically occurs 5–10 days postoperatively. Look for leakage of serosanguinous fluid from the wound (often after the patient coughs or strains), which is especially associated with wound infection. Treat with antibiotics (if secondary to infection) and reclosure of the incision.

EAR, NOSE, AND THROAT SURGERY

Rhinitis: edematous, vasodilated nasal mucosa and turbinates with clear nasal discharge. Causes include the following:

1. **Viral infection (common cold):** due to rhinovirus (most common), influenza, parainfluenza, adenovirus, or others. Treatment is symptomatic with short-term use of vasoconstrictors such as phenylephrine. Vasoconstrictors may cause rebound congestion, however.
2. **Allergy (hay fever):** associated with **seasonal** flare-ups, **boggy** and **bluish** turbinates, onset < 20 years old, **nasal polyps,** sneezing, pruritus, conjunctivitis, wheezing, asthma, eczema, family history, **eosinophils in nasal mucous,** and elevated IgE. Skin tests may identify an allergen. Treat with avoidance of any known antigen (e.g., pollen), **antihistamines,** cromolyn, and/or **intranasal steroid spray** for severe symptoms. Desensitization is also an option.
3. **Bacterial infection:** typically due to streptococci A (see figure), pneumococci, or staphylococci. Do streptococcal throat culture. Treat with antibiotics if appropriate (sore throat, fever, tonsillar exudate).

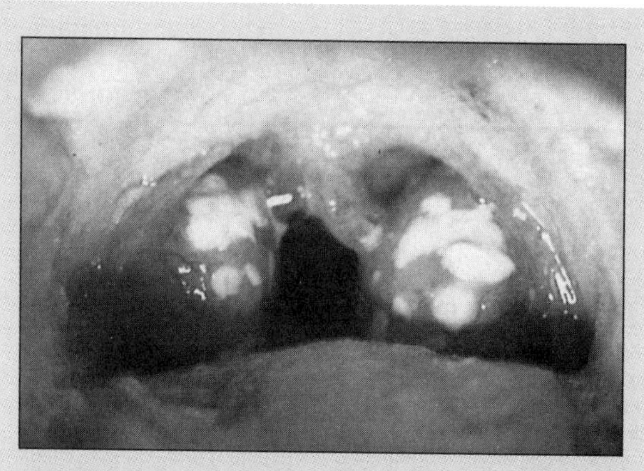

Acute streptococcal pharyngitis. Pus is present in the tonsillar crypts. (From Forbes CD, Jackson WF: Infections. In Forbes CD, Jackson WF (eds): Colar Atlas and Text of Clinical Medicine. St. Louis, Mosby, 1993, pp 9–86, with permisson.)

Sinusitis usually is due to *S. pneumoniae, Hemophilus influenzae, Moraxella* spp., other streptococci, or staphylococci. Look for **fever, tenderness over the affected sinus, headache,** and **purulent nasal discharge** (yellow or green). X-ray or CT scan shows opacification of the sinus, and CT is used to evaluate chronic sinusitis or suspected extension of infection outside the sinus (in patients with high fever and chills). Treat with antibiotics (amoxicillin or second-generation cephalosporin) for 10–14 days. Long-term antibiotics (6 weeks) or operative intervention usually is needed for chronic, resistant cases (e.g., drainage procedure, sinus obliteration). Remember that the frontal sinuses are not well developed until after the age of 10. Deviated nasal septum or other congenital defects are a rare cause of recurrent sinusitis; treat with surgical correction.

Otitis externa (swimmer's ear): most commonly due to *Pseudomonas aeruginosa*. **Manipulation of the auricle produces pain** (this sign is not present in otitis media), the skin of the auditory canal is erythematous and swollen, and patients may have a foul-smelling discharge and conductive hearing loss. Treat with topical antibiotics (neomycin/polymyxin B) and steroids to help reduce swelling and inflammation.

> ➤ ***CASE SCENARIO:*** What are the classic physical findings and bacterial cause for infectious myringitis? Otoscopy classically reveals vesicles on the tympanic membrane, and the classic cause is *Mycoplasma* spp. Other causes include *Streptococcus pneumoniae* and viruses. Treat with antibiotics.

Causes of hearing loss

1. **Aging (presbyacusis):** most common cause of **sensorineural hearing loss** in adults; a normal part of aging, not a disease.Patients can use hearing aids, if needed.
2. **Environmental noise:** prolonged or intense loud noise can permanently affect hearing. Advise earplugs for occupationally exposed patients.
3. **Otosclerosis:** most common cause of progressive **conductive hearing loss** in adults. Otic bones become fixed together and impede hearing. Treat with hearing aid or surgery.
4. **Meningitis or recurrent otitis media:** the classic causes in children. Screen for hearing loss after meningitis.
5. **Congenital hearing loss:** TORCH infection or inherited disability.
6. **Ménière disease:** usually occurs in middle-aged patients. The cause is unknown. Look for severe **vertigo, tinnitus,** nausea, and vomiting. Treat with anticholinergics, antihistamines (e.g., **meclizine**), or surgery (for refractory cases).
7. **Drugs:** aminoglycosides, aspirin (overdose causes tinnitus), quinine, loop diuretics, cisplatin.
8. **Tumor:** usually an acoustic schwannoma (schwannoma of the 8th cranial nerve).
9. **Labyrinthitis:** may have a viral etiology or follow or extend from meningitis or otitis media. Viral etiology often causes sudden deafness that develops over a few hours. Hearing usually returns within 2 weeks, but loss may be permanent. No treatment has proved effective, but empirical steroids often are used.

Causes of vertigo

1. **Meniere disease:** accompanied by tinnitus, hearing loss, and nausea/vomiting. See above.
2. **Benign positional/paroxysmal vertigo: induced by certain head positions** and may be accompanied by nystagmus without hearing loss. Cases often resolve spontaneously; the only treatment generally needed is to avoid the position that provokes symptoms.
3. **Acoustic schwannoma**
4. **Stroke**
5. **Infection**
6. **Multiple sclerosis:** a possible cause of any weird neurologic symptoms, usually in women of reproductive age.

Causes of facial paralysis

1. **Stroke:** commonly associated with older age, other deficits, and stroke risk factors.
2. **Bell's palsy:** one of the most common causes of facial paralysis, characterized by sudden unilateral onset, usually after an upper respiratory infection. The cause is thought to be a reactivation of **herpes simplex I** virus in most cases. Patients may have **hyperacusis** (everything sounds loud because the stapedius muscle in the ear is paralyzed). In severe cases, when patients are unable to close the affected eye, use artificial tears to protect the eye. Most cases resolve spontaneously in about 1–3 months, but some patients have permanent sequelae, thus consider giving antiherpes agents (e.g., **acyclovir**) to reduce the risk.
3. **Herpes zoster (Ramsay Hunt syndrome):** also causes ear pain. Look for ***vesicles on the pinna and inside the ear.*** Encephalitis or meningitis may be present.
4. **Lyme disease:** probably the most common causes of *bilateral* facial nerve palsy.
5. **Middle ear or mastoid infections/meningitis:** look for other symptoms of the infection.
6. **Temporal bone fracture:** patients may have Battle sign, bleeding from the ear, and deafness.
   - Perform CT/MRI scan if stroke, tumor, or fracture is suspected.
     - ➤ *CASE SCENARIO:* What tumor classically affects both the seventh and eighth cranial nerves? An acoustic schwannoma, which is located in the cerebellopontine angle. If present, consider neurofibromatosis.

Neck mass: 75% benign in children, 75% malignant in patients older than 40 years. Causes include the following:

1. **Branchial cleft cysts:** seen in children; ***lateral;*** may become infected.
2. **Thyroglossal duct cysts:** seen in children; ***midline;*** elevates with tongue protrusion.
3. **Cystic hygroma:** lymphangioma seen in children, classically in patients with ***Turner syndrome;*** treat with surgical resection.
4. **Cervical lymphadenitis:** may occur in children or adults, usually as a result of streptococcal pharyngitis, Epstein-Barr virus (very common in adolescents and young adults in their twenties), cat-scratch disease, or mycobacterial infection (***scrofula***).
5. **Neoplasm:** more common in adults than in children. The mass may be lymphadenopathy from primary (lymphoma) or metastatic neoplasm, or it may be the tumor itself.
   - ➤ *CASE SCENARIO:* What is the classic work-up for an "unknown cancer" (unknown primary) found in the neck? Random biopsy of the nasopharynx, palatine tonsils, and the base of the tongue as well as laryngoscopy, bronchoscopy, and esophagoscopy (with biopsies of any suspicious lesions)—the so-called "triple endoscopy with triple biopsy." CT/MRI also may help to detect lesions not apparent on physical exam.

Parotid swelling: classically due to mumps. The best treatment for mumps and the complication of infertility is prevention through immunization. Parotid swelling also may be due to alcoholism, neoplasm (the most common is benign pleomorphic adenoma), Sjögren syndrome, or sarcoidosis.

After a **nasal fracture** (seen on x-ray or CT scan), rule out a septal hematoma, which must be removed to prevent pressure-induced septal necrosis.

NEUROSURGERY

Intracranial bleeds: whenever an intracranial bleed is suspected, order a ***CT scan without contrast.*** Blood appears as white and may cause a shift of midline structures to the opposite side. Causes include the following:

1. **Subdural hematoma,** which is due to bleeding from veins that bridge the cortex and dural sinuses. On x-rays the hematoma is ***crescent-shaped.*** Subdural hematomas are common in alcoholics and after head trauma. They may present immediately after trauma or as long as 1–2 months later. If the question gives a history of head trauma, always consider the diagnosis of a subdural hematoma. Treat with surgical evacuation if significant or progressive symptoms present.

2. **Epidural hematoma** is due to bleeding from meningeal arteries (classically, the middle meningeal artery). On x-rays the hematoma is ***biconvex*** (see figure). Almost all epidural hematomas are associated with a ***temporal bone skull fracture,*** and roughly 50% of patients develop an ***ipsilateral "blown" pupil*** (see below). The classic history is head trauma with loss of consciousness, followed by a ***lucid interval*** of minutes to hours, then neurologic deterioration. Treat with surgical evacuation.

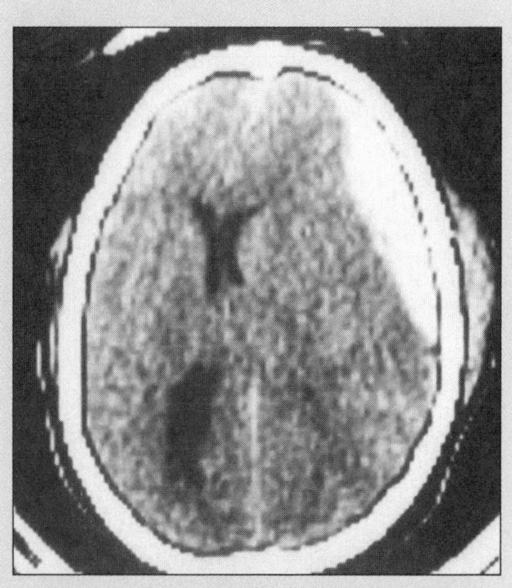

CT scan showing left-sided epidural hematoma. Note that blood shows up as white, lens-shaped collection. (From Waclawik AJ, Sutula TP: Neurology Pearls. Philadelphia, Hanley & Belfus, 2000, with permission.)

3. **Subarachnoid hemorrhage** is due to blood between the arachnoid and pia mater. The most common cause is ***trauma,*** followed by ***ruptured intracranial*** (typically berry) ***aneurysm.*** Blood is seen in ventricles and around (but not in) the brain or brainstem. The classic patient presents with the "***worst headache of my life,***" although many die before they reach the hospital or may be unconscious. If awake, patients have ***signs of meningitis*** (positive Kernig and Brudzinski signs) without significant fever. Remember the association between ***polycystic kidney disease*** and berry aneurysms. CT is the test of choice; if a lumbar tap is done, it shows ***grossly bloody cerebrospinal fluid.*** Treat with support, anticonvulsants, and observation. Once the patient is stable, do a cerebral angiogram or magnetic resonance angiogram to look for aneurysms and arteriovenous malformations (AVMs), which are usually treated with surgical clipping and ligation.

4. **Intracerebral bleed** is caused by bleeding into the brain parenchyma. The most common cause is hypertension; other causes include AVMs, coagulopathies, tumor, and trauma. Two-thirds of hypertensive bleeds occur in the basal ganglia (see figure), and patients often present in a coma. Awake patients may have contralateral hemiplegia and hemisensory deficits. Blood (white) is seen in the brain parenchyma and also may be seen in the ventricles. Surgery is reserved for large bleeds that are accessible (rare).

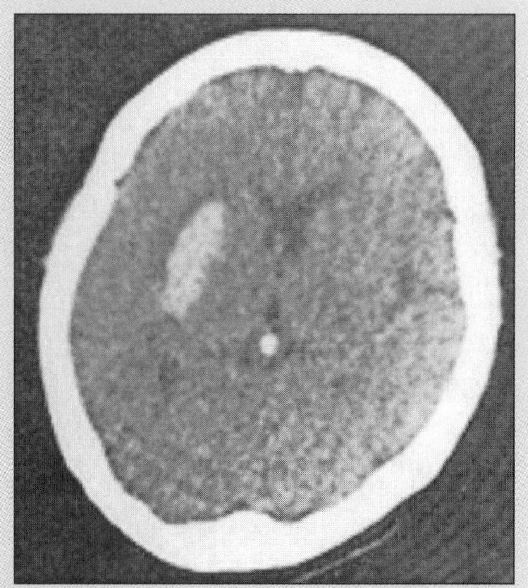

Basal ganglia hemorrhage. This is the classic and most common location for hypertension-related bleeds. (From Rolak LA: Neurology Secrets, 3rd ed. Philadelphia, Hanley & Belfus, 2001, p 192, with permission.)

After a history of trauma, a **dilated, unreactive pupil** (i.e. "blown" pupil) on only one side most likely represents impingement of the ipsilateral third cranial nerve and impending **uncal herniation** due to increased intracranial pressure. Of the different intracranial bleeds, this is most commonly seen with epidural bleeds.

> ➤ ***CASE SCENARIO:*** Why should you not do a lumbar puncture in the setting of trauma or evidence of increased intracranial pressure? You may cause uncal herniation and death. First do a CT scan without contrast. If it is negative and the diagnosis remains unclear, then consider lumbar puncture (rarely indicated).

Basilar (skull-base) fractures have four classic signs:

1. **Raccoon eyes:** periorbital ecchymosis.
2. **Battle sign:** postauricular ecchymosis.
3. **Hemotympanum:** blood behind the eardrum.
4. **Cerebrospinal fluid otorrhea/rhinorrhea:** clear fluid drains from ears or nose.

Skull fractures of the calvarium (top of skull) are seen on CT scan (preferred) or x-ray, generally as a linear or depressed fracture. Surgical repair is done only for contaminated fractures (cleaning and debridement), impingement on the brain parenchyma, or an open fracture with cerebrospinal fluid leak. Otherwise, such fractures can be observed and generally heal on their own.

Head trauma also may cause **cerebral contusion** or **shear injury** (i.e. **diffuse axonal injury**) of the brain parenchyma, both of which may not show up on a CT scan but may cause temporary or permanent neurologic deficits. They can be detected with MRI, but there is no treatment. MRI is used only for prognostic information in this setting.

Increased intracranial pressure (ICP), also known as intracranial hypertension (normal ICP = 5–15 mmHg), should be suspected in patients with **bilaterally dilated and fixed pupils.** Other symptoms include headache, **papilledema,** nausea and vomiting, and **mental status changes.** Look also for the classic **Cushing triad** (increasing blood pressure, bradycardia, respiratory irregularity), which indicates very high ICP. The first step is to put the patient in reverse Trendelenberg position (head up) and intubate. Once intubated, the patient can be hyperventilated to lower the ICP rapidly. Hyperventilation decreases intracranial blood volume by causing cerebral vasoconstriction. If this maneuver does not lower ICP, **mannitol** diuresis can be tried to lessen cerebral edema. Furosemide also is used, but it is less effective. Decompressive craniotomy (burr holes) is a last resort. Prophylactic anticonvulsants are controversial.

> ➤ ***CASE SCENARIO:*** How should hypertension be treated in the setting of increased intracranial pressure? It generally should not be treated! Cerebral perfusion pressure = blood pressure—ICP. The body, therefore, reflexively causes hypertension in the setting of increased ICP to maintain cerebral perfusion.

Spinal cord trauma often presents with "spinal shock" (loss of reflexes and motor function, hypotension). Order standard trauma x-rays (cervical spine, thorax, pelvis) as well as additional spinal x-rays or CT scans based on physical exam. Give IV **corticosteroids** immediately, which may improve outcome. Surgery is done for incomplete neurologic injury (with some residual function) with external bony compression of the cord (e.g., subluxation, bone chip).

Subacute spinal cord compression is often due to metastatic cancer but also may result from a primary neoplasm, subdural or epidural abscess or hematoma (especially after a lumbar tap or epidural/spinal anesthesia in patients with a bleeding disorder or taking anticoagulation). Patients present with **local spinal pain** (especially with bone metastases) and neurologic deficits below the lesion (e.g., hyperreflexia, positive Babinski sign, weakness, sensory loss). The first step is to give high-dose IV **corticosteroids.** Then order an MRI of the appropriate spinal level. Give **radiotherapy** if metastases are present. Alternatively, surgical decompression can be done for radioresistant tumors. For hematoma or subdural/epidural abscess (seen especially in diabetics, usually due to *Staphylococcus aureus*), surgery is indicated for decompression and drainage.

Syringomyelia is a central pathologic cavitation of the spinal cord, usually in the cervical or upper thoracic region. It may be idiopathic or result from trauma or congenital cranial base malformations (e.g., **Arnold-Chiari** malformation [see figure] and Dandy-Walker syndromes). The classic presentation is a ***bilateral loss of pain and temperature sensation below the lesion in the distribution of a "cape"*** because of involvement of the lateral spinothalamic tracts. The cavitation in the cord gradually widens to involve other tracts, causing motor and sensory deficits. MRI is the imaging study of choice, and treatment is typically surgical (creation of a shunt).

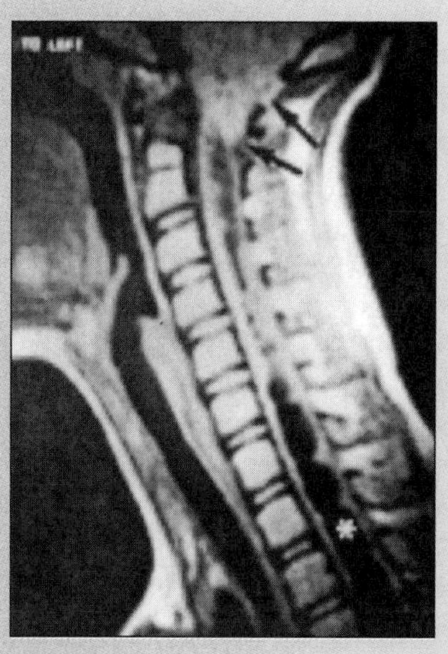

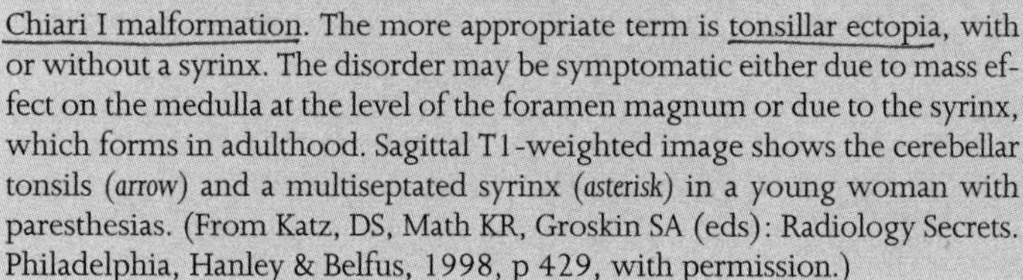

Chiari I malformation. The more appropriate term is tonsillar ectopia, with or without a syrinx. The disorder may be symptomatic either due to mass effect on the medulla at the level of the foramen magnum or due to the syrinx, which forms in adulthood. Sagittal T1-weighted image shows the cerebellar tonsils (*arrow*) and a multiseptated syrinx (*asterisk*) in a young woman with paresthesias. (From Katz, DS, Math KR, Groskin SA (eds): Radiology Secrets. Philadelphia, Hanley & Belfus, 1998, p 429, with permission.)

➤ ***CASE SCENARIO:*** In what condition of the elderly is the classic triad of ataxia, dementia, and urinary incontinence seen? Normal pressure hydrocephalus, which can be treated with a ventricular shunt.

OPHTHALMOLOGY

Conjunctivitis causes conjunctival vessel hyperemia and eye irritation. If vision loss occurs, think of more serious conditions. Classic causes:

ETIOLOGY	UNIQUE SIGNS/SYMPTOMS	TREATMENT
Allergic	Itching; bilateral, seasonal, long duration	Vasoconstrictors, if needed
Viral (especially adenovirus)	Periauricular adenopathy; highly contagious (history of infected contacts); clear, watery discharge	Supportive treatment; handwashing (prevents spread)
Bacterial	Purulent discharge; look for neonates	Topical and systemic antibiotics

Glaucoma is best thought of as ocular hypertension. Risk factors are ***age > 40 years, black race, diabetes,*** and ***family history.*** Two types:

1. **Open-angle glaucoma** accounts for 90% of the cases of glaucoma. It is **painless** and has no acute attacks. The only signs are elevated intraocular pressure (usually 20–30 mmHg), a **gradually progressive visual field loss** (starts in the periphery), and **optic nerve changes** (increased cup-to-disc ratio on funduscopic exam). Treat with several different types of medications (beta blockers, prostaglandins [latanoprost], acetazolamide, pilocarpine) and/or surgery.
2. **Closed-angle glaucoma** is the rare type that everyone worries about. It presents with **sudden ocular pain,** seeing **haloes around lights, red eye,** very high intraocular pressure (> 30 mmHg), **nausea and vomiting,** sudden decrease in vision, and a **fixed, mid-dilated pupil.** Treat immediately with pilocarpine drops and oral glycerin and acetazolamide to break the attack. Then use surgery to prevent further attacks (**peripheral iridectomy**). Very rarely, anticholinergic medications can cause an attack of closed-angle glaucoma in a susceptible, previously untreated patient. Medications do not cause attacks in patients with open-angle glaucoma or surgically treated closed-angle glaucoma.

Steroids, whether topical or systemic, can cause glaucoma and cataracts. Topical steroids can worsen ocular herpes and fungal infections. For board purposes, do *not* give steroid eye drops. Refer the patient to an ophthalmologist if you think that they are indicated.

> ***CASE SCENARIO:*** A patient has a branching ulcer over his cornea with terminal bulbs that stain green with fluorescein. What condition does the patient have? Ocular herpes keratitis. Refer to an ophthalmologist promptly for antiviral treatment (e.g., idoxuridine). The condition usually starts with conjunctivitis and vesicular lid eruption.

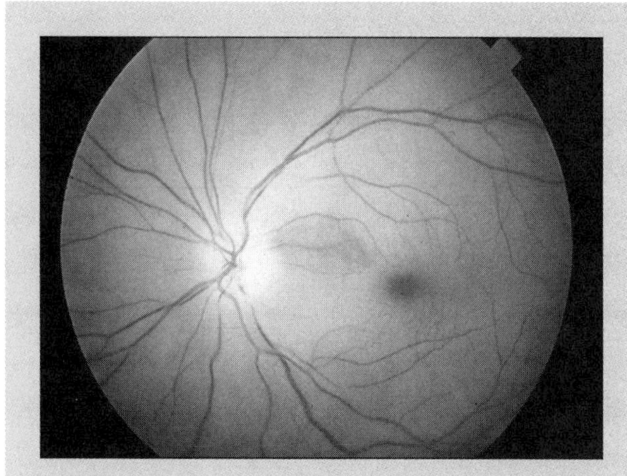

Central retinal artery occlusion. (From Vander JF, Gault JA: Ophthalmology Secrets. Philadelphia, Hanley & Belfus, 1998, with permission.)

Sudden unilateral, *painless* vision loss has a fairly short list of differential diagnoses:

1. **Central retinal artery occlusion** (see figure). The funduscopic appearance is classic. The most common cause is emboli (from carotid plaque or heart); treatment is generally supportive unless the cause is temporal arteritis (in which case you should give corticosteroids immediately).
2. **Central retinal vein occlusion.** The funduscopic appearance is classic. No satisfactory treatment is available. The most common causes are hypertension, diabetes, glaucoma, and increased blood viscosity (e.g., leukemia). Complications (vision loss, glaucoma) are related to neovascularization.
3. **Retinal detachment.** The history usually includes seeing "**floaters**" and **flashes of light.** Patients often describe the presentation as a "**curtain or veil coming down in front of my eye.**" This history should prompt immediate referral to an ophthalmologist, as prompt surgery (reattachment of the retina) may save the patient's sight.
4. **Vitreous hemorrhage.** The most common cause is bleeding from areas of neovascularization, classically in **diabetics.** The condition sometimes resolves or may improve after surgical vitrectomy.
5. **Optic neuritis/papillitis.** This condition usually takes at least a few hours to develop and is usually painful, but it may occur quickly and without pain. Sometimes symptoms are bilateral. Bilateral presentation in a 20–40-year-old woman should raise the suspicion of multiple sclerosis (or Lyme disease if appropriate history given). Worry about a tumor in male patients with signs of intracranial hypertension or other neurologic deficits. Disc margins may appear blurred on funduscopic exam, similar to papilledema.

6. **Stroke or transient ischemic attack:** see table on next page for visual pathway lesions.

Causes of sudden, unilateral *painful* loss of vision

1. **Trauma:** the history gives it away. Encourage use of goggles or safety glasses during athletics and work. With chemical burns to the eye (acid or alkaline), the key to management is **copious irrigation with the closest source of water** (tap water is fine). The longer you wait, the worse the prognosis; do not get additional history in this instance. ***Alkali burns have a worse prognosis,*** because they tend to penetrate more deeply into the eye.
2. **Closed-angle glaucoma:** see above for presenting signs and symptoms and treatment.
3. **Optic neuritis:** Usually painful, as described above.
4. **Migraine headache:** rare. Look for nausea, vomiting, and aura.

Sudden bilateral loss of vision is rare, but consider the following possible causes:

1. **Toxins:** the classic example is **methanol poisoning,** usually seen in alcoholics.
2. **Exposure to ultraviolet light** can cause keratitis (corneal inflammation) with resultant pain, foreign body sensation, red eyes, tearing, and decreased vision (usually some vision remains). Patients have a history of **welding, using a tanning bed or sunlamp, or snow-skiing** ("snow-blindness"). Treat with an eye patch (24 hours) and topical antibiotic, possibly also with an anticholinergic (cycloplegic) agent to reduce pain.
3. **Conversion reaction/hysteria**

Gradual-onset loss of vision, unilateral or bilateral, has a longer list of differential diagnoses but is more common than sudden-onset vision loss:

1. **Cataracts** are the most common cause of a painless, slowly progressive loss of vision. Often bilateral, but one side may be worse than the other. Look for **absent red reflex** or grossly opacified lens (see figure) and patient complains of "**looking through a dirty windshield.**" Treatment is surgical. Can delay surgery until patient's daily activities are affected.
2. **Open-angle glaucoma:** see above for specifics. Screen people over 40, especially if they are black or diabetic or have a positive family history. Open-angle glaucoma is the most common cause of blindness in blacks.
3. **Macular degeneration** is the most common cause of blindness in adults > 50 years. Blindness is often bilateral, but one side may be worse than the other. The appearance of the fundus (the yellow-white deposits of drusen in the macular area) makes the diagnosis. No good treatment is available for the most common (dry-type) form.

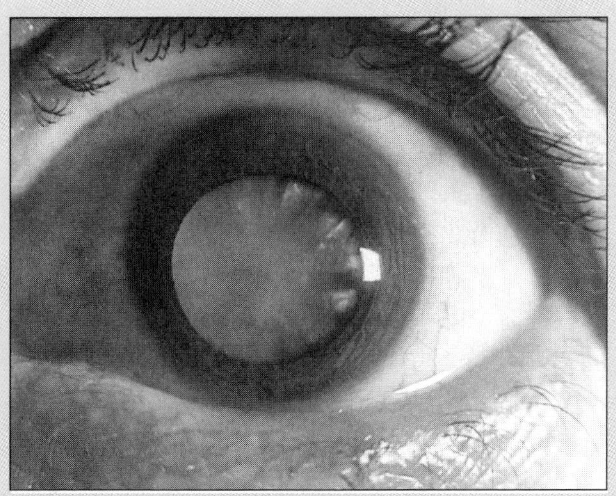

"Senile"-type cataract, which can occur at an earlier age in diabetic patients compared with the normal population. (From Forbes CD, Jackson WF: Endocrine, metabolic, and nutritional disorders. In Forbes CD, Jackson WF (eds): Color Atlas and Text of Clinical Medicine. St. Louis, Mosby, 1993, pp 303–352, with permission.)

4. **Diabetes** is the most common cause of blindness in adults < 50 years. Retinal/fundus changes include **dot-blot hemorrhages, microaneurysms, and neovascularization.** Proliferative diabetic retinopathy (with neovascularization) is treated by a laser applied to the periphery of the whole retina (**panretinal photocoagulation**). Focal laser treatment is often done for nonproliferative retinopathy with macular edema (the laser is applied only to the affected area).
5. **Uveitis:** look for association with autoimmune-type diseases. Screen children with **juvenile rheumatoid arthritis** regularly to detect uveitis. The usual treatment is corticosteroids (treated by an ophthalmologist).
6. **Papilledema** classically results from hypertension or other cause of increased intracranial pressure (e.g., brain tumor, **pseudotumor cerebri**).
7. **Optic neuritis** classically results from autoimmune-type conditions, infections (Lyme disease), or drugs (**ethambutol**).
8. **Infection of the cornea** (herpes keratitis, corneal ulcer) or retina (cytomegalovirus retinitis in AIDS), orbital cellulitis.
9. **Direct insult to brain:** stroke, tumor, meningitis (see table for visual pathway information).

VISUAL FIELD DEFECT	LOCATION OF LESION
Right anopsia (monocular blindness)	Right optic nerve
Bitemporal hemianopsia	Optic chiasm (classically due to pituitary tumor)
Left homonymous hemianopsia	Right optic tract
Left upper quadrant anopsia	Right optic radiations in the right temporal lobe
Left lower quadrant anopsia	Right optic radiations in the right parietal lobe
Left homonymous hemianopsia with macular sparing	Right occipital lobe (from posterior cerebral artery occlusion)

10. **Presbyopia:** between ages 40 and 50 years, the lens gradually **loses its ability to accommodate.** People need bifocals or reading glasses for near vision. This is a normal part of aging, not a disease.

Effects of hypertension on the fundus include arteriolar narrowing, copper/silver wiring, cotton-wool spots, and papilledema (with severe hypertension).

Hordeolum (stye) is a painful, red lump near the lid margin. Treat with warm compresses.

Chalazion is a painless lump away from the lid margin. Treat with warm compresses; if this approach fails, treat with incision and drainage.

Ophthalmic herpes zoster infection should be suspected with involvement of the tip of the nose and/or medial eyelid with a typical zoster dermatomal pattern. Treat with oral acyclovir. Complications include uveitis, keratitis, and glaucoma

Ophthalmologic cranial nerve (CN) palsies usually are due to **vascular complications of diabetes or hypertension** and resolve on their own within 2 months. In patients under 40, those without diabetes or hypertension, patients with other neurologic deficits or severe pain, and patients who fail to improve within 8 weeks, order an MRI; diabetes and hypertension are less likely to be the cause. Look for a **tumor** or **aneurysm** in this setting.

1. **Oculomotor (CN3):** eye is "**down and out,**" and cannot do anything but move laterally.
   - CASE SCENARIO: How can the pupil help you to decide between a serious and benign cause of a third cranial nerve palsy? If the palsy is due to hypertension or diabetes, the pupil is nor-

mal. A "blown" (dilated, nonreactive) pupil is a medical emergency. The most likely cause is an aneurysm or tumor. Order an MRI and/or magnetic resonance/cerebral angiogram.

2. **Trochlear (CN4):** when the gaze is medial, the patient ***cannot look down.***
3. **Abducens (CN6):** the patient ***cannot look laterally*** with the affected eye (see figure).
4. **CN5 and CN7 palsies** also affect the eye due to corneal drying (loss of corneal blink reflex). Use artificial tears and address the underlying cause, if possible.

➤ ***CASE SCENARIO:*** What cranial nerve palsy does the patient depicted in the figure above have? A left abducens nerve (cranial nerve VI) palsy.

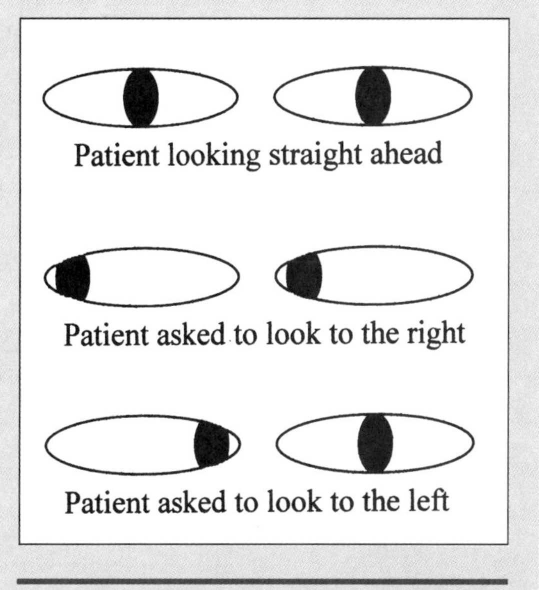

Left abducens palsy. (From Brochert A: Platinum Vignettes: Anatomy and Embryology. Philadelphia, Hanley & Belfus, 2003, p 73, with permission.)

ORTHOPEDIC SURGERY

With any fracture, do a neurologic and vascular exam distal to the fracture site to determine whether there is any compromise of nerves or blood vessels (either may be an emergency). With a suspected or obvious fracture, get ***two x-ray views*** (usually anteroposterior and lateral) of the site (see figure), and include the joint above and below the suspected fracture site.

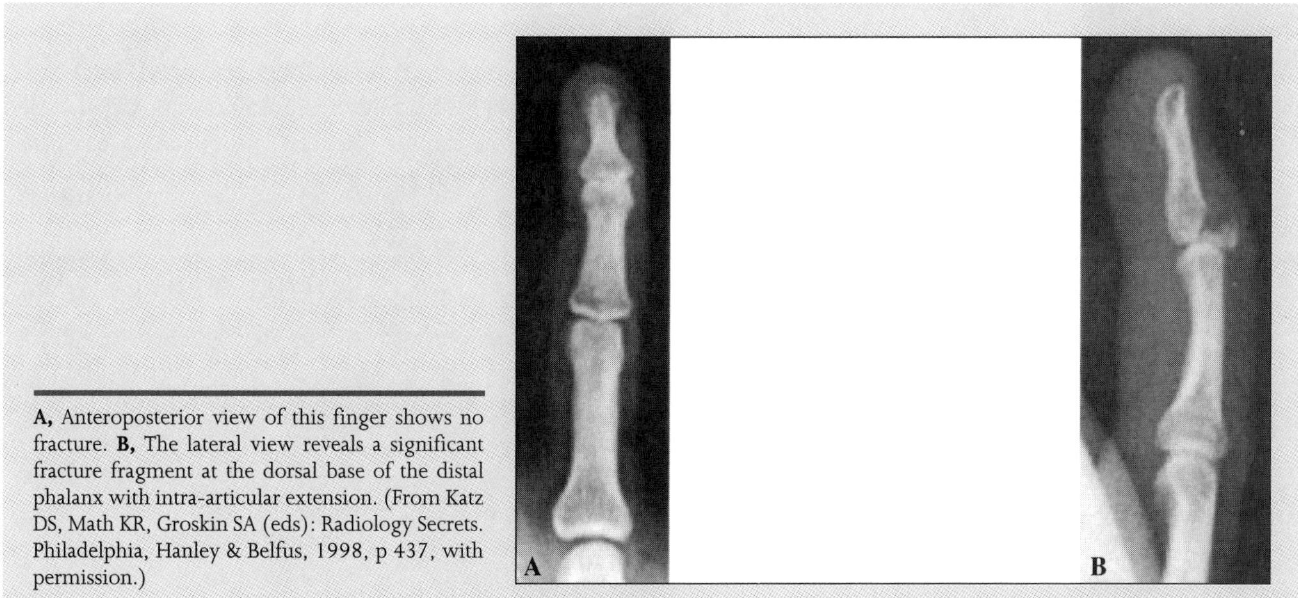

A, Anteroposterior view of this finger shows no fracture. **B,** The lateral view reveals a significant fracture fragment at the dorsal base of the distal phalanx with intra-articular extension. (From Katz DS, Math KR, Groskin SA (eds): Radiology Secrets. Philadelphia, Hanley & Belfus, 1998, p 437, with permission.)

When a fracture is suspected clinically (severe pain, point tenderness, swelling) but the x-rays are negative, ***treat conservatively as if the patient has a fracture.*** X-rays can be negative at first with smaller, nondisplaced fractures. Put the patient in a splint or even cast, and tell the patient not to use the affected limb (no weight-bearing) if symptoms are significant. If the suspected fracture is in the leg, the patient can use crutches. Repeat the x-ray in 1 week; evidence of a fracture is usually apparent by this time.

> ➤ **CASE SCENARIO:** What fractures are associated with the highest mortality rate? Pelvic fractures. Most pelvic fractures occur in elderly people who fall down and have many coexisting health problems. Young people, in whom pelvic fractures usually are due to severe trauma, may bleed to death. If patient is unstable, consider heroic measures such as military antishock trousers and external fixator.

In an **open (compound) fracture,** the skin is broken over the fracture site. In a **closed fracture,** the skin is intact. For open fractures, give broad-spectrum antibiotics, do surgical debridement, give tetanus, lavage fresh wounds (< 8 hours old), and do an **open reduction with internal fixation** (i.e., cut open the skin in the operating room to align the fracture fragments under more direct visualization). The main risk in open fractures is infection. Closed fractures often can be treated with **closed reduction and casting** (i.e., pull on the limb to align the fracture fragments without cutting open the skin).

Compartment syndrome usually occurs after fracture, crush injury, burn, or other trauma, or as a reperfusion injury (e.g., after revascularization procedure). The most common site is the **calf.** Symptoms and signs include **pain at rest, pain on passive movement** (out of proportion to injury), **paresthesias,** cyanosis or pallor, **firm-feeling muscle compartment,** hypesthesia or numbness (decreased sensation and two-point discrimination), paralysis (late, ominous sign), and **elevated compartment pressure** (> 30–40 mmHg). The diagnosis usually is made clinically without the need to measure compartment pressure, though this is fairly accurate and confirmatory. Compartment syndrome is an emergency, and quick action can save an otherwise doomed limb. **Pulses are usually palpable** (or detectable with Doppler ultrasound) at the time of diagnosis. Treatment is prompt **fasciotomy** (incising the fascial compartment relieves the pressure). Untreated, this condition progresses to permanent nerve damage and muscle necrosis.

- The classic clinical scenarios for compartment syndrome include supracondylar elbow fracture in children, proximal or midshaft tibial fractures, electrical burns, arterial or venous disruption, and revascularization procedures.

Reasons to do an open reduction (closed reduction should be done for all other fractures): intra-articular fractures or articular surface malalignment, open (compound) fractures, nonunion or failed closed reduction, compromise of blood supply or nerves, multiple trauma (to allow mobilization at earliest possible point), and extremity function requiring perfect reduction (e.g., professional athlete).

NERVE	MOTOR	SENSORY	WHEN CLINICALLY DAMAGED
Radial	Wrist extension	Back of forearm, back of hand (first 3 digits)	Humeral fracture (wrist drop)
Ulnar	Finger abduction	Front and back of last 2 fingers on hand	Elbow dislocation (claw hand)
Median	Pronation, thumb opposition	Palmar surface of hand (first 3 digits)	Carpal tunnel syndrome, humeral fracture
Axillary	Abduction/lateral rotation	Lateral shoulder	Upper humeral dislocation/fracture
Peroneal	Dorsiflexion/eversion	Dorsal foot and lateral leg	Knee dislocation (foot drop)

Ligament injuries in the knee commonly cause pain, joint effusions, instability of the joint, and history of the joint **"popping," "buckling," or "locking up."**

1. **Anterior cruciate ligament** (ACL). ACL tears are the most common. Watch for the **anterior drawer test.** The knee is placed in 90° of flexion and pulled forward (like opening a drawer). If the tibia

pulls forward more than normal (e.g., more than the unaffected side), the test is positive, and you have an ACL tear.

2. **Posterior cruciate ligament.** Watch for **posterior drawer test.** Push the tibia back with the knee in 90° of flexion. If the tibia pushes back more than normal, the test is positive and a PCL tear is present.
3. **Medial collateral ligament** (MCL). Watch for the **abduction or valgus stress test.** With the knee in 30° of flexion, abduct the ankle while holding the knee. If the knee joint abducts to an abnormal degree, the test is positive and a medical compartment injury is present.
4. **Lateral collateral ligament.** Watch for the **adduction or varus stress test.** Adduct the ankle while holding the knee. If the knee joint adducts to an abnormal degree, the test is positive, and lateral compartment injury is present.
   - MRI (see figure) or arthroscopy can be used to look for other injuries.

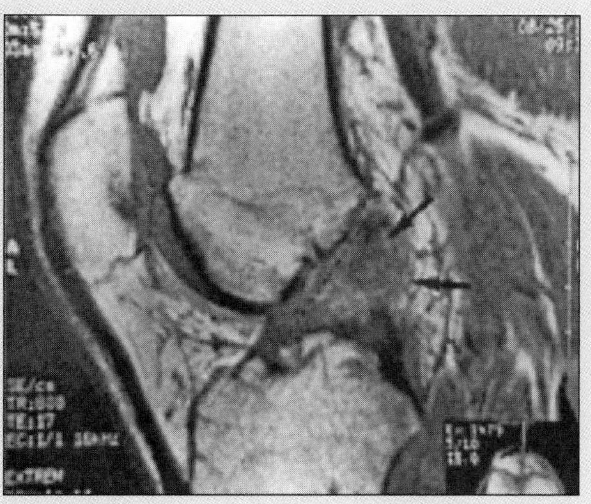

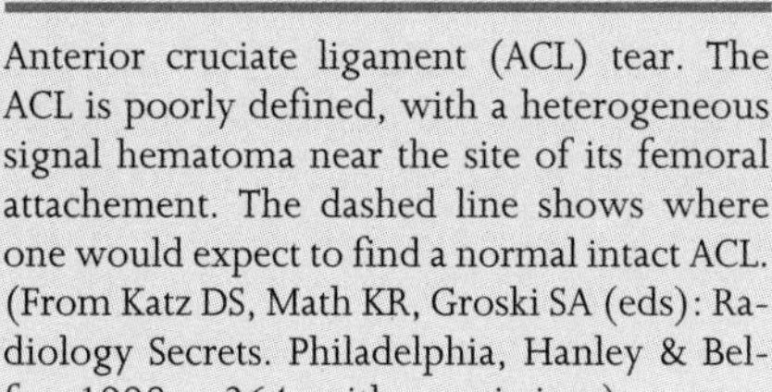

Anterior cruciate ligament (ACL) tear. The ACL is poorly defined, with a heterogeneous signal hematoma near the site of its femoral attachement. The dashed line shows where one would expect to find a normal intact ACL. (From Katz DS, Math KR, Groski SA (eds): Radiology Secrets. Philadelphia, Hanley & Belfus, 1998, p 264, with permission.)

   - Treatment may be nonsurgical (older patient, nonathlete, minor injury) or surgical (young patient, athlete, severe injury).
     - *CASE SCENARIO:* What is the "unhappy triad" knee injury? Damage to **ACL, MCL, and medial meniscus.** Classically this triad occurs when an extended knee joint is hit from the side and the knee is pushed medially while the foot is planted. For this reason, clipping is a 15-yard penalty in football.

Pain in the anatomic snuffbox after trauma (e.g., fall on an outstretched hand, especially in young adults) is usually a **scaphoid bone fracture.**

After a fall on an outstretched hand, the most likely fracture in older adults is a **Colles fracture** (distal end of radius).

Lumbar disc herniation is a common correctable cause of low back pain. Look for sciatica (not just back pain) with the straight leg raise test. The most common site is the L5–S1 disk; the second most common site is the L4–L5 disk.

1. **L5–S1 disk herniation** usually affects the S1 nerve root: **decreased ankle jerk, weakness of plantar flexors in the foot,** pain from **midgluteal area to the posterior calf** (i.e., **sciatica**).
2. **L4–L5 disk herniation** usually affects the L5 nerve root: **decreased biceps femoris reflex, weakness of foot extensors,** and pain in **hip** or **groin.**
   - Diagnosis is confirmed with CT/MRI or myelogram.

- **Conservative treatment** works in 90% of cases and includes short-term bed rest and analgesics, followed by physical therapy. Surgical treatment (diskectomy) is an option if conservative treatment fails.
- **Cervical disk disease** (classic symptom = neck pain) is less common than lumbar disk diseases. The C6–C7 disk is most commonly affected and typically causes C7 nerve root involvment. Look for **decreased triceps reflex/strength** and **weakness of forearm extension.**

Spinal stenosis is another cause of back pain that usually presents in the elderly and is due to degenerative changes in the spine. Patients may complain of pain with activity that is relieved by rest (sometimes called **"neurogenic" claudication**). Treatment is conservative with physical therapy and NSAIDs. Surgery (spinal decompression with laminectomy) is reserved for cases that fail conservative management.

Charcot joints and neuropathic joints most commonly are seen in **diabetes** and sometimes by other conditions causing peripheral neuropathy (e.g., tertiary syphilis). Lack of proprioception causes gradual arthritis/arthropathy and joint deformity. Order x-rays for any (even minor) trauma in neuropathic patients, who may not feel even a severe fracture.

With a **posterior knee dislocation,** worry about vascular injury. Consider an angiogram, especially if pulses asymmetric.

The **most common type of bone tumor** is metastatic (from the breast, lung, or prostate).

The **most common cause of a pathologic fracture** is **osteoporosis** (especially in elderly, thin women).

The most common cause of **osteomyelitis** is ***Staphylococcus aureus,*** but think of gram-negative organisms in immunocompromised patients and IVdrug abusers, and ***Salmonella* sp.** in sickle cell disease. Aspirate the bone and do Gram stain and culture and sensitivity of the sample, as well as blood cultures and complete blood cell count with differential if you are suspicious.

Septic arthritis also is most commonly due to ***S. aureus,*** but in a sexually active younger adult (especially if promiscuous), suspect ***Neisseria gonorrhoeae.*** Aspirate the joint (arthrocentesis) and do Gram stain and culture and sensitivity of the joint fluid, as well as blood cultures, complete blood cell count with differential, and urethral cultures when appropriate if you are suspicious.

UROLOGY

Testicular torsion vs. epididymitis:

	TESTICULAR TORSION	EPIDIDYMITIS
Age	< 30 years (classically adolescent)	> 30 years
Appearance	Testes may be elevated into inguinal canal; swelling	Swollen testis, overlying erythema, positive urinalysis, urethral discharge/urethritis, prostatitis
Prehn's sign	Pain stays the same or worsens	Pain decreases with testicular elevation
Ultrasound findings	No testicular blood flow	Normal testicular blood flow
Treatment	Immediate surgery to salvage testicle; orchiopexy for both testes	Antibiotics*

* In men < 50 years, commonly due to chlamydial infection or gonorrhea; treat accordingly. In men > 50 years commonly due to urinary tract infection; treat with trimethoprim-sulfamethoxazole or ciprofloxacin.

Testicular cancer usually presents as a ***painless mass in a young man*** (age 20–40 years). The main risk factor is ***cryptorchidism*** (40-fold higher risk). Roughly 90% are germ cell tumors; the most common type is ***seminoma.*** Testicular cancer generally is treated with orchiectomy and radiation; if the disease is widespread, use chemotherapy. Alpha fetoprotein is a tumor marker for yolk sac tumors, and human chorionic gonadotropin is a marker for choriocarcinoma. Leydig cell tumors may secrete androgens and cause precocious puberty. The first site of metastasis is often **retroperitoneal lymph nodes** (see figure), as the testicular veins (and accompanying lymphatics) drain to the inferior vena cava (right) or renal vein (left).

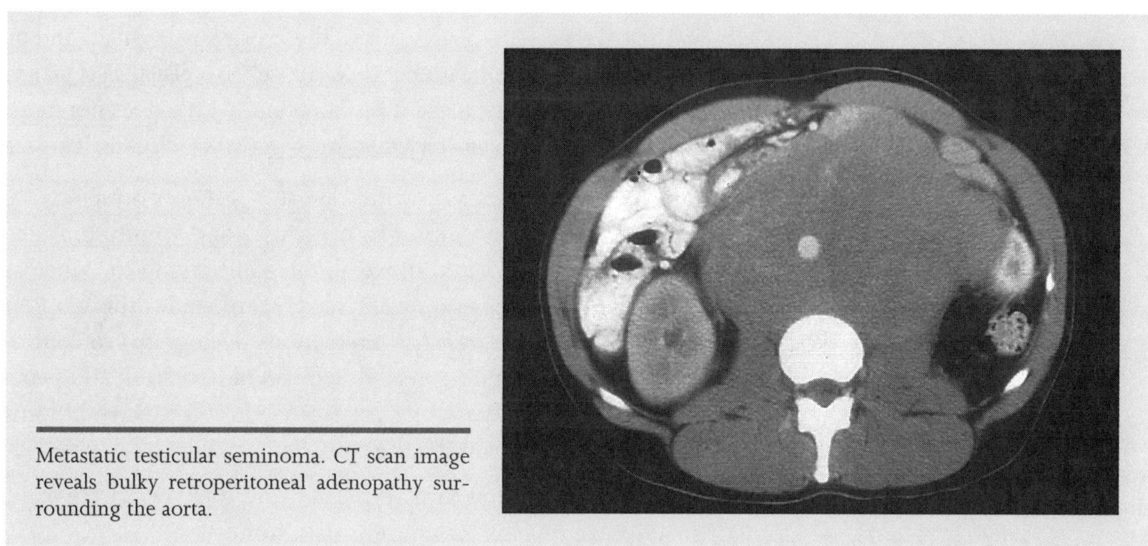

Metastatic testicular seminoma. CT scan image reveals bulky retroperitoneal adenopathy surrounding the aorta.

Remember mumps as a cause of orchitis (painful, swollen testis, usually unilateral, in a post-pubertal male). The best treatment is **prophylaxis** (immunization). Orchitis rarely causes sterility because it is usually unilateral.

Benign prostatic hypertrophy (BPH): symptoms include urinary hesitancy, intermittency, terminal dribbling, decreased size and force of stream, sensation of incomplete emptying, nocturia, urgency, dysuria, and frequency of urination. BPH may result in **urinary retention, urinary tract infections, hydronephrosis,** and even permanent kidney damage and/or failure in severe cases. Drug therapy for BPH is started when the patient becomes symptomatic and includes alpha-one blockade (e.g., **tamsulosin, prazosin**) and antiandrogens (e.g., **finasteride**). Transurethral resection of the prostate (TURP) is used for more advanced cases, especially those with repeated urinary tract infections, acute urinary retention, and hydronephrosis or kidney damage from reflux. Prostatectomy also may be used, but it carries a higher risk of morbidity and is usually not the preferred treatment.

With **acute urinary retention** (pain, palpation of full bladder on abdominal exam, history of BPH, no urination in past 24 hours), the first step is to **empty the bladder.** If you cannot pass a regular Foley catheter, do a suprapubic tap/place a **suprapubic Foley catheter.** Then address the underlying cause.

Impotence is most commonly caused by **vascular disease.** Medications are also a common culprit (especially **antihypertensives** and **antidepressants**). Diabetes can be a vascular (increased atherosclerosis) or neurogenic cause of impotence. Remember **p**oint and **s**hoot: **p**arasympathetic nerves mediate erection, **s**ympathetic nerves mediate ejaculation. Patients undergoing dialysis and patients with spinal cord injury are also commonly impotent.

- History often gives you a clue if the cause of impotence is **psychogenic.** Look for **selective dysfunction** (e.g., the patient has normal erections when masturbating, but not with his wife) and stress, anxiety, or fear.
  - ➤ ***CASE SCENARIO:*** What does a normal pattern of nocturnal erections mean in a patient with impotence? This finding essentially rules out a physical cause for the impotence.

In **all trauma patients,** look for signs of **urethral injury** (high-riding, ballottable prostate, blood at the urethral meatus, severe pelvic fracture, scrotal or perineal ecchymosis) before trying to pass a Foley catheter.

If any of these signs are present,do *not* try to pass a Foley catheter until you have ruled out a urethral injury, which is a contraindication to a Foley catheter.

> ➤ **CASE SCENARIO:** What test should be ordered in the setting of possible urethral injury? A **retrograde urethrogram.** A contrast agent is squirted backward through the urethra to look for a leak or tear.

Hydrocele vs. varicocele: hydrocele represents a remnant of the processus vaginalis and **transilluminates.** It generally causes no symptoms and requires no treatment. A varicocele is a **dilatation of the pampiniform venous plexus** (described as a "bag of worms" on physical exam, usually on the **left**), does not transilluminate, **disappears in the supine position,** and may be a cause of **male infertility** or pain (in which case, it is surgically treated).

Renal stones (nephrolithiasis): the risk is increased with *dehydration*. Patients present with **severe, intermittent, colicky, unilateral flank and/or groin pain** and, in most cases, nausea and vomiting. Patients with "renal colic" classically cannot get comfortable and often move about while trying to, whereas patients with peritonitis often lie very still. Look for **hematuria** on urinalysis; 85% of stones show up on abdominal x-ray. Use CT scan of the abdomen without contrast (or intravenous pyelogram) to confirm the presence of a stone. Most cases are idiopathic and should be treated with *lots* of hydration and pain control (to see if the stone will pass). If the stone does not pass, the patient needs shock wave lithotripsy or surgery (preferably endoscopic). Whenever possible, check stone composition, which can give a clue to the cause:

1. **Calcium stones** (75%): look for **hypercalcemia** (typically due to hyperparathyroidism or malignancy) or history of small bowel bypass (calcium oxalate stones).
2. **Struvite/magnesium-ammonium-phosphate stones** (15%): due to urinary tract infection (more common in women) with ammonia-producing bugs (*Proteus* spp., staphylococci). Look for staghorn calculi (see figure), which fill up the renal pelvis.

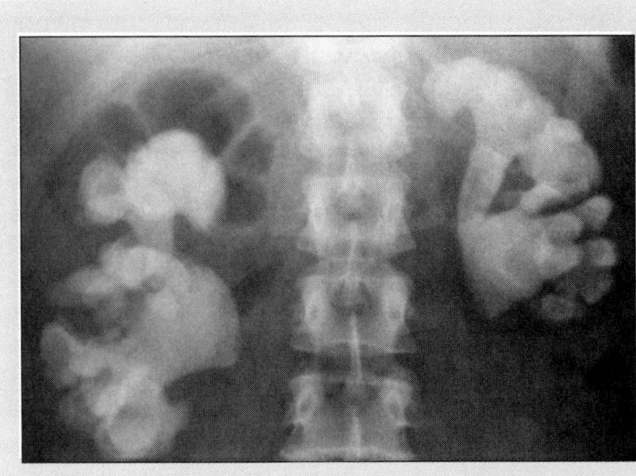

Plain abdominal radiograph in a woman with documented recurrent *Proteus* sp. urinary tract infections reveals bilateral staghorn calculi. (From Resnick MJ, Novick AC: Urology Secrets, 2nd ed. Philadelphia, Hanley & Belfus, 1999, with permission.)

3. **Uric acid stones:** due to **hyperuricemia;** thus associated with gout and leukemia treatment (allopurinol and IV fluids often are given before chemotherapy in leukemia to prevent stone formation). Uric acid stones usually dissolve with **alkalinization of the urine.**
4. **Cystine stones:** nearly diagnostic of **cystinuria**/aminoaciduria.

> ➤ **CASE SCENARIO:** Which type of stone classically cannot be seen on x-rays? Uric acid stones.

> ➤ **CASE SCENARIO:** A 32-year-old man has acute flank pain. An intravenous pyelogram reveals a small, 2-mm stone in the right ureter. How should you remove the stone? IV fluids and pain control. Let the patient pass the stone on his own. Do not be overly aggressive, because most small stones ($<$ 4–5 mm) pass spontaneously within 48 hours.

Renal Transplant Medicine

Renal transplant is an option for many patients with end-stage renal disease. Living, related donors are best (siblings or parents), especially when HLA similar, but cadaveric kidneys are more common because of availability. Before the transplant, perform an ABO blood type and lymphocytotoxic (HLA) cross-matching.

- A transplanted kidney is placed in the iliac fossa (for easy biopsy access in case of a problem as well as for technical reasons). Usually the recipient's kidneys are left in place to reduce morbidity.
- Unacceptable kidney donors: newborns, people older than 70, and people with a history of certain infections (e.g., AIDS, hepatitis), any disease with possible renal involvement (e.g., diabetes, hypertension, lupus eyrthematosus), or malignancy.

Rejection

1. **Hyperacute:** occurs within **minutes to hours** and is due to **preformed cytotoxic antibodies** against donor kidney (occurs with ABO mismatch as well as other preformed antibodies). Classic description: surgery is completed, vascular clamps are released, and the kidney quickly turns bluish-black. Treat by removing the kidney. Repeat transplant with new kidney.
2. **Acute rejection:** **T cell-mediated** rejection that presents within **days to weeks** with fever, oliguria, weight gain, tenderness and enlargement of the graft, hypertension, and/or renal function lab derangement. Treat by increasing steroids or using antithymocyte globulin (ATG) or other immunosuppressants. **Accelerated rejection** occurs over the **first few days** and is felt to reflect **reactivation of previously sensitized T cells.**
3. **Chronic rejection:** Occurs over **months to years** and is believed to be **T cell- and/or antibody-mediated.** Late cause of renal deterioration presenting with **gradual decline in kidney function, proteinuria, and hypertension.** Treatment is supportive and not effective, but the graft may survive for several years before it gives out completely. If possible, retransplant with a new kidney.
   - **Follow creatinine** to assess asymptomatic rejection.
   - **Immunosuppressive medications** include corticosteroids (inhibit interleukin [IL]-1 production), cyclosporine (inhibits IL-2 production), azathioprine (antineoplastic agent that is cleaved into mercaptopurine and inhibits DNA/RNA synthesis, which results in decreased B-cell/T-cell production), antithymocyte globulin, antilymphocyte globulin and OKT3 (antibody to CD3 receptor on T cells).
   - **Cyclosporine** causes nephrotoxicity, which can be difficult to distinguish from graft rejection clinically. When in doubt, drug levels are checked and a biopsy and/or ultrasound of the graft should be done. Practically speaking, if you increase the immunosuppressive dose, acute rejection should decrease, whereas cyclosporine toxicity will stay the same or get worse.
   - The **risks of immunosuppression** include infection (with common as well as strange organisms seen in patients witht AIDS) and cancer (especially lymphomas).

VASCULAR SURGERY

Carotid stenosis: the classic presentation is a transient ischemic attack (TIA), typically **amaurosis fugax** or sudden onset of transient, unilateral blindness, sometimes described as a "shade being pulled over one eye." Patients may have a **carotid bruit.** If a bruit is heard or the patient has a TIA, ultrasound of the carotid arteries should be done to determine whether carotid stenosis is present.

➤ **CASE SCENARIO:** What is the best treatment for a patient with a TIA and carotid stenosis less than 50%? Aspirin and medical management of atherosclerosis risk factors.

> ➤ **CASE SCENARIO:** What is the best treatment for a patient with a TIA and carotid stenosis more than 70%? Carotid endarterectomy (CEA). Between 50% and 70% stenosis is a controversial area and treatment depends on degree of symptoms, type of plaque and experience of local surgeons. Carotid stenting may become the treatment of choice in the future, but is not currently the standard of care.

- Patients should not undergo CEA after a stroke that leaves them severely disabled because they will receive no benefit; the damage is already done. Nor should patients undergo CEA during a TIA or stroke in evolution; CEA is an elective, not emergent, procedure.
- Carotid stenosis and peripheral vascular disease (PVD) are generalized markers for atherosclerosis. Almost all patients have significant coronary artery disease (CAD). In fact, peri-operative myocardial infarction (MI) is the most common cause of death in patients undergoing vascular surgery. Make sure to evaluate and medically manage risk factors for atherosclerosis in all "vasculopaths."

Abdominal aortic aneurysm (AAA): look for a **pulsatile abdominal mass** (see figure), which may cause abdominal pain. If pain is present, suspect possible rupture of the AAA, although an unruptured AAA may cause some pain. CT scan usually is used for initial evaluation. If the AAA is $\leq$ 5 cm, you can follow it with serial ultrasound exams to make sure that it is not enlarging. If the AAA is $\geq$ 5 cm or you are told that it is rapidly enlarging, surgical correction is generally advised.

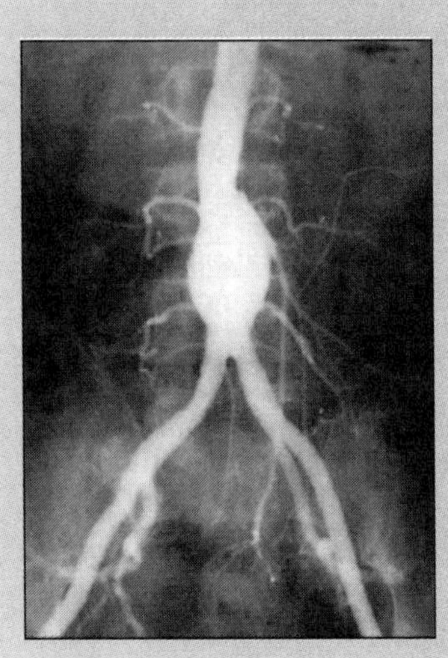

Small abdominal aortic aneurysm as visualized by angiography. (From Forbes CD, Jackson WF: Cardiovascular disorders. In Forbes CD, Jackson WF (eds): Color Atlas and Text of Clinical Medicine. St. Louis, Mosby, 1993, pp 209–264, with permission.)

> ➤ **CASE SCENARIO:** What should you do with a patient who has a pulsatile abdominal mass and hypotension? Send the patient for emergent laparotomy. This combination of findings indicates a ruptured AAA (mortality rate = roughly 90%).
>
> ➤ **CASE SCENARIO:** Can dissection of a AAA be managed medically? Yes. It can be managed with **antihypertensive agents** if it is not ruptured, and this approach is common in sick patients. However, elective AAA repair should be considered if the patient is in good health.

Claudication: pain in the lower extremity (usually) brought on by exercise and relieved by rest. Claudication is an indicator of severe atherosclerotic disease. Associated physical findings include **cyanosis** (with dependent rubor), atrophic changes (**thickened nails, loss of hair, shiny skin**), **decreased temperature,** and **decreased (or absent) distal pulses.** The best treatment is conservative (smoking cessation, exercise, control of cholesterol, diabetes, and hypertension). Beta blockers sometimes worsen claudication (due to $beta_2$ receptor blockade).

- If claudication progresses to rest pain (forefoot pain, generally at night, relieved by hanging the foot over the edge of the bed) or the patient cannot continue current lifestyle or work obligations, advise revascularization procedure.

- Severe pain in the foot that has a sudden onset with no previous history of foot pain, trauma, or any associated chronic physical findings is generally more serious and may represent an embolus. Look for atrial fibrillation.

  ➤ ***CASE SCENARIO:*** What is **Leriche syndrome**? Claudication in the buttocks, buttock atrophy, and impotence in men. It is a classic marker for aortoiliac occlusive disease. Patients usually benefit from an aortoiliac bypass graft.

Chronic mesenteric ischemia: the classic patient has a long history of postprandial abdominal pain (i.e. "***intestinal angina***"), which causes a "fear" of food that results in weight loss. This is a difficult diagnosis because it classically presents in patients over 50, who have other problems that may be cause similar symptoms (e.g., ulcers, pancreatic or stomach cancer). Look for a history of extensive atherosclerosis (previous MI or stroke, known coronary artery disease or peripheral vascular disease with several risk factors), ***abdominal bruit,*** and no jaundice (which should steer you toward pancreatic cancer). Most patients get a CT scan of the abdomen, which is negative and should make you more suspicious of ischemia. The diagnosis is confirmed with angiography. Patients should be treated surgically with revascularization because of the risks of bowel infarction and malnutrition.

After penetrating trauma in an extremity (or iatrogenic damage), patients may develop an **arteriovenous fistula.** Watch for a ***bruit*** over the area or a ***palpable pulsatile mass*** (pseudoaneurysm). Arteriovenous fistulas can be left alone if they are small; otherwise, surgical correction is needed.

Venous insufficiency: generally refers to the lower extremities. Look for a history of deep venous thrombosis; chronic swelling in the extremity; pain, fatigability, and heaviness, all of which are ***relieved by elevating the leg;*** and/or ***varicose veins.*** Patients may have increased skin pigmentation around the ankles with skin breakdown and ulceration (venous stasis ulcer, classically over the ***medial malleolus***). The initial treatment is conservative: elastic compression stockings, elevation with minimal standing, and treatment of any ulcers with cleaning, wet-to-dry dressings, and antibiotics (if cellulitis present).

Superficial thrombophlebitis: Patients have ***localized leg pain with superficial, cordlike induration, reddish discoloration,*** and mild fever. This should not be confused with deep venous thrombosis, as superficial thrombophlebitis generally does not cause pulmonary emboli and patients do not need anticoagulation. Many patients have associated varciose veins. Treatment is often thrombectomy under local anesthesia. Medical therapy may be used if the pain is mild or the patient does not want surgery; use **NSAIDs.** The pain generally subsides in a few days on its own.

Subclavian steal syndrome: usually due to left subclavian artery obstruction proximal to the vertebral artery. To get blood to an exercising arm, blood is "stolen" from the vertebrobasilar system. Blood flows backward through the vertebral artery into the distal subclavian artery instead of forward into the brainstem. The patient develops ***central nervous system symptoms*** (syncope, vertigo, confusion, ataxia, dysarthria) and unilateral ***upper extremity claudication.*** Treat with surgical bypass.

Thoracic outlet syndrome: May be due to a **cervical rib** (a normal variant) or muscular hypertrophy that compromises subclavian vessel blood flow. Patients have unilateral ***upper extremity claudication.*** Confirm diagnosis with angiography. Treat with surgery (e.g., rib resection).

  ➤ ***CASE SCENARIO:*** What is the easy way to tell the difference between thoracic outlet syndrome and subclavian steal syndrome using only the patient history? Subclavian steal causes central nervous system symptoms; cervical rib does not. Both can cause unilateral upper extremity claudication.

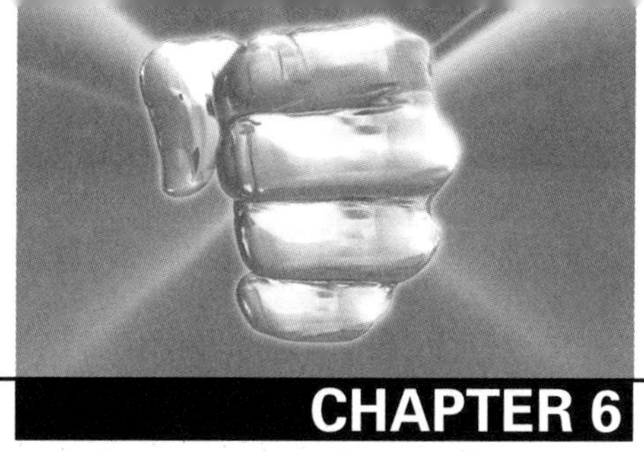

CHAPTER 6

Internal Medicine and Medical Subspecialties

INTERNAL MEDICINE

Hypertension

Health maintenance: screening for hypertension (HTN) should be done roughly every 2 years starting at the age of three, although blood pressure is typically measured routinely during any health encounter.

New patient management issues: hypertension is diagnosed when the average blood pressure from two separate measurements is greater than 140/90 mmHg (lower values are used in children; typically the 95th percentile for age is used in pediatric patients).

Hypertension classification and management in people ≥ 18 years of age (2003 JNC guidelines):

SYSTOLIC BP* (mmHg)	DIASTOLIC BP* (mmHg)	CLASSIFICATION	INITIAL DRUG TREATMENT (ALL PATIENTS SHOULD MAKE LIFESTYLE MODIFICATIONS)
< 120	< 80	Normal	None
120–139	80–89	Prehypertension	None unless compelling indications[†]
140–159	90–99	Stage 1 hypertension	Thiazides preferred. Use other agents for comorbidities or combination treatment.
≥ 160	≥ 100	Stage II hypertension	Thiazide plus at least one other agent (if tolerated) typically needed.

*__Classification is based on the worst number__ (e.g., 168/60 mmHg is considered stage II hypertension even though diastolic pressure is normal).

†Compelling indications are **diabetes** and **chronic kidney disease.** Such patients should be treated with a goal of **< 130/80** mmHg.

After the first abnormal blood pressure measurement, prescribe lifestyle modifications as indicated: **weight reduction, exercise, low salt and cholesterol diet, moderation of alcohol intake,** and **smoking cessation.** If these measures fail after a 1- to 2-month observation period, start medications. Lifestyle modifications should continue to be prescribed once drug therapy is initiated.

Basic studies and evaluation in a new hypertensive patient include **urinalysis, basic blood chemistry panel** (i.e., basic metabolic profile [BMP] or Chem-7 panel), **electrocardiogram, complete blood count,** and a **fasting lipid profile.** These tests, along with the history, help to screen for secondary causes of HTN and check for end-organ damage and associated cardiovascular risk factors.

General management issues: the goal of treatment is to **maintain a blood pressure < 140/90 mmHg** (<130/80 mmHg for patients with diabetes or chronic renal disease). There are five primary first-line agents for the treatment of HTN: **thiazide diuretics** (preferred agent in patients without additional comorbidities/indications), **beta blockers, angiotensin-converting enzyme inhibitors (ACE-Is), angiotensin-receptor blockers (ARBs),** and **calcium channel blockers.** The choice is often made because of coexisting conditions:

DRUG CLASS	USE IN PATIENTS WITH:	AVOID IN PATIENTS WITH:
Thiazides	Heart failure, diabetes, high-risk for coronary artery disease or stroke, osteoporosis	Gout, electrolyte disturbances (e.g., hyponatremia), pregnancy
Beta blockers	Stable angina, acute coronary syndrome/unstable angina, acute or prior myocardial infarction, high-risk for coronary artery disease, atrial tachycardia/fibrilliation, thyrotoxicosis (short-term), essential tremor, migraines	Asthma, chronic obstructive pulmonary disease, heart block, sick sinus syndrome
ACE inhibitors	Heart failure, diabetes, acute coronary syndrome/unstable angina, acute or prior myocardial infarction, high-risk for coronary artery disease or stroke, chronic kidney disease	Pregnancy, angioedema, renovascular hypertension (may cause renal failure)
ARBs (e.g., losartan, irbesartan)	Heart failure, diabetes, chronic kidney disease	Pregnancy, renovascular hypertension (may cause renal failure)
Calcium channel blockers	Raynaud syndrome, atrial tachyarrhythmias	Heart block, sick sinus syndrome, congestive heart failure (all related to central-acting agents), pregnancy
Aldosterone receptor blockers (e.g., spironolactone, eplerenone)	Heart failure, prior myocardial infarction	Hyperkalemia, pregnancy

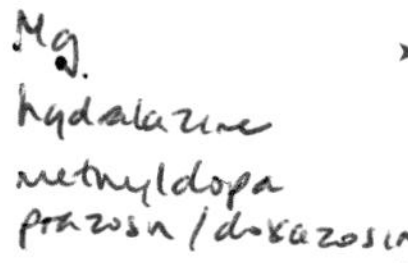

- **CASE SCENARIO:** What antihypertensive agents are appropriate for pregnant patients? Use hydralazine, alpha-methyldopa, or beta blockers, typically labetolol. Remember that in preeclamptic patients, **magnesium sulfate** (used for seizure prophylaxis) lowers blood pressure.
- **CASE SCENARIO:** Which agent is the best for a 32-year-old woman with hypertension? Any agent that is not teratogenic! Do not forget to counsel women of reproductive age about the risks of pregnancy. Always do a pregnancy test before starting a standard HTN drug (or any other possible teratogen).
- **CASE SCENARIO:** What antihypertensive agents are good for men with coexisting benign prostatic hypertrophy (BPH)? Alpha antagonists (e.g., prazosin, doxazosin)

Secondary HTN: clues are onset before age 30 or after age 55, very high or hard-to-control blood pressure, and other history or lab values.

1. **Birth control pills:** the most common secondary cause in young women. Discontinue their use to see if HTN resolves.
2. **Renovascular HTN:** may be due to **fibromuscular dysplasia** in young women or **atherosclerosis** in elderly persons. Watch for renal bruit or renal failure after taking an ACE inhibitor. Consider ultrasound, CT, MRI, or arteriogram to diagnose. Treatment typically with angioplasty.
3. **Excessive alcohol intake:** a common cause, especially in young men.
4. **Pheochromocytoma:** watch for **intermittent severe HTN, dizziness,** and **diaphoresis.** Check 24-hour urinary catecholamines (e.g., vanillylmandelic acid, metanephrine) as a screening test.
5. **Polycystic kidney disease:** flank mass, family history, renal insufficiency.
6. **Cushing disease:** patient taking steroids or with Cushingoid appearance. Use 24-hour urine cortisol level or dexamethasone suppression test as screening tool.

7. **Conn syndrome:** aldosterone-secreting adrenal adenoma causes high aldosterone, **low renin,** and hypokalemia.
8. **Coarctation of the aorta:** upper extremity HTN only, unequal pulses, radiofemoral delay, associated with **Turner syndrome,** rib notching on X-ray.

Hypertensive urgency and emergency: Exact cut-off number varies between textbooks, but a systolic BP >200 mmHg and/or diastolic BP >120 mmHg is defined as a hypertensive urgency if the patient is **asymptomatic** and an emergency if there is **evidence of acute end-organ damage.** Signs of end-organ damage include: acute left ventricular failure/pulmonary edema; unstable angina; myocardial infarction; encephalopathy (i.e., headaches, mental status changes, vomiting, blurry vision, dizziness, and/or papilledema); stroke; life-threatening arterial bleeding; aortic dissection; and/or acute renal insufficiency/failure. Admit affected patients and treat with IV **nitroprusside, nitroglycerin,** or **labetalol** emergently.

Epidemiology facts

1. Lowering HTN lowers the risk for **stroke** (HTN is the most important risk factor), **congestive heart failure, myocardial infarction, renal failure, atherosclerosis,** and **aortic dissection.**
2. Coronary disease is the most common cause of death among untreated hypertensive patients
3. The risk of cardiovascular disease doubles with each blood pressure increment of 20/10 mm Hg starting at 115/75 mm Hg.
4. People who are normotensive at age 55 have a 90% lifetime risk of developing hypertension.

Diabetes Mellitus

Screening: universal screening is generally not recommended. Screening in patients who are obese or older than 45 years, have a family history, or are members of certain ethnic groups (black, American Indian, Hispanic) is more accepted, but not uniformly.

Diagnosis: the diagnosis is made when a **fasting plasma glucose is ≥ 126 mg/dl** (after an overnight fast) or a **random glucose** (no fasting) is **≥ 200 mg/dl.** If needed, an oral glucose tolerance test can be done and DM is diagnosed when levels ≥ 200mg/dl are reached within or at 2 hours after a 75-gm oral glucose load.

New patient management issues: classic symptoms of diabetes mellitus (DM) are **polydipsia, polyuria, polyphagia,** and **weight loss.** Patients also may have a classic infection, such as **candidiasis,** and sometimes complain or near-sightedness or improvement of far-sightedness due to osmotic lens swelling (goes away with treatment).

Classic differences between type I and type II diabetes mellitus*:

	TYPE I	TYPE II
Age at onset	Most commonly < 30 years	Most commonly > 30 years
Associated body habitus	Thin	Obese
Develop ketoacidosis	Yes	No
Develop hyperosmolar state	No	Yes
Level of endogenous insulin	Low to none	Low to high (insulin resistance)
Twin concurrence	< 50%	> 50%
HLA association	Yes	No
Respond to oral hypoglycemics	No	Yes
Antibodies to insulin	Yes (at diagnosis)	No
Risk for diabetic complications	Yes	Yes
Islet cell pathology	Insulitis (loss of most B cells)	Normal number, but with amyloid deposits

*Some overlap exists.

Routine health maintenance issues in diabetic patients

1. Measure **urine microalbumin** annually to monitor for early renal disease. Consider ACE-inhibitor in all diabetics to delay nephropathy.
2. Schedule annual visit to ophthalmologist to monitor for vision problems.
3. Patients should wash and inspect their own feet daily and wear comfortable, properly-fitting shoes.
4. Do a formal foot exam and assess for **neuropathy** with monofilament or tuning fork roughly every 6 months.
5. Follow compliance with **hemoglobin A1c** level. The goal is generally a level ≤ 7. This parameter is an accurate measure of overall control for the previous 3 months. To get a very crude estimate of average glucose level, multiply the hemoglobin A1c level by 20.
6. Screen for and treat coexisting modifiable risk factors for atherosclerosis (e.g., HTN, cholesterol) aggressively.

General management issues

The **goal of treatment** is to keep postprandial glucose less than 200, fasting glucose less than 130. Stricter control may result in too many episodes of hypoglycemia.

> ➤ **CASE SCENARIO:** A 42-year-old woman who takes three insulin injections daily and is very compliant complains of episodes of sweating and palpitations with confusion. What is the cause? Episodes of hypoglycemia from overaggressive glucose control.

> ➤ **CASE SCENARIO:** A 31-year-old male nurse who is histrionic has episodes of severe hypoglycemia. What lab value should you measure? **C-peptide level.** If the C-peptide level is low immediately after an episode, the patient has factitious disorder and is secretly taking insulin. If C-peptide is high, the patient has an insulinoma.

Diabetic ketoacidosis: primarily seen in type I diabetics. Patients have **hyperglycemia, hyperketonemia** with **ketonuria,** and **metabolic acidosis.** Give fluids and IV regular insulin, closely monitor electrolytes and glucose level, and give **potassium** and **phosphorus** replacement. Do not give bicarbonate unless the pH is ≤ 7.0. Remember to search for the cause, which often is infection or noncompliance. Can be fatal.

Nonketotic hyperglycemic hyperosmolar state: seen in type II diabetics. Patients have **hyperglycemia** and **hyperosmolarity** *without* ketonemia. Treatment involves aggressive IV fluids, IV insulin, and electrolyte replacement. Can be fatal.

Long-term complications of DM

1. **Atherosclerosis,** including coronary artery disease and peripheral vascular disease with their associated risks and complications.
2. **Retinopathy:** DM is one of the leading causes of acquired blindness.
3. **Nephropathy:** use ACE inhibitors to help prevent renal complications. DM causes 30% of end-stage renal disease.
4. **Neuropathy:** the classic example is sensory neuropathy leading to numb feet, infection, **gangrene,** and/or **Charcot joints.** In addition, diabetics classically have "silent" heart attacks (i.e., no chest pain) due to sensory loss. Autonomic peripheral neuropathy can lead to **gastroparesis** (early satiety and nausea), resting tachycardia, orthostatic hypotension, and **impotence.** Gastroparesis can be treated with **metoclopramide.**
5. **Increased risk of infections:** hyperglycemia interferes with neutrophil function. Vascular disease and neuropathy contribute to infection and delayed patient detection.

➤ **CASE SCENARIO:** What is the treatment for proliferative diabetic retinopathy? Pan-retinal laser photocoagulation helps to prevent progression and blindness. The laser is used to make multiple burns in the peripheral retina.

➤ **CASE SCENARIO:** How should doses of regular and neutral protamine Hagedorn (NPH) insulin be adjusted in the following cases?

1. Patient has high (low) 7 AM glucose? Increase (decrease) NPH insulin at dinner the night before.
2. Patient has high (low) noon glucose? Increase (decrease) morning dose of regular insulin.
3. Patient has high (low) 5 PM glucose? Increase (decrease) morning dose of NPH.
4. Patient has high (low) 9 PM glucose? Increase (decrease) dinner-time dose of regular insulin.

➤ **CASE SCENARIO: Somogyi effect** vs. **dawn phenomenon.** How do you treat a 52-year-old man with 7 am glucose of 220? Measure the 3 am glucose. If it is 40, the patient has the Somogyi effect due to hypoglycemia. You should decrease the pm dose of NPH. If the 3 am glucose is 160, the patient has the dawn phenomenon due to normal morning surge of growth hormone and cortisol. You should increase the pm dose of NPH.

➤ **CASE SCENARIO:** What is the best insulin regimen on the day of elective surgery? Because patients do not eat before surgery, give one-third to one-half of the normal insulin dose. The glucose should be monitored throughout surgery and postoperatively; typically, 5% dextrose in water (D5W) and IV regular insulin are used to maintain glucose control.

➤ **CASE SCENARIO:** A 47-year-old diabetic woman takes metoprolol for prior heart attack and hypertension. She keeps passing out without warning. What should you do? Have the patient check the glucose level after the next attack. If it is low, decrease the amount of diabetes medications. Do not stop the beta blocker if you can avoid doing so, because it has been shown to prolong survival after an infarct. Counsel the patient that a beta blocker can eliminate warning signs of hypoglycemia.

➤ **CASE SCENARIO:** A 59-year-old diabetic man taking metformin gets a CT scan with contrast and subsequently develops lactic acidosis. How could this complication have been prevented? Stop metformin after the contrast is given and restart it 2 days later if creatinine level is stable. Also, consider aggressive intravenous hydration before and after giving the contrast in patients with diabetes and/or renal disease.

Cholesterol

Health maintenance: Screen all people by measuring a fasting lipoprotein profile (total cholesterol, LDL, HDL, and triglycerides) every 5 years (unless abnormal) starting at age 20. Consider earlier and more aggressive screening for a strong family history and/or obesity. Screen all family members of a patient with familial hyperlipidemia. Total cholesterol goal is less than 200 mg/dL with >240 considered high and normal triglyceride levels are <150 mg/dL with >200 considered high, but LDL is usually the main player for treatment decisions (see below).

Cholesterol is important mainly because it is a risk factor for atherosclerosis. To keep the importance in perspective, atherosclerosis is involved in about one-half of all deaths in the United States and one-third of deaths in people between ages 35 and 65. Atherosclerosis is the most important cause of permanent disability and accounts for more hospital days than any other illness.

New patient management issues: look for ***xanthelasma, xanthomas*** (see figures) and ***corneal arcus*** in younger people as well as lipemic-looking serum and obesity (markers of possible familial hypercholesterolemia). Also look for pancreatitis with no risk factors (e.g., no alcohol or gallstones) as a marker for familial hypertriglyceridemia.

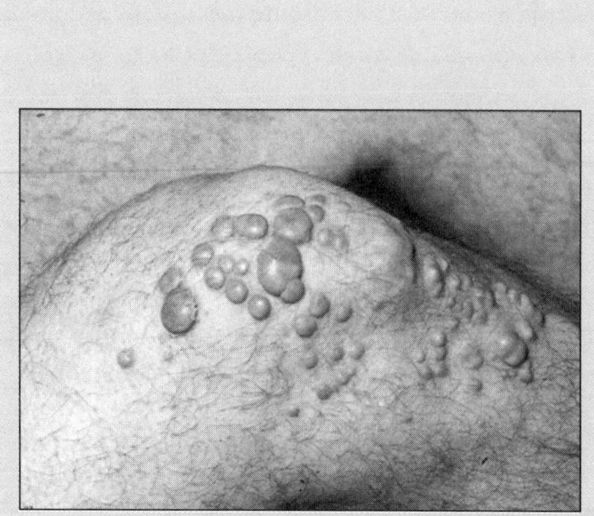

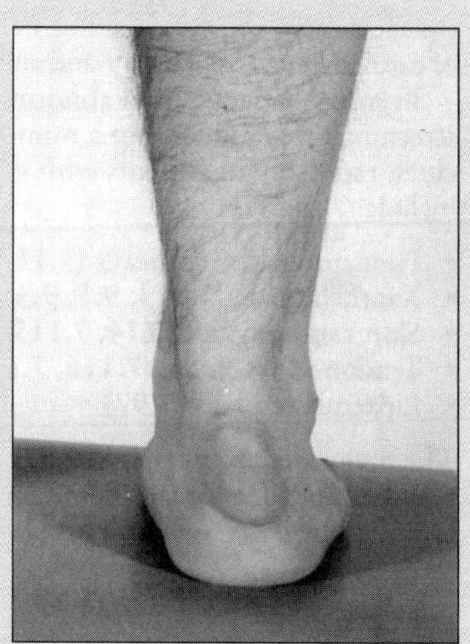

Xanthomata of the knee **(left)** and Achilles tendon **(right),** two classic and common locations. Most are located along tendons and extensor surfaces of joints. (From Forbes CD, Jackson WF: Endocrine, metabolic, and nutritional disorders. In Forbes CD, Jackson WF (eds): Color Atlas and Text of Clinical Medicine. St. Louis, Mosby, 1993, pp 303–352, with permission).

Lipoprotein analysis involves measuring total cholesterol, HDL, and triglycerides. Low-density lipotprotein (LDL) cholesterol can be calculated from the formula LDL = total cholesterol − HDL − (triglycerides/5).

Standard management guide for cholesterol levels (mg/dl):

NO CHD RISK FACTORS	≥2 CHD RISK FACTORS*	KNOWN CAD/ EQUIVALENT**	VERY HIGH RISK†	INTERVENTION
LDL < 160	LDL < 100	LDL < 100	LDL < 70	None (meets goal)
LDL 160-189	LDL 100-129		LDL 70-99	Diet +/− medications‡
LDL ≥ 190	LDL ≥ 130	LDL ≥ 100	LDL ≥ 100	Medications (+ diet)

*CHD = coronary heart disease. Risk factors for CHD are listed on the next page.

**CAD = coronary artery disease. CHD equivalents include diabetes mellitus, peripheral arterial atherosclerotic disease, symptomatic carotid artery disease, and abdominal aortic aneurysm.

†"Very" high-risk patients are those with CAD who have a heart attack, diabetes or other severe and poorly controlled risk factors (e.g., metabolic syndrome, heavy smoking).

‡"Diet" includes general lifestyle modifications such as eating less and healthier, decreasing alcohol intake, exercising, etc. The trend is toward more aggressive intervention, so you will not be faulted for initiating medications at these "gray area" LDL levels, particularly in higher risk people.

Risk factors for CHD

1. **Age** (men ≥ 45, women ≥ 55, or women with premature menopause and no hormone replacement therapy).
2. **Family history of premature CHD** (defined as definite MI or sudden death in first-degree male relative $<$ 55 years old or first-degree female relative $<$ 65 years old).
3. **Current cigarette smoking** ($>$ 10 cigarettes per day)
4. **Hypertension** (BP ≥ 140/90 mmHg or taking antihypertensive medications)
5. **Low HDL** ($<$ 40 mg/dL)

   NOTE: HDL ≥ 60 mg/dl is considered to be protective and **negates one risk factor.**

"Softer" risk factors and other information:

- **Obesity, stress, physical inactivity,** and **"type A" personality** are not independent risk factors for board purposes. However, watch for these clues in a clinical case scenario describing CHD.
- **Male sex** is a risk factor for CHD because men develop CHD earlier than women. Postmenopausal women quickly catch up to age-matched men, however. If you give a man one risk factor for male gender, do not give him a second risk factor for age.
- **High LDL** and **total cholesterol** are risk factors for CHD, but don't count them when deciding to treat or not treat hyperlipidemia using the above table. **Hypertriglyceridemia** alone is not considered a risk factor, but in association with high cholesterol it causes more CHD than high cholesterol alone.

Give a patient at least 3 months to try lifestyle modifications (**decrease in calories, cholesterol, and saturated fat in diet; decrease in alcohol intake and smoking; exercise**) before initiating drug therapy. If levels are still higher than guidelines, prescribe medication.

General management issues

HMG CoA-reductase inhibitors (e.g., lovastatin) are the most effective drugs and are the first-line agents for management of elevated LDL. Order baseline liver function tests and periodically **monitor liver enzymes** in people taking these agents. HMG CoA-reductase inhibitors should not be used in patients with liver disease and can also cause muscle damage (watch for sore muscles and/or elevated creatine phosphokinase [CPK] levels).

Second-line agents for cholesterol are **niacin** (poorly tolerated, but effective and also raises HDL) and **bile-acid binding resins** (e.g., cholestyramine). **Gemfibrozil** lowers only triglycerides.

HDL is protective against atherosclerosis and is increased by **moderate (not high) alcohol consumption** (1–2 drinks/day), **exercise,** and **estrogens.** HDL is decreased by smoking, androgens, progesterone, and hypertriglyceridemia.

Secondary causes of hyperlipidemia include diabetes, hypothyroidism, uremia, nephrotic syndrome, obstructive liver disease, excessive alcohol intake (increases triglycerides), and medications (birth control pills, glucocorticoids, thiazides, and beta-blockers). If the underlying problem is corrected in such cases, no other treatment may be needed.

> ➤ ***CASE SCENARIO:*** Patient has high cholesterol and is diabetic. Diabetes is poorly controlled. How should you manage cholesterol? First, get diabetes under control, then re-measure cholesterol.

Smoking

Smoking is the **single most significant source of preventable morbidity and premature death** in the United States. Whenever you are not sure which risk factor is most responsible for death, gloom, or doom, smoking is a safe guess on the boards.

> ➤ **CASE SCENARIO:** In a 58-year-old male smoker with no exercise, high stress, high cholesterol, and a drinking problem, what is the best way to reduce mortality? Quit smoking.

Smoking is the best risk factor to eliminate to prevent deaths due to **heart disease** (responsible for 30–45% of coronary heart disease deaths). The risk is decreased by 50% within 1 year after quitting compared with continuing smokers, and the risk decreases to that of people who have never smoked in 15 years.

Smoking increases the risk for the following cancers: **lung** (causes 85–90% of cases), **oral cavity** (90% of cases), **esophagus** (70–80% of cases), **larynx, pharynx, bladder** (30–50% of cases), **kidney** (20–30% of cases), **pancreas** (20–25%), **cervix, vulva, penis** and **anus.** It may also increase the risk of **stomach** cancer.

Emphysema and **chronic bronchitis** (i.e., COPD) are almost always due to smoking. Although the changes associated with emphysema are irreversible, the risk of death still decreases after quitting smoking.

Smoking retards the healing of **peptic ulcer disease.**

Smoking by a pregnant woman increases the risk of **low birth weight, prematurity, spontaneous abortion, stillbirth,** and **infant mortality.**

> ➤ **CASE SCENARIO:** A 27-year-old woman has smoked 5 cigarettes per day for the last 2 years and now has emphysema. What is the cause? Alpha-one antitrypsin deficiency. The patient has not smoked enough cigarettes to cause emphysema (usually need at least 5–10 pack years).

> ➤ **CASE SCENARIO:** A 3-year-old child has asthma and recurrent otitis media. Both parents smoke. What is the best initial treatment? Persuade the parents to quit smoking around the child and in the house.

> ➤ **CASE SCENARIO:** A 29-year-old man who is a heavy smoker gets painful red fingers and cold toes. What should you do? The patient has **Buerger disease.** If he stops smoking, the disease should resolve.

> ➤ **CASE SCENARIO:** Is it acceptable for a 36-year-old female smoker to take birth control pills? No.

> ➤ **CASE SCENARIO:** Is it acceptable for a 58-year-old female smoker to take estrogen replacement therapy? Yes.

Alcohol

Health maintenance: alcohol abuse is more common in men. Roughly 10–15% of people abuse alcohol. Alcoholism has a heritable component and is especially passed from **fathers to sons.**

Alcohol increases the risk for the following cancers: **oral, larynx, pharynx, esophagus,** and **liver.** It may increase the risk for gastric, pancreatic, and **breast** cancer as well.

Alcohol is the most common cause of cirrhosis and esophageal varices and is involved in roughly **50% of fatal car accidents, 67% of drownings and homicides, 70–80% of deaths in fires,** and **35% of suicides.**

Patient management issues

1. **Alcohol withdrawal**

   Can be fatal and should be treated on an inpatient basis.

   - Give **benzodiazepines** and gradually taper the dose over days.

- Classic withdrawal stages and symptoms. First comes the **acute withdrawal syndrome** (12–48 hours after last drink), in which the person develops tremors, sweating, hyperreflexia, and **seizures** ("rum fits"). Next is **alcoholic hallucinosis,** which consists of hallucinations (auditory/visual) and illusions without autonomic symptoms. Finally comes **delirium tremens** (usually 2–4 days after the last drink), which involves hallucinations and illusions plus confusion, poor sleep, and autonomic lability (e.g., sweating, increased pulse and temperature). Occasionally delirium tremens is fatal.

  ➤ **CASE SCENARIO:** About 24 hours after surgery, a middle-aged patient becomes delirious and shaky. He has no hypoxia, no obvious infection, and no abnormal electrolytes. He is taking no medications, has never taken corticosteroids, and is on a regular surgery floor (not the intensive care unit). Why is he delirious? The patient most likely is a closet alcoholic going into withdrawal.

2. Know the **stigmata of chronic liver disease and cirrhosis** in alcoholics: varices, hemorrhoids, caput medusae, jaundice, ascites, palmar erythema, spider angiomas, gynecomastia, testicular atrophy, encephalopathy, **asterixis,** prolonged prothrombin time, hyperbilirubinemia, spontaneous bacterial peritonitis, hypoalbuminemia, and anemia.

3. Know the **various diseases associated with alcohol:** gastritis, Mallory-Weiss tears, pancreatitis (acute and chronic), peripheral neuropathy, dilated cardiomyopathy, fatty change in the liver, hepatitis, cerebellar degeneration/ataxia, and rhabdomyolysis (acute and chronic).

   ➤ **CASE SCENARIO:** In a patient with hepatitis, the aspartate aminotransferase (AST) level is 250 and the alanine aminotransferase (ALT) level is 110. What is the cause of the hepatitis? Alcohol (AST $\geq$ 2 times the ALT value, versus a 1:1 ratio or higher ALT with viral and other forms of hepatitis).

   ➤ **CASE SCENARIO:** What is the best treatment for alcoholics who want to quit? Alcoholics Anonymous or another support group.

4. Alcohol is a **definite teratogen** and can cause **fetal alcohol syndrome,** which includes mental retardation, microcephaly, microphthalmia, short palpebral fissures, midfacial hypoplasia, and cardiac defects. No alcohol is good alcohol during pregnancy. An estimated 1 in 3000 births are affected by fetal alcohol syndrome.

   ➤ **CASE SCENARIO:** What is the most common cause of preventable mental retardation? Maternal alcohol consumption.

   ➤ **CASE SCENARIO:** A "skid-row" alcoholic is found combative with low glucose. He gets glucose and starts acting confused, ataxic, and cannot move his eyes. What happened? Wernicke encephalopathy precipitated by giving glucose before thiamine. Give thiamine first, then glucose in alcoholics.

   ➤ **CASE SCENARIO:** A chronic alcoholic patient can't form new memories and makes up stories. Why? Chronic thiamine deficiency has led to Korsakoff syndrome, which is chronic and irreversible.

5. Watch for **aspiration pneumonia** with enteric organisms such as *Klebsiella* spp. (currant-jelly sputum), anaerobes, *Escherichia coli*, streptococci, and staphylococci.

6. Alcoholics can have just about any **vitamin or mineral deficiency** but are especially prone to deficiencies of **folate, magnesium,** and **thiamine.**

   ➤ **CASE SCENARIO:** A known alcoholic with jaundice, ascites, and caput medusae vomits large quantities of blood. What should you do? First, stabilize the patient with IV fluids and blood and assess baseline lab values. Then do upper endoscopy and sclerotherapy with cauterization, banding, or vasopressin if esophageal varices are the cause. Other possible causes include gastritis and peptic ulcer disease. The mortality rate with varices is high, and rebleeding is common, especially early after the initial episode. If possible, choose a **transjugular intrahepatic portosystemic shunt (TIPS)** over open surgical portocaval shunting. The splenorenal shunt is the most physiologic type.

Acid-Base Disorders

- **CASE SCENARIO:** What is the primary disturbance in the following settings?
  1. pH high, carbon dioxide low? Respiratory alkalosis.
  2. pH high, bicarbonate high? Metabolic alkalosis.
  3. pH high, carbon dioxide high? Metabolic alkalosis (with respiratory compensation).
  4. pH high, bicarbonate low? Respiratory alkalosis (with metabolic compensation).
- **CASE SCENARIO:** A patient takes "a handful of pills" and has tinnitus, near-normal pH, low carbon dioxide, and low bicarbonate. What did she take? Aspirin, which causes primary metabolic acidosis and primary metabolic alkalosis. Alkalinization of the urine (with bicarbonate) speeds excretion.
- **CASE SCENARIO:** Early asthma causes hyperventilation and respiratory alkalosis, with no time for metabolic compensation in an acute attack. If the pH changes to normal, the patient becomes sleepy, and carbon dioxide starts to rise, what should you do? Prepare to intubate!
- **CASE SCENARIO:** A 68-year-old woman with emphysema who takes 2 liters of oxygen by nasal cannula 24 hours/day at home presents with increased shortness of breath. She receives 6 liters via nasal cannula to maintain oxygen saturation above 93%, but carbon dioxide starts to rise and the pH falls on repeat blood gas analysis. What should you do? Turn down the oxygen. High oxygen levels may shut down the respiratory drive of patients with severe chronic obstructive pulmonary disease.
- **CASE SCENARIO:** What do you expect the blood gas analysis to show in patients with a heroin overdose? Respiratory acidosis, with high carbon dioxide, low pH, and near-normal bicarbonate (due to lack of time for metabolic compensation).
- **CASE SCENARIO:** A 32-year-old woman presents with severe dyspnea, 100% oxygen saturation, high pH, low carbon dioxide, normal bicarbonate, and a normal chest x-ray and EKG. She is also afebrile and has no wheezing. What is happening? Probably a **panic attack** causing primary respiratory alkalosis.
- **CASE SCENARIO:** In an obese, tired 36-year-old man whose wife says that he snores a lot, why does the blood gas analysis show high pH, high bicarbonate, and normal carbon dioxide during an office visit? The patient has sleep apnea. Chronic respiratory acidosis during sleep causes chronic metabolic compensation. During the day, the patient is awake and blows off enough carbon dioxide. Alkalosis develops because the bicarbonate is still high (i.e. the compensation becomes the primary disturbance).
- **CASE SCENARIO:** In a 37-year-old woman with new-onset hypertension, the chemistry panel shows hypokalemia and high bicarbonate. Why? Aldosterone-secreting adenoma (**Conn syndrome**).
- **CASE SCENARIO:** What is the difference in the acid-base disturbance caused by diarrhea and vomiting? Diarrhea usually results in metabolic acidosis, whereas vomiting usually results in metabolic alkalosis (and hypokalemia).

Note: Avoid using bicarbonate to treat low pH unless the pH is < 7.0 and other measures have failed. First try to correct the underlying problem and/or give normal saline.

Hyponatremia

Watch for confusion, lethargy, mental status changes, anorexia, **seizures,** disorientation, cramps, and coma.

The first step in determining the cause of hyponatremia is to ensure that the patient does not have "false" hyponatremia due to **hyperglycemia.** The most important next step is to check the volume status.

	HYPOVOLEMIC	EUVOLEMIC	HYPERVOLEMIC
Think of	Dehydration, diuretics, diabetes, Addison's disease, hypoaldosteronism	Syndrome of inappropriate antidiuretic hormone, psychogenic polydipsia, oxytocin use	Congestive heart failure, nephrotic syndrome, cirrhosis, toxemia, renal failure

The **syndrome of inappropriate antidiuretic hormone (SIADH)** commonly results from head trauma, surgery, meningitis, **small cell cancer of the lung,** postoperative or other painful states, pulmonary infections (pneumonia or tuberculosis), opioids, or chlorpropamide.

- **CASE SCENARIO:** A patient has head trauma and needs neurosurgery. Postoperatively the patient has a lot of pain and needs meperidine. The sodium level was normal preoperatively but 3 days after surgery is very low. What should you do? Restrict water intake. The patient has SIADH.
- **CASE SCENARIO:** A patient with small cell lung cancer develops severe hyponatremia. Water restriction does not help. What drug can you try? **Demeclocycline,** which causes renal diabetes insipidus and counteracts the SIADH.
- **CASE SCENARIO:** A patient with history of severe asthma undergoes an uncomplicated appendectomy and develops hypotension turning into shock as well as hyponatremia and hyperkalemia that doesn't respond to IV fluids. What should you do? Give IV corticosteroids. The patient probably has acute adrenal insufficiency from taking steroids in the past.
- **CASE SCENARIO:** A nursing home patient taking furosemide presents with marked tenting of skin, hyponatremia, and hypokalemia. What should you do? Give normal saline—the treatment for hypovolemic hyponatremia. Do not give hypertonic saline!
- **CASE SCENARIO:** What is the treatment for euvolemic and hypervolemic hyponatremia? Free water restriction and possible diuretics in the case of hypervolemia.
- **CASE SCENARIO:** An alcoholic patient presents with very low sodium. He is given hypertonic saline, and the sodium becomes normal within 12 hours. The patient goes into a coma. What happened? Brainstem damage (**central pontine myelinolysis**). Hypertonic saline should be avoided on the boards (used only when a patient has seizures from hyponatremia and even then only briefly and cautiously). Normal saline is a better choice 99 times out of 100 for board purposes.
- **CASE SCENARIO:** A 27 year-old woman (G1P0) is in labor and is given **oxytocin** for failure to progress. After a few hours, she has a seizure. The sodium level is low. What should you do first? Stop the oxytocin, which caused the hyponatremia.

Note: In a surgical patient, the most common cause of hyponatremia is inappropriate or excessive fluid administration.

Hypernatremia

Signs and symptoms are similar to those of hyponatremia: confusion, mental status changes, hyperreflexia, seizures, and coma.

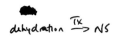

- **CASE SCENARIO:** A demented patient is found unconscious at home. He has marked tenting of the skin. The sodium level is extremely high. What should you do? Give normal saline, because the patient is dehydrated. Do not give 1/2 normal saline or D5W. The patient needs volume.
- **CASE SCENARIO:** Pituitary vs. nephrogenic diabetes insipidus. In a patient with diabetes insipidus, how do you know if the cause is nephrogenic or pituitary? Give **vasopressin.**

Pituitary causes respond appropriately (i.e. urine becomes more concentrated); nephrogenic causes do not.

- **CASE SCENARIO:** A manic-depressive patient taking lithium has fatigue and polyuria. The serum sodium level is very high, and glucose is normal. What is the problem? Nephrogenic diabetes insipidus due to lithium.
- **CASE SCENARIO:** What drug can be used to treat a patient with nephrogenic diabetes insipidus? A **thiazide diuretic** (paradoxical effect decreases urine formation).
- **CASE SCENARIO:** A 29-year-old woman has severe postpartum hemorrhage and goes into shock. She recovers after aggressive resuscitation. Later she cannot breastfeed and produces 20 L/day of urine. What happened? The patient developed Sheehan syndrome (pituitary infarction), which may result in central diabetes insipidus and other endocrine problems (e.g., in this case, lack of prolactin, thus she can't breastfeed).

Hypokalemia

Look for **muscular weakness,** which can lead to paralysis and ventilatory failure. Also affects the smooth muscles; the patient may have an adynamic **ileus** and/or hypotension.

- **CASE SCENARIO:** A 58-year-old woman taking furosemide develops palpitations. The EKG shows loss of T wave, U waves, and multiple premature ventricular contractions. Cardiac enzymes are normal. What is the problem? Hypokalemia.
- **CASE SCENARIO:** A 22-year-old man presents with diabetic ketoacidosis and has severe acidosis with a normal potassium level. Why should you give potassium? Because acidosis causes hyperkalemia, thus the normal potassium level will become low once you start treating the acidosis with fluids and insulin. To make matters worse, insulin drives potassium from the extracellular space and plasma into the intracellular space. The end result is that if you don't start potassium replacement now, you'll probably get into trouble with hypokalemia later.

The heart is particularly sensitive to hypokalemia when **digitalis** is present.

Do not replace potassium too quickly. The best replacement route is oral, but if potassium is given IV, use EKG monitoring and do not exceed 20 mEq/hr.

Hyperkalemia

The classic symptom of hyperkalemia is **weakness** or paralysis.

EKG changes (in order of increasing potassium value) include **tall, peaked T waves;** widening of QRS; PR interval prolongation; loss of P waves; and a sine-wave pattern. Arrhythmias include asystole and ventricular fibrillation.

Common causes of hyperkalemia are **renal failure** (acute or chronic) and **medications** (potassium-sparing diuretics, NSAIDs, and ACE inhibitors). Other causes include severe tissue destruction, hypoaldosteronism (watch for hyporeninemic hypoaldosteronism in diabetes), and adrenal insufficiency (patients also have low sodium levels and low blood pressure).

- **CASE SCENARIO:** A patient has a high potassium level but is asymptomatic and has a normal EKG. What is the best treatment? Oral sodium polystyrene resin.
- **CASE SCENARIO:** What should you give to a severely hyperkalemic patient with EKG changes? First, give **calcium gluconate** (cardioprotective), then **sodium bicarbonate** (alkalosis causes potassium to shift inside cells). Also consider giving IV glucose with insulin (also forces potassium inside cells). Dialysis can be used in an emergency or in patients with renal failure.

Hypocalcemia

The classic sign of hypocalcemia is **tetany,** which can be elicited by tapping on the facial nerve to elicit contraction of the facial muscles (**Chvostek sign**). Other symptoms and signs include depression, encephalopathy, dementia, laryngospasm, and convulsions. The EKG shows **QT-interval prolongation.**

> ➤ **CASE SCENARIO:** A nurse checks a patient's blood pressure and the patient's hand goes into spasm. She tries the other arm, and the same thing happens. What does the patient have? Hypocalcemia. This is a positive **Trousseau sign.**

> ➤ **CASE SCENARIO:** A neonate born with low-set ears, cleft palate, and ventricular septal defect develops irritability and facial muscle contractions when the face is touched. The child then goes into convulsions. What rare syndrome might the child have? **DiGeorge syndrome.**

> ➤ **CASE SCENARIO:** What surgery classically results in iatrogenic hypocalcemia? Thyroidectomy, when all four parathyroids are accidentally removed.

Other causes of hypocalcemia include **renal failure** (remember the kidney's role in vitamin D metabolism), vitamin D deficiency, pseudohypoparathyroidism (short fingers, short stature, mental retardation, and normal levels of parathyroid hormone with end-organ unresponsiveness to parathyroid hormone), and acute pancreatitis (hypocalcemia is one of Ranson's criteria for poor outcome).

> ➤ **CASE SCENARIO:** When a patient has a low calcium level, what other lab test do you have to check to interpret the low calcium level? An albumin level. **Hypoalbuminemia** of any etiology can cause hypocalcemia because the protein-bound fraction of calcium is decreased. In this instance, however, the patient is asymptomatic, because the ionized/unbound, biologically active fraction of calcium is unchanged.

Rickets and **osteomalacia** are the skeletal effects of vitamin D deficiency in children and adults, respectively.

Alkalosis can cause symptoms similar to hypocalcemia because of its effects on the ionized fraction of calcium. Treat by correcting the pH.

Remember that phosphorus and calcium levels are usually in opposite directions. Derangements in one can cause problems with the other. In patients with renal failure, you must try not only to raise calcium, but also to restrict phosphorus.

Hypercalcemia

Hypercalcemia is usually asymptomatic and discovered by routine lab tests. When symptoms are present, remember "**bones, stones, groans,** and **psychiatric overtones**" ("bones" = bone changes such as osteopenia and pathologic fractures; "stones" = kidney stones and polyuria; "groans" = abdominal pain, anorexia, constipation, ileus, nausea, and vomiting; and "psychiatric overtones" = depression, psychosis, delirium, confusion).

The EKG shows **QT-interval shortening.**

> ➤ **CASE SCENARIO:** Hypercalcemia is discovered on routine lab tests in an outpatient. What is the most likely cause? Hyperparathyroidism.

Other causes of hypercalcemia include **malignancy,** vitamin A or D intoxication, sarcoidosis, thiazide diuretics, familial hypocalciuric hypercalcemia (look for low urinary calcium, which is rare with hypercalcemia), and immobilization.

Hyperproteinemia of any cause can cause hypercalcemia because of an increase in the protein-bound fraction of calcium, but the patient is asymptomatic because the ionized/unbound, active fraction is unchanged.

Severe prolonged hypercalcemia can cause **nephrocalcinosis** and **renal failure** from calcium salt deposits in the kidney.

> ➤ **CASE SCENARIO:** A patient has severe hypercalcemia. What is the first step in treatment? IV normal saline. After the patient is well hydrated, you can give **furosemide.**

Other possible hypercalcemia treatments include oral phosphorus administration (IV phosphorus is rarely used because it is dangerous), calcitonin, diphosphonates (e.g., etidronate in Paget disease), plicamycin, and prednisone (for malignancy-induced hypercalcemia).

Other Electrolyte Disturbances and Fluid Administration

Hypomagnesemia often is seen in alcoholics. The signs and symptoms (including EKG changes and tetany) are similar to those of hypocalcemia. Hypomagnesemia is notorious because it **makes hypokalemia and hypocalcemia difficult to correct.** Treat with oral replacement.

Hypermagnesemia is common in patients with renal failure.

> ➤ **CASE SCENARIO:** A woman treated with magnesium sulfate for severe pre-eclampsia develops low blood pressure and trouble with breathing. Deep tendon reflexes are markedly decreased bilaterally. What should you do first? Stop the magnesium, because the patient has developed hypermagnesemia.

Hypophosphatemia is seen primarily in patients with diabetic ketoacidosis and alcoholics. Signs and symptoms include neuromuscular disturbances (encephalopathy, weakness), rhabdomyolysis, and anemia.

Hyperphosphatemia usually is seen in patients with renal failure. Treat with phosphate restriction, dialysis, and phosphate-binding resins (calcium carbonate).

> ➤ **CASE SCENARIO:** In a hypotensive trauma patient, what is the IV fluid of choice? Ringer's lactate. The second choice is normal saline.

In **hypovolemic** patients, normal saline or Ringer's lactate is often the best choice for IV fluid, regardless of other electrolyte problems.

> ➤ **CASE SCENARIO:** What is the best choice of maintenance fluid in patients who are not allowed to eat? D5 $^{1}/_{2}$ normal saline (NS). In younger pediatric patients, use D5 $^{1}/_{4}$ NS or D5 $^{1}/_{3}$ NS because of renal differences. Do not forget to monitor potassium levels (and replace as needed) if the patient is not going to be eating.

Shock

Look for the classic history of hypotension, oliguria/anuria, and, usually, tachycardia. To keep things simple (and pragmatic), remember four basic clinical types of shock:

1. Hypovolemic
2. Cardiogenic
3. Septic
4. Neurogenic

In most cases, the first step in management should be to give an IV fluid bolus (using normal saline), unless the patient is clearly in congestive heart failure (i.e. bilateral pulmonary rales, peripheral edema, etc.). If the patient does not respond to a fluid bolus and you are given the choice, use invasive hemodynamic monitoring (Swan-Ganz catheter) to help make diagnostic and therapeutic decisions.

TYPE OF SHOCK	CO	PCWP	SVR	SVO_2
Septic (early)	High	Low	Low	High
Hypovolemic	Low	Low	High	Low (also the parameters for late septic shock)
Cardiogenic	Low	High	High	Low
Neurogenic	Low	Low	Low	Low

CO = cardiac output, PCWP = pulmonary capillary wedge pressure, SVR = systemic vascular resistance, SvO_2 = systemic venous oxygen saturation.

Classic findings help to determine the cause of shock:

1. **Neurogenic shock:** history of severe central nervous system trauma or hemorrhage; flushed skin; heart rate may be normal or bradycardic.
2. **Septic shock:** fever, high white blood cell count, flushed skin warm to the touch, and extremes of age. Use broad-spectrum antibiotics after "pan-culturing" the patient (blood, sputum, and urine cultures plus others if history dictates).
3. **Cardiogenic shock:** history of myocardial infarction, chest pain, heart failure, or several risk factors for coronary artery disease. Patients have cold, clammy skin and look pale, with **distended neck veins** and **pulmonary congestion** (on exam and x-ray).
4. **Hypovolemic shock:** history of fluid loss (blood, diarrhea, vomiting, sweating, diuretics, inability to drink water). Patients have cold, clammy skin and look pale. Remember that fluid loss can be internal, as in patients with a ruptured aortic aneurysm or spleen, patients with pancreatitis, or after surgery. **Orthostatic hypotension, tachycardia, sunken eyes,** or **tenting of skin** may be seen (also **sunken fontanelle** in children). tenting of skin = dehydration
5. **Anaphylaxis:** look for **bee stings, peanuts, shellfish, penicillins, sulfa drugs,** or other medications. Treat with **epinephrine** and fluids, administer oxygen, and intubate if necessary. Do a tracheostomy or cricothyroidotomy if laryngeal edema prevents intubation. Antihistamines are of help only when the reaction is mild or cutaneous (worthless for shock or airway compromise). Corticosteroids are not first-line drugs in the treatment of anaphylaxis. Monitor all patients for at least 6 hours after an initial reaction.
6. **Pulmonary embolus:** look for risk factors for deep venous thrombosis (**Virchow triad** = endothelial damage, stasis, hypercoagulable state); history of recent childbirth (amniotic fluid embolus); fractures (fat emboli); positive **Homan sign** with painful, swollen leg; and postoperative status (especially after orthopedic or pelvic surgery). Patients classically have **chest pain, tachypnea,** and **shortness of breath.** Order a ventilation/perfusion nuclear scan or CT angiogram. Give heparin to prevent further clotting and emboli.
7. **Pericardial tamponade:** history of stab wound in the left chest and **distended neck veins.** Perform pericardiocentesis emergently. **Tension pneumothorax** is also classically seen in the traumatic setting and causes **hypertympany to percussion** and **absent breath sounds** on the affected side. Perform needle thoracentesis emergently.
8. **Toxic shock syndrome:** the classic patient is a woman of reproductive age who leaves tampons in place for too long. Look for skin desquamation. The cause is *Staphylococcus aureus* toxin.

The ABCs come first. Patients often need heroic measures to survive. Intubate at the drop of a hat, do not let patients eat, and avoid narcotics if possible. Mental status changes are often an important clue to impending doom. Monitor EKG, vital signs, Swan-Ganz parameters, urine output, arterial blood gases, complete blood counts, and, in some cases, lactate levels.

➤ *CASE SCENARIO:* A 30-year-old patient is brought in after a car wreck and is hypotensive. How much IV fluid should you give? Start with 1 liter of Ringer's lactate or normal saline (10–20 cc/kg). After the bolus, reassess the patient (i.e., check vital signs) to determine whether the bolus helped. Do not be afraid to repeat the bolus if the first bolus produces no improvement—but, of course, watch for fluid overload, which may cause heart failure.

IV medications in hypotensive shock

1. **Dobutamine:** $beta_1$ agonist used to increase cardiac output by increasing contractility (ICU equivalent of digoxin).
2. **Dopamine:** at low doses, hits dopamine receptors in renal vasculature and keeps kidney perfused; at higher doses, has $beta_1$ agonist effects to increase contractility. At highest doses, dopamine has $alpha_1$ agonist effects and causes vasoconstriction. Although some authorities debate this differential effect, it still comes up on exams.
3. **Norepinephrine:** used for its $alpha_1$ agonist effects; given to patients with hypotension to increase peripheral resistance so that perfusion to vital organs can be maintained.
4. **Phenylephrine:** also used for its $alpha_1$ agonist effects.
5. **Epinephrine:** used for ***cardiac arrest*** and ***anaphylaxis.***
6. **Milrinone/amrinone:** phosphodiesterase inhibitors used in refractory heart failure (*not* first-line agents) because they have a positive inotropic effect; may cause tachyarrhythmias.

CARDIOLOGY

Chest Pain and Myocardial Infarct

With **acute chest pain,** the main question is whether the pain is related to the heart. Always order a *chest x-ray, EKG, and cardiac enzymes* at a minimum.

Use **pretest probability** to help you through the process. A 30-year-old patient with no risk factors for atherosclerosis who develops chest pain after eating a spicy meal does not have ischemic cardiac pain. A 65-year-old heavy smoker with high cholesterol, hypertension, diabetes, and a strong family history of heart attacks has cardiac pain until you prove otherwise.

Look for key clues to suggest a ***myocardial infarction* (MI):**

1. **EKG:** after an MI, you should see flipped or flattened T waves, ST-segment elevation, and/or Q waves in a *segmental* distribution (e.g., leads II, III, and aVF for an inferior infarct).
2. **Pain characteristics:** pain usually is described as crushing, poorly localized substernal pain that may ***radiate to the shoulder, arm,*** or ***jaw;*** it is not reproducible on palpation. Pain usually does not resolve with nitroglycerin (as it often does with angina) and usually lasts at least 15–30 minutes.
3. **Lab tests:** assays for myocardial-associated ***creatine kinase* (CK-MB)** or ***troponin* I/P** usually are performed every 8 hours times 3 before MI is ruled out. Lactate dehydrogenase (LDH)elevation and flip ($LDH_1 > LDH_2$) are now rarely used for late presentation (> 24 hours), since troponins stay elevated for days. Chest x-ray may show cardiomegaly, pulmonary congestion, and/or congestive heart failure; echocardiography may show ventricular wall motion abnormalities.
4. **Physical exam:** bilateral pulmonary rales in the absence of other pneumonia-like symptoms, distended neck veins, S3 or S4, new murmurs, hypotension, and/or shock should make you think along the lines of an MI. Patients are classically ***diaphoretic, tachycardic*** (unless the conduction system has been damaged), and ***pale;*** nausea and vomiting may be present.

5. **History:** patients with MI often have a history of angina or previous chest pain, murmurs, arrhythmias, and/or risk factors for coronary artery disease. They also may be taking heart medications (digoxin, furosemide, hypertension or cholesterol medications).

Treatment for probable MI

1. EKG monitoring: if ventricular tachycardia occurs (see figure), give **amiodarone** or **lidocaine.** Do not use lidocaine prophylactically.

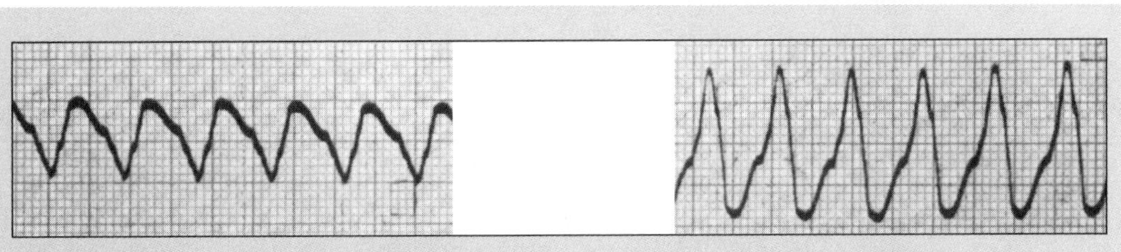

Two examples of ventricular tachycardia, which can have a range of appearances. The QRS complexes are broad, and the heart rate is often in the range of 150–200 beats/minute. (From Forbes CD, Jackson WF: Cardiovascular disorders. In Forbes CD, Jackson WF (eds): Color Atlas and Text of Clinical Medicine. St. Louis, Mosby, 1993, pp 209–264, with permission.)

2. Give oxygen to maintain oxygen saturation > 90%.
3. **Nitroglycerin**
4. **Beta blocker** (give indefinitely in the absence of contraindications; proven to reduce incidence of second MI)
5. **Aspirin**
6. Control pain with **morphine** (which may help with pulmonary edema if present).
7. Thrombolysis or angioplasty should be considered if the patient presents early; consider a cardiology consultation.
8. Consider **ACE inhibitor** and **HMG-CoA reductase inhibitor** acutely (becoming standard treatments).

   Note: Begin anticoagulation with IV heparin if the patient has cardiac thrombus, large area of dyskinetic ventricle, or severe heart failure.

   Note: Remember that patients can re-infarct on the same hospital visit even with good medical management.

Other causes of chest pain and clues to diagnosis:

1. **Reflux or peptic ulcer disease:** related to certain foods (spicy, chocolate), **smoking, caffeine,** or lying down flat; relieved by antacids or acid-reducing medications. Patients with ulcers test positive for **Helicobacter pylori.**
2. **Stable angina:** pain begins with exertion or stress and remits with rest or calming down; pain is relieved by nitroglycerin. The EKG shows **ST-segment depression** with the pain, then reverts to normal when the pain stops. Pain lasts < 20 minutes.
3. **Chest wall pain** (costochondritis, bruised or broken ribs): pain reproducible on palpation and localized.
4. **Esophageal problems** (achalasia, nutcracker esophagus, or esophageal spasm): difficult differential. The question probably will give you a negative work-up for MI; look for barium swallow with **bird's beak tapering** distally (achalasia) or esophageal manometry abnormalities. Treat achalasia with

pneumatic dilatation or botulinum toxin injection; treat nutcracker/esophageal spasm with calcium channel blockers. Surgical myotomy can be used if other treatments are ineffective.

5. **Pericarditis:** look for viral upper respiratory infection prodrome. The EKG shows **diffuse ST-segment elevation.** Other clues include elevated sedimentation rate and low-grade fever. The most common cause is viral (Coxsackievirus); others include uremia, tuberculosis, malignancy, and lupus or other autoimmune diseases.
6. **Pneumonia:** chest pain is due to pleuritis. Patients also have cough, fever, and/or sputum production. Look for possible sick contacts.
7. **Aortic dissection:** don't forget the "other" cardiovascular emergency! Watch for severe pain **radiating to the back, hypertension,** and widened mediastinum on chest x-ray. Get a CT scan with intravenous contrast (or conventional angiography). If the ascending aorta or proximal arch is involved in the dissection, prompt surgery is indicated (Stanford type A dissection).

Unstable angina often presents with normal cardiac enzymes and EKG changes (ST depression) with prolonged chest pain that does not respond to nitroglycerin initially (like MI). Pain often begins at rest. Treat like an MI, but use IV heparin to anticoagulate and consider an emergent cardiology consultation for angioplasty if the pain fails to resolve. Patients usually have a history of stable angina and cardiac risk factors. By strict definition, unstable angina is defined as a change from previous stable angina. Thus, if a patient used to experience angina once per week and now experiences it once a day, he or she has unstable angina.

Variant (Prinzmetal) angina is rare and associated with anginal pain at rest with **ST elevation** (cardiac enzymes, however, are normal). The cause is coronary artery spasm. Variant angina responds to nitroglycerin and usually is treated over the long term with **calcium channel blockers.**

Twenty-five percent of MIs are "silent." They present without chest pain (especially in **diabetics,** who have neuropathy). Patients present with heart failure, shock, or confusion and delirium (especially elderly patients).

Valvular Heart Disease

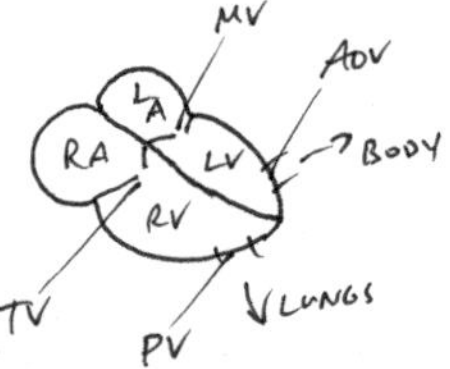

Murmur characteristics:

VALVE PROBLEM	PHYSICAL CHARACTERISTICS (BEST HEARD HERE)	OTHER FINDINGS
Mitral stenosis	Late diastolic blowing murmur (at apex)	Opening snap, loud S1, atrial fibrillation, LAE, PHT
Mitral regurgitation	Holosystolic murmur (radiates to axilla)	Soft S1, LAE, PH, LVH
Aortic stenosis	Harsh systolic ejection murmur (aortic area, radiates to carotids)	Slow pulse upstroke, S3/S4, ejection click, LVH, cardiomegaly; syncope, angina, CHF
Aortic regurgitation	Early diastolic descrescendo murmur (apex)	Widened pulse pressure, LVH, LV dilatation, S3
Mitral prolapse	Mid-systolic click/late systolic murmur	Panic disorder

LAE = left atrial enlargement, PH = pulmonary hypertension, LVH = left ventricular hypertrophy, CHF = congestive heart failure.

Endocarditis prophylaxis: use for people with known valvular heart disease or prosthetic valves. For patients with mitral valve prolapse, use prophylaxis only if a murmur is heard on physical exam or the patient has a previous history of endocarditis.

1. **For oral surgery,** use amoxicillin before the procedure; use clindamycin or azithromycin if the patient is allergic to penicillin.

2. **For gastroinestinal/genitourinary procedures,** use ampicillin plus gentamicin before and amoxicillin after the procedure; use vancomycin if the patient is allergic to penicillin.

Deep Venous Thrombosis, Pulmonary Embolus, and Anticoagulation

Virchow triad (***endothelial damage, stasis,*** and ***hypercoagulable state***) is a clue to the presence of deep venous thrombosis (DVT).

Common causes or situations in which DVT occurs: surgery (especially orthopedic, pelvic, or abdominal), neoplasms, trauma, immobilization, pregnancy, birth control pills, lupus anticoagulant/antiphospholipid syndrome, factor V Leyden, thrombin variant, and/or deficiency of antithrombin III, protein C, or protein S.

The **classic symptoms** are unilateral leg swelling, pain and tenderness, and/or ***Homan sign*** (present in 30% of patients and unreliable, but classic).

The **best way to diagnose DVT** is ***Doppler ultrasound*** or impedance plethysmography. The gold standard test is venography, but this invasive test usually is reserved for situations in which the diagnosis is not clear. A ***negative D-dimer*** test helps exclude DVT with a fairly high degree of accuracy, but a positive D-dimer test is less specific (does not necessarily indicate thrombosis).

Superficial thrombophlebitis (erythema, tenderness, edema and palpable clot in a superficial vein) is *not* a risk factor for pulmonary embolism and is generally considered a benign condition. Treat with NSAIDs or aspirin.

If a patient has DVT, **systemic anticoagulation** is necessary. Use some form of heparin, followed by gradual crossover to oral warfarin. Patients are maintained on warfarin for at least 3–6 months and possibly permanently if they have more than one episode.

The **best DVT prophylaxis** for surgery is pneumatic compression boots and early ambulation postoperatively. Use low-dose heparin if ambulation is not possible. Warfarin is an alternative choice, especially for orthopedic hip and knee surgery.

Pulmonary embolus (PE) follows DVT, delivery (amniotic fluid embolus), or fractures (fat emboli). Symptoms include ***tachypnea, dyspnea, chest pain, hemoptysis*** (with lung infarct), and hypotension, syncope, or death in severe cases. Rarely, on a chest x-ray you may see a wedge-shaped defect due to a pulmonary infarct.

Left-sided heart clots (from atrial fibrillation, ventricular wall aneurysm, severe CHF, or endocarditis) that embolize cause arterial-sided infarcts (stroke; renal, GI, or extremity infarcts), *not* PEs. **Right-sided clots** that embolize (DVTs) cause PEs, *not* arterial infarcts.

> ➤ ***CASE SCENARIO:*** A 58-year-old woman with atrial fibrillation, taking no medications, presents with a *cold*, swollen, painful right leg. What probably happened? An intracardiac thrombus embolized to the leg.

Use a **ventilation-perfusion nuclear scan** or CT angiogram to screen for PE. If the scan is positive, PE is diagnosed and treated. If the screening test is indeterminate, order a conventional pulmonary angiogram (the gold standard, but invasive) if clinical suspicion remains significant. If scan is negative or indicates a low probability of PE, it is unlikely that patient has a significant PE.

Treat PE with IV heparin or low-molecular weight heparin to prevent further clots and emboli, then gradually switch to oral warfarin, which patient should take for at least 3–6 months.

> ➤ ***CASE SCENARIO:*** A woman has DVT with PE. She is put on heparin/warfarin and 1 month later develops a second DVT and PE. What should you do? Place an inferior vena cava filter (e.g., Greenfield filter) to prevent further PE.

➤ ***CASE SCENARIO:*** Four days after a patient is put on heparin, his platelet count is very low. What should you do? Stop the heparin, which can cause thrombocytopenia and even arterial thrombosis in some patients.

Heparin is followed by determination of the **partial thromboplastin time** (**PTT;** internal pathway) and **warfarin** by determination of the **prothrombin time** (**PT;** external pathway), whereas **aspirin** affects the **bleeding time.** In emergencies, reverse heparin with protamine, reverse warfarin with fresh frozen plasma and/or vitamin K, and reverse aspirin with platelet transfusion.

➤ ***CASE SCENARIO:*** In a patient receiving enoxaparin, how often should you check the PTT? You shouldn't. Low-molecular-weight heparin does not affect the PT, PTT, or bleeding time. Its effects are not monitored with lab values; in fact, one of the reasons for its popularity is that no monitoring is required. In the rare cases when monitoring is needed, an **anti-factor Xa** assay can be used to measure the effects.

Other conditions affecting coagulation tests:

DISEASE	PROLONGS THIS TEST	OTHER AIDS TO DIAGNOSIS
Hemophilia A	PTT	Low levels of factor 8; normal PT and bleeding time; X-linked
Hemophilia B	PTT	Low levels of factor 9; normal PT and bleeding time; X-linked
VFW deficiency	Bleeding time and PTT	Normal levels of factor 8; normal PT; autosomal dominant
Disseminated intravascular coagulation	PT, PTT, bleeding time	Positive d-dimer or FDPs; postpartum, infection, malignancy; schistocytes/fragmented cells on peripheral smear
Liver disease	PT	PTT normal or prolonged; all factors but 8 are low; stigmata of liver disease; no correction with vitamin K
Vitamin K deficiency	PT, PTT (slight)	Normal bleeding time; low levels of factors 2, 7, 9, and 10, proteins C and S; look for neonate (who did not receive prophylactic vitamin K), malabsorption, alcoholism, or prolonged use of antibiotics (which kill vitamin K-producing bowel flora)

VWF = von Willebrand factor, PTT = partial thromboplastin time, PT = prothrombin time, FDPs = fibrin degradation products.

Note: Uremia causes a qualitative platelet defect, and vitamin C deficiency or chronic corticosteroid therapy can cause a petechial-type bleeding tendency with normal coagulation tests.

Congestive Heart Failure

Health maintenance: most cases of congestive heart failure (CHF) are due to atherosclerosis and its effects on the adult heart. Aggressive management of risk factors for atherosclerosis is the key to prevention.

➤ ***CASE SCENARIO:*** In a 54-year-old man with sudden-onset signs and symptoms of CHF, what condition should you rule out first? A myocardial infarct.

Symptoms and signs of CHF:

LEFT-SIDED FAILURE	RIGHT-SIDED FAILURE
Fatigue, dyspnea, cardiomegaly	Fatigue, dyspnea, cardiomegaly
Left-sided S3/S4	Right-sided S3/S4
Orthopnea	Peripheral edema
Paroxysmal nocturnal dyspnea	Jugular venous distention
Pulmonary congestion/rales	Hepatomegaly/ascites

New patient management issues

1. First make sure that the patient is stable (ABCs).
2. Check EKG and cardiac enzymes to rule out myocardial infarct.
3. Check chest x-ray to look for pulmonary edema, cardiomegaly, or chronic obstructive pulmonary disease (which may cause right-sided failure/cor pulmonale).
4. Check complete blood count to rule out anemia.
5. Check levels of thyroid-stimulating hormone (TSH) to rule out hyperthyroidism (the patient's history should give away this cause of CHF).
6. Echocardiography is used to estimate ejection fraction, check for valvular dysfunction, and rule out pericardial effusion or tamponade.

Treat new patients with sodium restriction and an ***ACE inhibitor*** (first-line agent proven to reduce mortality in CHF); add a ***beta blocker*** once the patient is stable. Diuretics, usually ***furosemide,*** may help to reduce symptoms but have no effect on mortality rates.

- Digoxin and vasodilators (arterial and venous) are second-line agents.
- IV sympathomimetics (dobutamine, dopamine, amrinone) plus furosemide and oxygen can be used for inpatients with severe CHF.

> ➤ ***CASE SCENARIO:*** A 25-year-old man has an upper respiratory infection. Ten days later he develops chest pain and then CHF. What condition does he probably have? Myocarditis, usually from a virus (e.g., coxsackievirus). Treatment is supportive with NSAIDs for pain.

Cor pulmonale: right ventricular enlargement, hypertrophy, or failure due to primary lung disease. Watch for tachypnea, ***cyanosis, clubbing, parasternal heave,*** loud P2, and right-sided S4 in addition to signs and symptoms of pulmonary disease. The most common cause is chronic obstructive pulmonary disease. Chronic sleep apnea also can cause cor pulmonale.

> ➤ ***CASE SCENARIO:*** What condition should you worry about if signs and symptoms of right-sided heart failure develop suddenly in a younger patient without cardiac history or risk factors? Pulmonary embolus. Cardiac tamponade would be another consideration.

> ➤ ***CASE SCENARIO:*** A 28-year-old woman with gradually worsening dyspnea over a few months develops peripheral edema, clubbing, hypoxia, and a right-sided S4. Pulmonary embolus tests are negative, and she takes no medications and has no risk factors for heart disease. What condition does she probably have? Primary pulmonary hypertension. Consider treatment with calcium channel blockers while awaiting heart-lung transplantation.

Dilated cardiomyopathy: classically due to ***alcohol, myocarditis,*** or ***doxorubicin,*** since by definition ischemia is not considered a cardiomyopathy (although coronary artery disease/ischemia is the most common cause of a dilated, poorly functioning heart). Heart is enlarged, with thin, "flabby" walls. Manage like regular CHF.

Arrhythmias

Atrial fibrillation and flutter

- With atrial fibrillation, consider hyperthyroidism (check TSH) as the cause. Alcohol is another classic cause; tell the patient to stop drinking.
- If the patient is asymptomatic acutely, no specific treatment is needed. Consider anticoagulation for chronic cases.
- If the patient is symptomatic but stable, slow the ventricular rate with medication, such as verapamil, diltiazem, beta blocker, or digoxin.

- If the patient is symptomatic and unstable (i.e., decreased blood pressure, chest pain, hypoxia), use DC cardioversion.

Be able to recognize the following EKG abnormalities and know their treatments. Always check for ischemia and electrolyte disturbances as the cause.

ARRHYTHMIA	TREATMENT AND WARNINGS
Heart block	
First degree (see figure)	No treatment, but avoid beta blockers and central calcium channel blockers (both slow conduction). 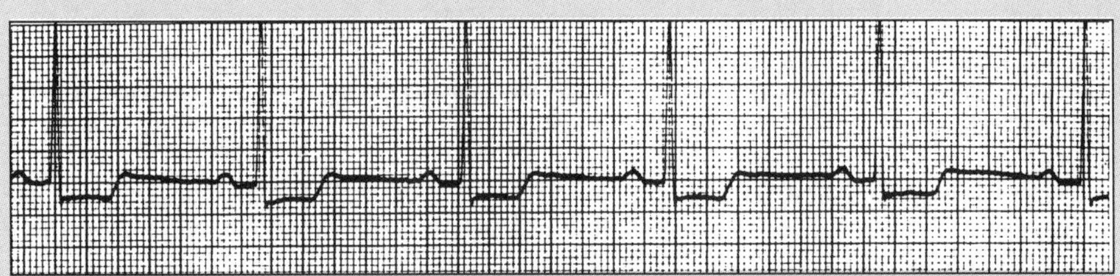 First-degree block (PR interval = 0.26 seconds). (From Seelig CB: Simplified EKG Analysis. Philadelphia, Hanley & Belfus, 1992, with permission.)
Second degree	Pacemaker or atropine only if symptomatic in Mobitz type I (see figure). 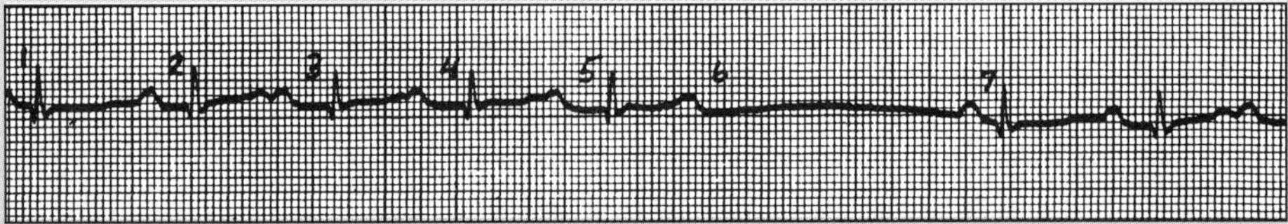 Mobitz type I second-degree AV block (Wenckebach). Note the gradual prolongation of the PR interval (1–5), the missing QRS complex after the sixth P wave, and the return of the PR interval to its shortest duration (7). (From Seelig CB: Simplified EKG Analysis. Philadelphia, Hanley & Belfus, 1992, with permission.)
	Use pacemaker for all Mobitz type II (see figure). 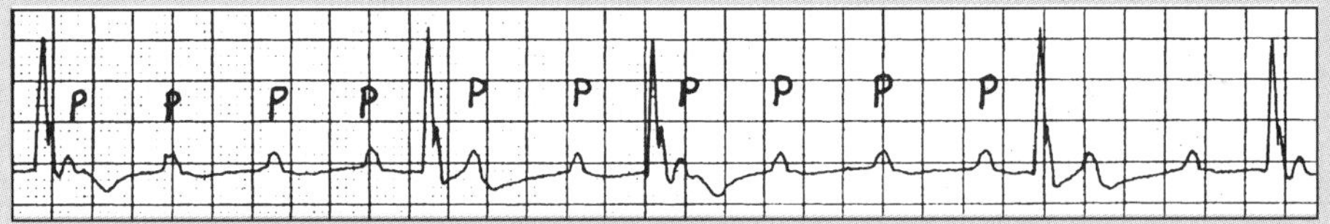 Mobitz type II second-degree AV block. Note that when beats are conducted, the PR interval is unvarying. (From Seelig CB: Simplified EKG Analysis. Philadelphia, Hanley & Belfus, 1992, with permission.)
Third degree (see figure)	Pacemaker 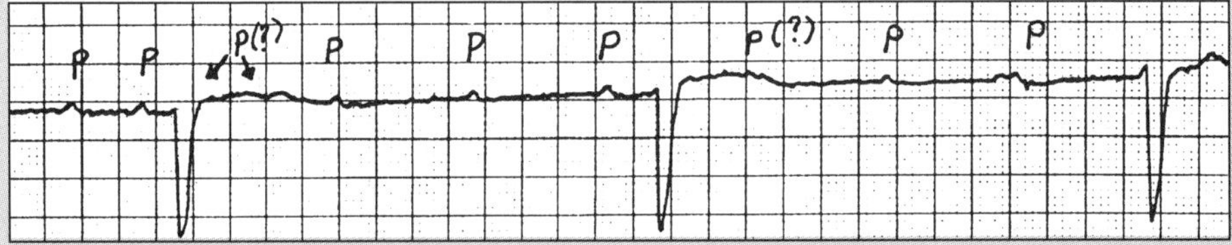 Third-degree AV block with a ventricular escape rhythm at 32 bpm. P-wave activity is somewhat irregular. (From Seelig CB: Simplified EKG Analysis. Philadelphia, Hanley & Belfus, 1992, with permission.)

(*Table continued on next page.*)

ARRHYTHMIA	TREATMENT AND WARNINGS
WPW syndrome	Use procainamide or quinidine; avoid digoxin and verapamil.
VTach (see figure)	Amiodarone or lidocaine 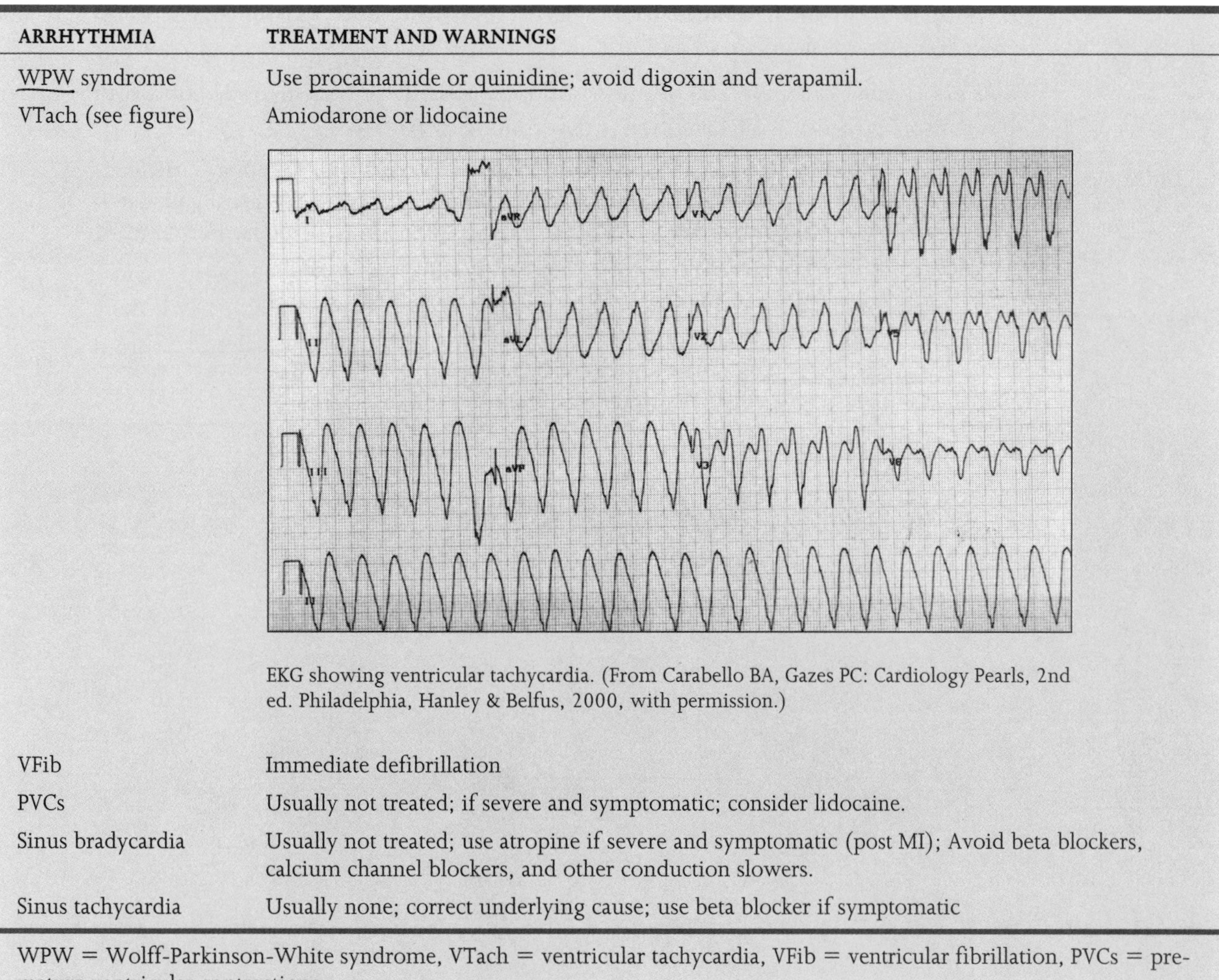 EKG showing ventricular tachycardia. (From Carabello BA, Gazes PC: Cardiology Pearls, 2nd ed. Philadelphia, Hanley & Belfus, 2000, with permission.)
VFib	Immediate defibrillation
PVCs	Usually not treated; if severe and symptomatic; consider lidocaine.
Sinus bradycardia	Usually not treated; use atropine if severe and symptomatic (post MI); Avoid beta blockers, calcium channel blockers, and other conduction slowers.
Sinus tachycardia	Usually none; correct underlying cause; use beta blocker if symptomatic

WPW = Wolff-Parkinson-White syndrome, VTach = ventricular tachycardia, VFib = ventricular fibrillation, PVCs = premature ventricular contractions

Note: Sinus tachycardia and atrial fibrillation are common presentations for hyperthyroidism. Check TSH.

ENDOCRINOLOGY

Hypothyroidism

Classic symptoms: fatigue, bradycardia, depression, menstrual disturbances (usually menorrhagia), slow speech, cold intolerance, constipation, carpal tunnel syndrome, decreased reflexes, anemia of chronic disease, and/or coarse hair. Hypothyroidism may cause hypercholesterolemia, which resolves with treatment. Check thyroid function labs (TSH, free thyroxine [T_4]). Usually TSH is *high* and T_4 is *low* (i.e. primary gland disturbance). Treat with ***thyroxine*** **(T_4)**.

Causes of hypothyroidism

1. **Hashimoto thyroiditis:** most common cause; autoimmune disease. Remember association with other autoimmune diseases (e.g., pernicious anemia, vitiligo, lupus). Look for positive ***antimicrosomal antibodies.*** Histology shows lymphocyte infiltration of the gland.
2. **Subacute thyroiditis:** acute viral inflammation with fever and enlarged, ***tender*** thyroid gland. A history of upper respiratory infection is common. Give NSAIDs for symptom relief. Patients often recover without treatment.

3. **Hypothyroidism due to treatment of hyperthyroidism** (iodine-131 for Graves disease): second most common cause of hypothyroidism in the United States.

4. **Sick euthyroid syndrome:** can be caused by any illness. Treatment is needed only for the underlying disorder, because the condition is self-limiting.

   ➤ ***CASE SCENARIO:*** A 52-year-old man is hospitalized for 2 weeks with pneumonia. He feels tired 2 days after leaving the hospital. Triiodothyronine (T_3) and T_4 levels are slightly low. What lab value will confirm sick euthyroid syndrome? TSH, which should be near-normal.

   ➤ ***CASE SCENARIO:*** A 29-year-old woman has a goiter. Is she hyper- or hypothyroid? You cannot know until you have a more detailed history and check the lab tests. She may be hypo-, hyper- or euthyroid. A goiter simply means the thyroid gland is enlarged and can be due to many different conditions (see x-ray figure). Significant thyroid enlargement can cause dysphagia or respiratory symptoms due to local mass effect.

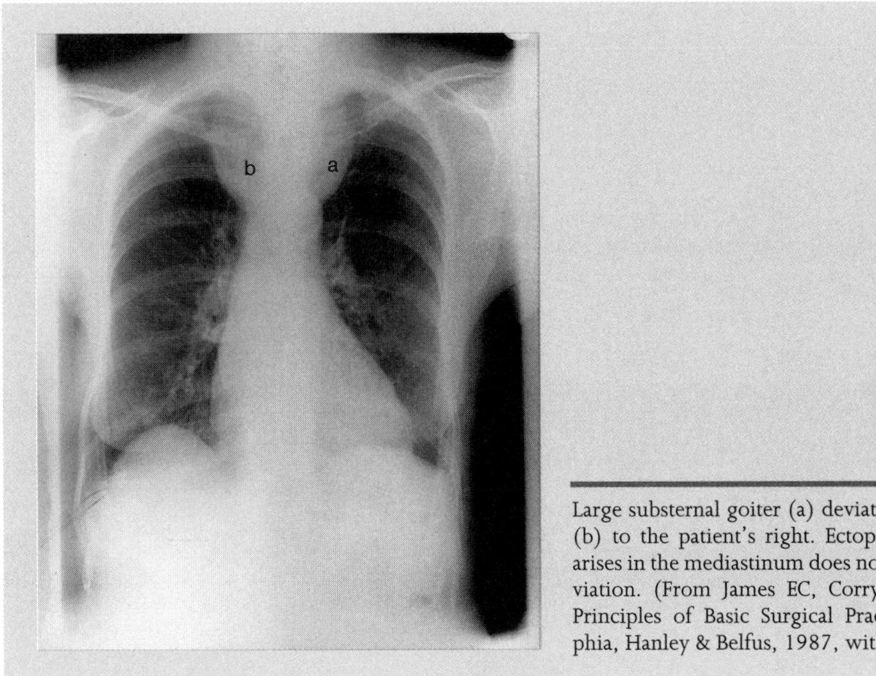

Large substernal goiter (a) deviating the trachea (b) to the patient's right. Ectopic thyroid that arises in the mediastinum does not cause this deviation. (From James EC, Corry RJ, Perry JF: Principles of Basic Surgical Practice. Philadelphia, Hanley & Belfus, 1987, with permission.)

Hyperthyroidism

Classic symptoms: nervousness, anxiety, insomnia, tachycardia, palpitations, **atrial fibrillation,** heat intolerance, weight loss, diarrhea, menstrual irregularities (hypomenorrhea), increased appetite, and "thyroid stare." Usually TSH is *low* and T_4 is *high* (i.e. primary gland disturbance).

Causes of hyperthyroidism

1. **Graves disease:** by far the most common cause. ***Exophthalmos*** and ***pretibial myxedema*** are specific for Graves disease. Patients have positive ***thyroid-stimulating immunoglobulins*** and ***antibodies,*** which activate the TSH receptor. They also have a non-tender, diffuse goiter. The whole gland takes up excessive radioactive iodine (RAI) on a thyroid nuclear scan.

2. **Plummer disease/toxic multinodular goiter:** hyperfunctioning nodules cause a lumpy goiter without positive antibodies or exophthalmos/pretibial myxedema. RAI uptake is high in nodules but decreased in the rest of the gland.

3. **Toxic adenoma:** one nodule is palpable and has high RAI uptake; the rest of the gland has decreased uptake (thyroid cancer is almost never hyperfunctional).
4. **Thyroiditis:** Hashimoto or subacute thyroiditis may have a transient hyperthyroidism from inflammation before converting to hypothyroidism.

Treatment of hyperthyroidism: you can start with antithyroid drugs (**propylthiouracil** or **methimazole**), but these don't fix the underlying problem. Most patients eventually require further therapy; radioactive iodine is usually the treatment of choice. Surgery is considered for young patients and pregnant women (i.e. avoid radiation to fetus) but is not used very often. Propranolol (or another beta blocker) is used for **thyroid storm** (when patients decompensate, physically and mentally, from very high thyroid hormone levels) and symptomatic tachycardia, palpitations, or arrhythmias.

> ➤ ***CASE SCENARIO:*** A 29-year-old woman feels anxious about her pregnancy. Total T_4 is high, but other thyroid tests are normal. What type of hyperthyroidism does she probably have? None. Pregnancy and other factors (birth control pills, estrogens, infections) can cause elevation of thyroid-binding globulin, which causes elevation of total thyroid hormone levels. However, free (active) thyroid levels are not elevated, and the TSH is normal. No treatment needed!

Hypoadrenalism

Primary hypoadrenalism (also known as ***Addison disease*** or primary adrenal insufficiency) is usually idiopathic (probably of autoimmune origin). Look for ***increased skin pigmentation,*** weight loss, dehydration, anorexia, nausea and vomiting, dizziness and syncope, hyponatremia, and hyperkalemia. Under metabolic stress (e.g., infection, surgery), patients may have an adrenal crisis characterized by abdominal pain, hypotension or cardiovascular collapse, renal shutdown, and death. Give hydrocortisone and IV fluids to avoid this complication.

- The diagnosis of hypoadrenalism can be made by administering adrenocorticotropic hormone (ACTH) and determining whether there is an appropriate increase in plasma cortisol over baseline. *Do not delay* giving steroids to do this test if the patient is crashing—he or she may die while you are waiting for the results.

Secondary adrenal insufficiency is more common (and more commonly tested). It is due most often to previous administration of steroids. Once patients take steroids for more than a few weeks, they may not be able to mount an appropriate increase in ACTH for ***up to 1 year***! The classic example is a surgery patient with a history of severe asthma (implied use of steroids) who develops hypotension and electrolyte disturbances after surgery. Give corticosteroids. Other secondary causes of adrenal insufficiency are ***Sheehan syndrome*** (i.e. pituitary infarction; history of postpartum hypotension, inability to breast-feed, and other endocrine insufficiencies typically present) and neoplasms (e.g., pituitary tumor).

- In secondary hypoadrenalism, mineralocorticoid (aldosterone) secretion is not affected, because it is not directly under pituitary control. Thus, electrolyte disturbances are not as severe.

> ➤ ***CASE SCENARIO:*** What physical finding may help to differentiate between primary and secondary hypoadrenalism? Skin hyperpigmentation, which is seen only in primary cases. This symptom is thought to be due to excessive melanocyte-stimulating hormone, which is secreted with ACTH. In secondary cases, ACTH is decreased.

Hyperadrenalism

Hyperadrenalism (**Cushing syndrome**) usually is due to administration of steroids (see figure). Look for moon facies, truncal obesity, "buffalo hump," striae, poor wound healing, hypertension, osteoporosis,

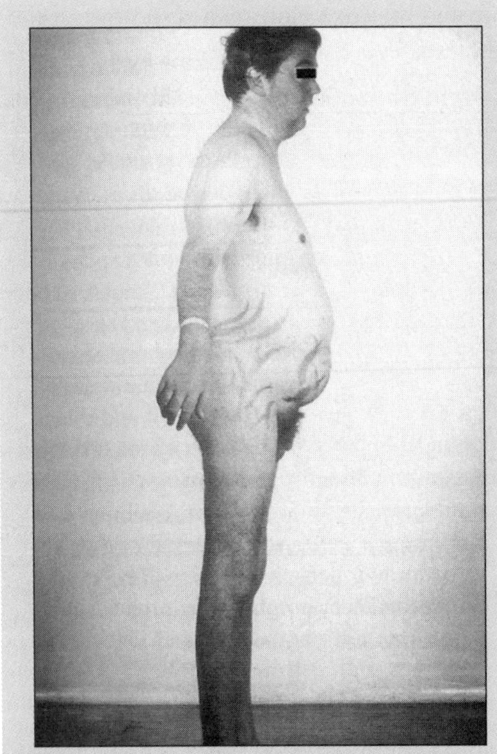

Cushing syndrome. Note the red face and obese torso with prominent striae. (From du Vivier A: The skin and systemic disease. In du Vivier A (ed): Atlas of Clinical Dermatology, 3rd ed. New York, Churchill Livingstone, 2002, pp 509–561, with permission.)

secondary diabetes or glucose intolerance, proximal muscle weakness, menstrual abnormalities, and psychiatric disturbances (depression, psychosis). **Cushing disease** is Cushing syndrome caused by pituitary overproduction of ACTH (i.e., pituitary adenoma). Order an MRI of the brain if the patient has no history of taking steroids and reports headaches or visual disturbances. Other causes include an adrenal neoplasm that secretes steroids and small cell cancer of the lung, which may produce ACTH.

➤ ***CASE SCENARIO:*** A patient presents with fatigue, moon facies, and abdominal striae. What screening test should you order for hyperadrenalism? A 24-hour urine collection for assessment of free cortisol. Plasma cortisol level is not a good test because of wide inter- and intrapatient fluctuation. The second choice is a dexamethasone suppression test.

Watch for side effects of steroids in patients on long-term therapy. Classic questions ask about **secondary diabetes,** hypertension, **osteoporosis,** psychiatric disturbances, and **proximal muscle weakness.**

Miscellaneous Topics

Primary vs. secondary endocrine disorders: remember basic physiology!

- In **primary endocrine disorders,** the gland itself is the problem, and the pituitary gland and hypothalamus react normally. For example, TSH is low in Graves disease because the gland is overproducing thyroid hormone. The appropriate response is for the pituitary to secrete less TSH because of feedback inhibition.
- In **secondary endocrine disturbances,** the gland is normal, but the pituitary or hypothalamus is malfunctioning. For example, if the pituitary secretes low levels of TSH or the hypothalamus secretes low levels of TRH, hypothyroidism occurs even though the thyroid gland is normal.

  ➤ ***CASE SCENARIO:*** What gland is the problem?

  1. Low TRH, high TSH, high free T_4? Pituitary gland (probable adenoma).
  2. Low corticotropin-releasing hormone, low ACTH, high free cortisol? Adrenal gland (or iatrogenic).
  3. Low gonadotropin-releasing hormone, low follicle-stimulating hormone and luteinizing hormone, low testosterone? Hypothalamus.

Primary hyperaldosteronism is known as **Conn syndrome** and is due to an adrenal adenoma. Look for hypertension, hypernatremia, hypokalemia, and **low renin** levels. Order a CT scan of the abdomen. **Secondary hyperaldosteronism** is much more common and is often related to renovascular hypertension (i.e. renal artery stenosis) and edematous disorders (e.g., heart failure, cirrhosis, nephrotic syndrome). Look for the underlying cause and **high renin** levels. Treat the underlying cause.

1° hyperaldosteronism = Conn Syn

Pheochromocytoma: look for intermittent severe hypertension and wild swings in blood pressure, tachycardia, postural hypotension, headaches, sweating, dizziness, mental status changes, and/or feeling of impending doom. Patients also may have glucose intolerance due to high catecholamines. If pheochromocytoma is suspected, first screen with a 24-hour urine test to look for catecholamines and their breakdown products (vanillylmandelic acid, homovanillic acid, or metanephrines). If the screen is positive, order an abdominal CT to confirm adrenal mass (usual location). Treat with surgery after stabilizing the patient with alpha and beta blockers.

Diabetes insipidus (DI): patients have severe **polydipsia** and **polyuria** (urinary volume may be 25 L/day!). DI has no relation to blood sugar. When access to water is restricted, patients rapidly develop dehydration and hypernatremia, which can cause death. Administration of antidiuretic hormone (ADH) determines whether the cause is central or nephrogenic. Central DI responds to ADH; nephrogenic DI does not.

1. **Nephrogenic DI:** look for medications as the cause (e.g., **lithium,** methoxyflurane, demeclocycline). Treat with **thiazide diuretics** (paradoxical effect); ADH does not help!
2. **Central DI:** look for trauma, neoplasm, or sarcoidosis, although central DI often is idiopathic. Treat with ADH/vasopressin, and treat the underlying cause, if possible.

> ➤ **CASE SCENARIO:** What is the relationship of serum to urine osmolarity when DI is present? Serum osmolarity is high, and urine osmolarity inappropriately low (due to lack of ADH or its effects).

Syndrome of inappropriate antidiuretic hormone (SIADH) causes hyponatremia as well as low levels of every other electrolyte (and lab value) because of dilution from excessive water retention. Look for medications (e.g., morphine) and watch for a pregnant patient (oxytocin effect). Other causes include small cell lung cancer, postoperative status (watch for all electrolytes to fall after surgery), trauma, lung infections, and pain. Treat with **water restriction.** For board purposes, avoid hypertonic saline, and do not attempt aggressive or quick correction of hyponatremia (which may cause brainstem damage).

> ➤ **CASE SCENARIO:** What is the relationship between serum and urine osmolarity in SIADH? Serum osmolarity is low, and urine osmolarity is inappropriately high (due to excessive ADH).

> ➤ **CASE SCENARIO:** What drug can be given in SIADH if conservative treatment (water restriction) fails? Demeclocycline, which at controlled doses induces mild nephrogenic DI to counteract the SIADH.

Obesity increases the risk of the following problems:

1. Overall mortality (at any age)
2. Insulin resistance and diabetes mellitus
3. Hypertension
4. Hypertriglyceridemia (also weakly associated with hypercholesterolemia)
5. Heart disease and coronary artery disease
6. Gallstones (cholesterol stones)
7. Hypoventilation, Pickwickian syndrome, and sleep apnea
8. Osteoarthritis
9. Cancer—especially endometrial cancer
10. Thromboembolism
11. Varicose veins

GASTROENTEROLOGY

Gastroesophageal Reflux Disease

High-yield pearls

- Due to inappropriate, intermittent lower esophageal sphincter relaxation.
- Incidence greatly increased in patients with a sliding hiatal hernia. Obesity can aggravate.
- Classically presents as "heartburn," often related to eating and lying supine. However, it also may present as chest pain, regurgitation, cough and asthma, sore throat, dysphagia, laryngitis and hoarseness, or recurrent pneumonia.
- The initial treatment is to elevate the head of the bed and avoid coffee, alcohol, tobacco, chocolate, spicy and fatty foods, and medications with anticholinergic properties. If this approach fails, antacids, H_2 blockers, and proton-pump inhibitors may be tried; often they are started empirically at the initial presentation.
- Surgery is reserved for severe and resistant cases (Nissen fundoplication or similar procedure).
- Sequelae include esophagitis, esophageal stricture (which may mimic esophageal cancer), esophageal ulcer, hemorrhage, and ***Barrett's metaplasia/esophageal adenocarcinoma.***
- In cases that are atypical or do not respond to medical therapy, consider endoscopy. The gold standard for diagnosis is 24-hour esophageal pH monitoring (a probe is inserted into the esophagus).

Hiatal hernia, as commonly used, implies a ***sliding*** hiatal hernia. The entire gastroesophageal junction moves above the diaphragm, pulling the stomach with it—a common and benign finding associated with gastroesophageal reflux diseases (GERD). In a ***paraesophageal*** hiatal hernia, the gastroesophageal junction stays below the diaphragm, but the stomach herniates through the diaphragm into the thorax. This uncommon, serious type of hernia can become strangulated and should be repaired surgically if detected.

Peptic Ulcer Disease

Peptic ulcer disease (PUD) classically presents with chronic, intermittent, epigastric burning, gnawing, or aching pain that is localized and often relieved by antacids or milk. Look for epigastric tenderness. PUD also can cause atypical chest pain. Patients may have occult blood in the stool, nausea, and vomiting. PUD is more common in men. There are two types: gastric and duodenal.

	DUODENAL	GASTRIC
Percentage of cases	75	25
Acid secretion	Normal to high	Normal to low
Main cause	*Helicobacter pylori*	Use of nonsteroidal anti-inflammatory drugs
Peak age	40s	50s
Blood type	O	A
Eating food	Pain gets better, then worse 2–3 hours later	Pain often not relieved or made worse

Other pearls

- Endoscopy is becoming the first-line diagnostic study, because it is more sensitive and specific (but more expensive) than x-rays. It also allows biopsy and *H. pylori* testing.
- Biopsy all gastric ulcers to exclude malignancy if given the option. Always worry about gastric cancer if a stomach ulcer fails to heal after 2 months of treatment. Duodenal ulcers are almost never malignant and do not need biopsy.
- The classic complication is perforation. Look for peritoneal signs, history of PUD, and free air under the diaphragm on abdominal x-ray. Treat with antibiotics and laparotomy with repair of perforation.
- If duodenal ulcers are severe, atypical (e.g., located in distal duodenum), or nonhealing, think about **Zollinger-Ellison syndrome,** and check the gastrin level.
- Diet changes (e.g., avoidance of spicy foods) do not help to heal ulcers, but reduced usage of alcohol and tobacco does.
- For initial treatment, use H_2 blockers or proton-pump inhibitors. Use antibiotics to eliminate *H. pylori* if demonstrated by culture or serum or breath testing. Three- or four-drug therapy is commonly used, with many possible regimens. A classic regimen consists of a proton-pump inhibitor with two other antibiotics, such as ampicillin/amoxicillin, clarithromycin, or metronidazole. Bismuth (Pepto-Bismol) also can be used.
- Surgical options are considered after failure of medication or development of complications (perforation, bleeding). Commonly done are antrectomy, vagotomy, and Bilroth I and II procedures. After surgery (especially with Billroth procedures), watch for dumping syndrome (weakness, dizziness, sweating, nausea and vomiting after eating). Patients with dumping syndrome also develop hypoglycemia 2–3 hours after the meal, which causes the same symptoms to recur. Also watch for afferent loop syndrome (bilious vomiting after a meal relieves abdominal pain), bacterial overgrowth, and vitamin deficiencies (B_{12} and/or iron deficiency, which causes anemia).

Gastrointestinal Bleeding

Upper vs. lower GI bleeds:

	UPPER GI	LOWER GI
Location	Proximal to ligament of Treitz	Distal to ligament of Treitz
Common causes	Gastritis, peptic ulcer disease, varices	Vascular ectasia, diverticulosis, colon cancer, colitis, inflammatory bowel disease, hemorrhoids
Stool	Tarry, black stool (melena)	Red blood seen in stool (hematochezia)
Nasogastric tube aspirate	Positive for blood	Negative for blood

Management issues

- The first step is to make sure that the patient is stable. Check vital signs and hemoglobin level (and recheck frequently). Remember the ABCs, and give IV fluid or blood, if needed; then get a diagnosis once the patient is stabilized. Monitor blood counts every 4–8 hours on an inpatient basis until hemoglobin is stable for at least 24 hours.
- Endoscopy is the first test performed (upper or lower, depending on symptoms). Endoscopically treatable lesions include polyps, vascular ectasias, and varices.

- Radionuclide scans can detect slow or intermittent bleeds if the source cannot be found with endoscopy. Angiography can detect more rapid bleeds and allows embolization of bleeding vessels.
- Surgery is reserved for severe or resistant bleeds and usually involves resection of affected bowel (usually colon).
- ***A lower GI bleed (or just a positive occult blood test of the stool) in an adult over age 40 is colon cancer until proved otherwise.*** A complete work-up is required.

Diverticulosis is extremely common, and the incidence increases with age (present in roughly 50% of people over age 60). It is thought to be caused in part by a low-fiber, high-fat diet. Complications are **GI bleeding** (common cause of lower GI bleeds) and **diverticulitis** (inflammation of a diverticulum). In patients with diverticulitis, look for lower left quadrant pain and tenderness, fever, diarrhea/constipation, and an elevated white blood cell count.

Diarrhea

Diarrhea can have multiple causes and is best broken down into categories:

1. **Systemic:** any illness can cause diarrhea as a systemic symptom (e.g., hyperthyroidism, flu), especially in children.
2. **Osmotic:** nonabsorbable solutes remain in the bowel, where they retain water (e.g., lactose or other sugar intolerances). When the person stops eating the offending substance (e.g., no more milk or a trial of NPO status [nothing by mouth]), the diarrhea stops.
3. **Secretory:** bowel secretes fluid because of bacterial toxins (cholera, some strains of *Escherichia coli*), VIPoma (pancreatic islet cell tumor), or bile acids (after ileal resection). Diarrhea continues with NPO status.
4. **Malabsorption** (e.g., celiac sprue, Crohn disease). In patients with celicac sprue, look for **dermatitis herpetiformis,** and stop gluten in the diet. Diarrhea stops with NPO status.
5. **Infectious:** look for fever, recent history of travel (Montezuma's revenge caused by *E. coli*), and white blood cells in stool (not with toxigenic bacteria; only with invasive bacteria such as *Shigella, Salmonella, Yersinia,* and *Campylobacter* spp.).

   > **CASE SCENARIO:** A hiker presents with steatorrhea (fatty, greasy, malodorous stools that float) and crampy abdominal pain. What should you look for in the stool? Giardial protozoal cysts. Steatorrhea is due primarily to small bowel involvement. Treat with metronidazole.

6. **Exudative:** inflammation in bowel mucosa causes seepage of fluid; classically due to inflammatory bowel disease or cancer.
7. **Altered intestinal transit:** after bowel resections or medications that interfere with bowel function.

Management issues

- Watch for dehydration and check for electrolyte disturbances (metabolic acidosis, hypokalemia), a common and preventable cause of death in underdeveloped areas.
- Do a rectal exam, check for occult blood in stool, and examine stool for bacteria, ova, parasites, fat content (steatorrhea), and white blood cells.
- If the cause is not obvious, a trial of NPO status is helpful to see if the diarrhea stops.
- If the patient has a history of antibiotic usage, think of *Clostridium difficile* and test the stool for toxin. If the test is positive, treat with metronidazole; if metronidazole fails or or is not a choice, use vancomycin.
- Remember diabetes mellitus (diabetic diarrhea), factitious diarrhea (secret laxative abuse, usually by medical personnel), hyperthyroidism, and colorectal cancer as causes of diarrhea.

- After bacterial diarrhea (especially if due to *E. coli* or *Shigella* spp.) in children, watch for **hemolytic uremic syndrome (HUS).** Symptoms include thrombocytopenia, hemolytic anemia (schistocytes, helmet cells, fragmented red blood cells), and acute renal failure. Treat supportively. Patients may need dialysis and/or transfusions.

Irritable bowel syndrome (IBS) is a common cause of GI complaints. Classic patients are anxious or neurotic and have a history of **symptoms aggravated by stress,** often **alternating between diarrhea and constipation,** with bloating, **abdominal pain relieved by defecation,** and/or **mucous in the stool.** Look for psychosocial stressors in the history and normal physical findings and diagnostic tests. IBS is a diagnosis of exclusion; you must do at least basic lab tests, rectal and stool examination, and sigmoidoscopy. Because it is extremely common, it is the most likely diagnosis if the question gives you no positive findings, especially in young adults (three times more common than in women than in men).

Liver Disease

Acute liver disease: elevated liver function tests (LFTs), jaundice, nausea and vomiting, right upper quadrant pain and tenderness, and/or hepatomegaly.

1. **Alcoholic hepatitis:** elevated LFTs with aspartate aminotransferase (AST) more than twice as high as alanine aminotransferase (ALT).
2. **Viral hepatitis:** acute symptoms are similar in all types; use serology to determine type.
   - **Hepatitis A:** look for outbreaks from foodborne source. No long-term sequelae. Serology: IgM anti-HAV-positive during jaundice or shortly thereafter.
   - **Hepatitis B:** prevention (vaccination) is the best treatment. The virus is acquired through needles, sex, or perinatal transmission. Transfused blood now screened, but a history of transfusion years ago is still a risk factor. Use hepatitis B immunoglobulin for exposed neonates. Serology: HBsAg-positive with any unresolved infection (acute or chronic). HBeAg is a marker for infectivity (i.e., a person with a positive HBeAb has a low likelihood of spreading disease). The first antibody to appear is IgM anti-HBc, which appears during the "window phase," when the patient presents with acute symptoms; both HBsAg and HBsAb are negative. Positive HBsAb means that the patient is immune (due either to recovery from infection or vaccination) and never appears if the patient has chronic hepatitis. Sequelae are cirrhosis and hepatocellular cancer (only with chronic infection).
   - **Hepatitis C:** the new king of chronic hepatitis. The hepatitis C virus is the most likely cause of hepatitis after a blood transfusion (replacing the hepatitis B virus). Hepatitis C can also progress to chronic hepatitis, cirrhosis, and cancer. Serology: HCV Ab shows prior exposure but does *not* indicate recovery. The hepatitis C quantitative RNA test can detect virus in patients with chronic hepatitis C; donated blood is now screened. Order RNA test in any patient with hepatitis C-antibody positive serum and elevated liver enzymes.
   - **Hepatitis D:** seen only in patients with hepatitis B. Infection can become chronic. The virus is acquired in the same ways as the hepatitis B virus. IgM antibody to hepatitis D antigen shows recent resolution of infection; presence of the hepatitis D antigen indicates chronicity
   - **Hepatitis E:** similar to hepatitis A (food- or water-borne, no chronic state). Often fatal in **pregnant women.**
3. **Drug-induced hepatitis:** look for acetaminophen, isoniazid (and other tuberculosis drugs), or HMG-CoA reductase inhibitors. Stop the drug!
4. **Reye syndrome:** look for child given *aspirin* for a fever.
5. **Acute fatty liver of pregnancy:** occurs in third trimester. Treat with immediate delivery.
6. **Ischemia/shock:** look for history of shock.

7. **Idiopathic autoimmune hepatitis:** look for a 20–40-year-old woman with **anti-smooth muscle** or **antinculear antibodies** and no risk factors or lab markers of other causes for hepatitis. Treat with steroids.
8. **Biliary tract disease:** see below; look for markedly elevated **alkaline phosphatase** and **direct** (i.e., **conjugated**) **bilirubin.**

Chronic liver disease usually results from alcohol, viral hepatitis, or metabolic diseases (hemochromatosis, Wilson disease, alpha$_1$ antitrypsin deficiency). Classic signs include gynecomastia, testicular atrophy, palmar erythema, spider angiomas on skin, ascites, and varices.

1. **Hemochromatosis:** the primary form is **autosomal recessive;** look for a family history. Excessive iron is absorbed through gut and deposited in the liver (cirrhosis, liver cancer), pancreas (diabetes), heart (dilated cardiomyopathy), skin (pigmentation; classically called "bronze diabetes"), and joints (arthritis). Men are symptomatic earlier and more often because women lose iron with menstruation. Treat with **phlebotomy.** Secondary iron overload can also cause a hemochromatosis-like picture; this is why you should *not* give iron to patients with thalassemia or other anemia-causing hemoglobinopathy!
2. **Wilson disease: autosomal recessive** disease characterized by the presence of excessive copper. Serum **ceruloplasmin is low,** and serum copper may be normal or elevated, but liver biopsy reveals excessive copper. Patients also have **Kayser-Fleischer rings** in the eyes and have central nervous system or psychiatric manifestations due to copper deposits in the basal ganglia. Another name for this disease is hepatolenticular degeneration. Treat with **penicillamine** (copper chelator).
3. **Alpha$_1$ antitrypsin deficiency:** a younger adult develops **cirrhosis** and/or **emphysema** without risk factors for either. **Autosomal recessive** pattern of inheritance.

Remember all of the **metabolic derangements** that accompany liver failure (classically seen in chronic liver disease, but most also can occur acutely).

1. **Coagulopathy:** prolonged prothrombin time (PT); with severe disease, partial thromboplastin time (PTT) also may be prolonged. Vitamin K is *ineffective* because it cannot be utilized by a damaged liver. Coagulopathy must be treated with **fresh frozen plasma** (FFP).
2. **Jaundice/hyperbilirubinemia:** elevated conjugated and unconjugated bilirubin with hepatic damage (vs. biliary tract disease with elevation primarily of direct bilirubin).
3. **Hypoalbuminemia:** a damaged liver cannot make albumin.
4. **Ascites:** due to portal hypertension and/or hypoalbuminemia. Ascites can be detected on physical exam by **shifting dullness** or a **positive fluid wave.** A possible complication is **spontaneous bacterial peritonitis;** infected ascitic fluid can lead to sepsis. Look for fever and/or change in mental status in a patient with known ascites. Do a paracentesis and examine the ascitic fluid for white blood cells (especially neutrophils). Other lab tests include Gram stain with culture and sensitivities, glucose level (low with infection), and protein level (high with infection). The usual cause is *Escherichia coli, Streptococcus pneumoniae,* or other enteric bugs. Treat with broad-spectrum antibiotics.
5. **Portal hypertension:** causes ascites, hemorrhoids, esophageal varices, and caput medusae.
6. **Hyperammonemia:** the liver clears ammonia. Treat with decreased intake of protein (source of ammonia) and **lactulose,** which prevents absorption of ammonia. The last choice is neomycin, which kills bowel flora so they cannot make ammonia.
7. **Hepatic encephalopathy:** at least in part due to hyperammonemia; often precipitated by protein, GI bleed, or infection.
8. **Hepatorenal syndrome:** liver failure causes kidney failure (idiopathic).
9. **Hypoglycemia:** the liver stores glycogen.
10. **Disseminated intravascular coagulation:** because activated clotting factors are usually cleared by the liver.

Biliary Tract Disease

Jaundice also can be caused by **bile duct obstruction.** Look for marked elevation of **alkaline phosphatase** (or *gamma-glutamyl* **transpeptidase** [GGT] or 5'-*nucleotidase*). Conjugated (i.e., direct) bilirubin is more elevated than unconjugated bilirubin. Other symptoms include pruritus, **clay-colored stools,** and **dark urine,** which is strongly bilirubin-positive. Unconjugated bilirubin is *not* excreted in the urine because it is tightly bound to albumin.

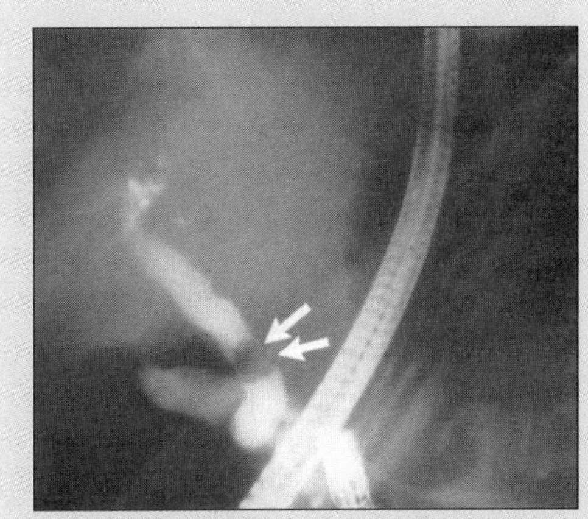

ERCP reveals a single common bile duct stone (*arrows*). (From Katz dS, Math KR, Groski SA (eds): Radiology Secrets. Philadelphia, Hanley & Belfus, 1998, with permission.)

1. **Common bile duct obstruction with gallstone** (i.e. choledocholithiasis): look for history of gallstones or the four Fs (female, forty, fertile, fat). Ultrasound may be able to image the stone; if not, use endoscopic retrograde cholangiopancreatography (ERCP; see figure) or MRCP (MRI scan).
2. **Common bile duct obstruction from cancer:** usually pancreatic cancer (painless jaundice and palpable gallbladder = **Courvoisier sign**), occasionally cholangiocarcinoma or bowel cancer.
3. **Cholestasis:** often from medications (birth control pills, phenothiazines, androgens) or pregnancy.
4. **Primary biliary cirrhosis:** middle-aged woman with no risk factors for liver or biliary disease, marked **pruritus, jaundice,** and **positive antimitochondrial antibodies** (the rest of the work-up is negative). Cholestyramine helps with symptoms, but no treatment is available other than liver transplantation.
5. **Primary sclerosing cholangitis:** seen in young adults with **ulcerative colitis;** presents like cholangitis.
6. **Cholangitis:** infected bile, usually under pressure. Treat with antibiotics, and remove stones /obstruction surgically or endoscopically.

   ➤ *CASE SCENARIO:* A 39-year-old woman with a history of gallstones develops right upper quadrant pain, fever, shaking chills, and jaundice. What happened? An impacted gallstone in the common bile duct has led to cholangitis. **Charcot's triad** of cholangitis is jaundice, fever, and right upper quadrant pain.

Foreshortened colon from longstanding ulcerative colitis. Note stricture of sigmoid colon from carcinoma (*arrows*). (From James EC, Corry RJ, Perry JF: Principles of Basic Surgical Practice. Philadelphia, Hanley & Belfus, 1987, with permission.)

Inflammatory Bowel Disease

Crohn disease vs. ulcerative colitis (see figure):

	CROHN DISEASE	ULCERATIVE COLITIS
Site of origin	Distal ileum, proximal colon	Rectum
Thickness of pathology	Transmural	Mucosa/submucosa only
Progression	Irregular (skip lesions)	Proximal, continuous from rectum; no skipped areas
Location	From mouth to anus	Involves only colon; rarely extends to ileum
Bowel habits change to	Obstruction, abdominal pain	Bloody diarrhea
Classic lesions	Fistulas/abscesses, cobblestoning, string sign on barium x-ray	Pseudopolyps, lead-pipe colon on barium x-ray, toxic megacolon
Colon cancer risk	Slightly increased	Markedly increased
Surgery cures bowel disease?	No (may make worse)	Yes (proctocolectomy with ileoanal anastomosis)

Patients with either form of inflammatory bowel disease (IBD) may develop **uveitis, arthritis, ankylosing spondylitis, erythema nodosum** or **multiforme, primary sclerosing cholangitis** (more common in ulcerative colitis), failure to thrive or grow (children), anemia of chronic disease, and fever. Both conditions are treated with some form of ***5-ASA*** (aspirin derivative) with or without a sulfa drug (e.g., sulfasalazine). Corticosteroids and other immunosuppresants are used for severe disease flare-ups.

Although **toxic megacolon** is classically seen with ulcerative colitis, it also can occur in infectious colitis (especially with *Clostridium difficile*) or Crohn disease. It may be precipitated by the use of antidiarrheal medications. Patients have high fever, leukocytosis, abdominal pain, severe tenderness, and a very **dilated colon on x-ray with "thumbprinting"** (i.e. wall thickening with mucosal irregularity). Toxic megacolon is an emergency! Start treatment by discontinuing all antidiarrheal medications; then place the patient on NPO status, insert a nasogastric tube, and administer intravenous fluids and antibiotics to cover bowel flora (e.g., ampicillin or cefazolin), and give steroids (if the cause is IBD). Go to surgery if perforation (as indicated by free air on x-ray and rebound tenderness) occurs.

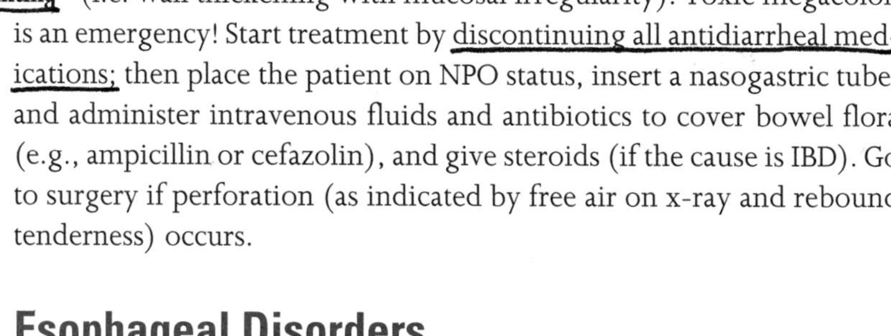

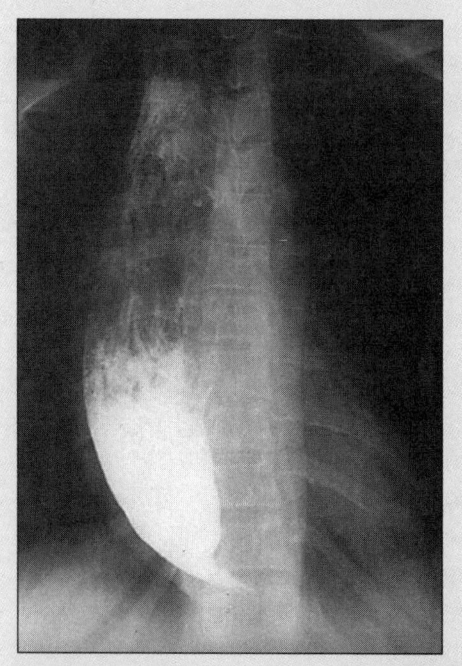

Anteroposterior radiograph from a barium esophagram, demonstrating the marked esophageal dilatation with "beaked" narrowing distally that is characteristic of achalasia. Note lucency within the barium column, representing undigested food. (Courtesy of Dr. Beth Wadler. From Katz DS, Math KR, Groskin SA (eds): Radiology Secrets. Philadelphia, Hanley & Belfus, 1998, with permission.)

Esophageal Disorders

Patients usually present with dysphagia or atypical chest pain.

1. **Achalasia:** hypertensive lower esophageal sphincter (LES), incomplete relaxation of LES and loss or derangement of peristalsis. Achalasia is usually idiopathic but may be secondary to **Chagas disease** (South America). Patients have dysphagia for both solid foods and liquids. Barium swallow reveals dilated esophagus with **distal "bird-beak" narrowing** (see figure). The diagnosis can be made with esophageal manometry. Treat with calcium channel blockers, botulinum toxin injections, pneumatic balloon dilatation, and, as a last resort, surgery (myotomy).

   ➤ ***CASE SCENARIO:*** A 32-year-old woman has dysphagia for solids and liquids, atypical chest pain, and severe heartburn. Can you rule out achalasia? Essentially, yes. Patients with achalasia do not have heartburn because the LES will not open to allow reflux.

2. **Diffuse esophageal spasm/nutcracker esophagus:** both have irregular, forceful, painful esophageal contractions that cause intermittent chest pain. Diagnose with esophageal manometry. Treat with calcium channel blockers and, if needed, surgery (myotomy).

3. **Scleroderma:** may cause aperistalsis due to fibrosis and atrophy of smooth muscle. Look for positive antinuclear antibody (ANA), mask-like facies, and other autoimmune symptoms (**CREST** = **c**alcinosis, **R**aynaud's, phenomenon, **e**sophageal dysmotility, **s**clerodactyly, **t**elangiectasias).
   - ➤ ***CASE SCENARIO:*** A 32-year-old woman has positive ANA and heartburn. Should you worry about scleroderma? Yes, because the LES usually becomes incompetent and patients develop severe reflux.
4. **Barrett esophagus:** columnar metaplasia due to acid reflux. Once detected, it must be followed with periodic endoscopy and biopsies to rule out progression to adenocarcinoma.
5. **Mallory-Weiss tears:** superficial esophageal erosions that may cause a GI bleed. They are usually seen with ***vomiting and retching (alcoholism, bulimia)***. Diagnosis and treatment are done endoscopically; sclerose any bleeding vessels.
6. **Boorhave tears:** full-thickness esophageal ruptures. If not iatrogenic (from endoscopy), they are usually due to ***vomiting and retching (alcoholism, bulimia)***. Diagnose with endoscopy or water-soluble contrast (i.e., Gastrografin) x-ray study, and treat with immediate surgical repair and drainage.

Pancreatitis

Causes: more than 80% of cases of acute pancreatitis are due to ***alcohol*** or ***gallstones.*** Other causes include hypertriglyceridemia, viral infections (mumps, coxsackievirus), trauma, and medications (steroids, thiazide diuretics).

Symptoms: watch for abdominal pain radiating to the back, nausea and vomiting that fail to relieve the pain, leukocytosis, and ***elevated amylase*** and ***lipase.*** Perforated peptic ulcers also have elevated amylase and present similarly, but amylase elevation is mild, free air is classically seen on x-rays and patients often have a history of ulcer disease. Lipase is often normal with ulcer disease.

Grey Turner sign: blue-black flanks; **Cullen sign:** blue-black umbilicus. Both result from hemorrhagic exudate, and both indicate severe pancreatitis.

Diffuse calcifications within the pancreas may be seen on plain x-ray in patients with **chronic** pancreatitis. Gallbladder disease is not associated with chronic pancreatitis.

Treatment: NPO status, nasogastric tube, intravenous fluids, and narcotics (***meperidine,*** not morphine, as morphine may cause sphincter of Oddi spasm and worsen pain). Treat chronic pancreatitis with alcohol abstinence, oral pancreatic enzyme replacement, and fat-soluble vitamin supplements.

Complications: ***pseudocyst*** (drain surgically if symptomatic), ***abscess*** or infection (antibiotics and surgical abscess drainage), and diabetes (with chronic pancreatitis).

GERIATRICS

The most rapid increase in the U.S. population (percentage-wise) is in people over 65. Within this subgroup, the over-85 group is increasing most rapidly. About 15% of the population is over age 65.

At age 80, elderly patients have half the lean body mass of a 30-year-old. Since basal metabolic rate depends on lean body mass, the elderly need fewer calories.

Normal changes in elderly people: slightly impaired immune response, visual (***presbyopia***) and hearing (***presbyacusis***) impairment, decreased muscle mass, increased fat deposits, osteoporosis, brain changes (decreased weight, enlarged ventricles and sulci), and slightly decreased ability to learn new material (which is why "you can't teach an old dog new tricks.")

Normal sexual function changes in men: longer time to get an erection; increased refractory period (after ejaculation, it takes longer before the patient can have another erection); and delayed ejaculation (the patient may ejaculate only 1 out of every 3 times he has sex). ***Impotence and lack of sexual desire are not normal*** and should be investigated. Look for psychiatric (depression) as well as physical causes. Medications, especially antihypertensives, are notorious culprits.

Normal sexual function changes in women: decreased lubrication may require use of a water-soluble lubricant; atrophy of clitoris, labia, and vaginal tissues may cause dyspareunia (treat with estrogen cream); and orgasm may be delayed. ***Lack of sexual desire is not normal*** and should be investigated (psychiatric or physical causes).

Sleep changes in elderly people: the elderly sleep less deeply, wake up more frequently during the night, and awaken earlier in the morning. They take longer to fall asleep (longer sleep latency) and have less stage 3, 4, and rapid-eye-movement (REM) sleep.

Depression in the elderly can present as dementia (known as ***pseudodementia***). Look for a history that would trigger depression (e.g., loss of a spouse, terminal or debilitating disease).

Dementia affects 15% of people over age 65 . The most common causes of dementia (in order): ***Alzheimer disease*** (gradually progressive, neurofibrillary tangles), ***multiple cerebral infarcts*** (step-wise, risk factors for stroke), and others (e.g., HIV, Pick disease).

Only 5% of people over the age of 65 live in **nursing homes.**

More than 90% of **hip fractures** are associated with falls. Most occur in patients over 70. Decrease the risk of falls in the elderly with mobility problems by "fall-proofing" the home (e.g., repair broken hand rails or steps and slippery floors, remove items that can be tripped over) and watching for medications that decrease the patient's sense of balance (the classic offenders are sedatives and anticholinergic drugs).

HEMATOLOGY

Anemia

Definition: hemoglobin < 12 mg/dl in women or < 14 mg/dl in men.

Symptoms include fatigue, dyspnea on exertion, light-headedness, dizziness, syncope, palpitations, angina, and claudication. Signs include tachycardia, pallor (especially of the conjunctival and mucous membranes), systolic ejection murmurs (from high flow), and signs of the underlying cause (e.g., jaundice in hemolytic anemia, positive stool guaiac in GI bleed).

Important clues in the history

1. **Medications:** many medications can cause anemia through various mechanisms. For example, ***methyldopa*** causes red blood cell (RBC) antibodies and hemolysis, chloroquine and ***sulfa drugs*** cause hemolysis in patients with glucose-6-phosphate dehydrogenase (G6PD) deficiency, ***phenytoin*** causes megaloblastic anemia, and ***chloramphenicol*** causes aplastic anemia.
2. **Blood loss:** trauma, surgery, GI bleed, menstrual blood loss.
3. **Chronic diseases:** anemia of chronic disease, seen especially in patients with inflammatory and debilitating conditions, such as autoimmune diseases, infections, and cancer. Conditions such as osteoarthritis do not cause anemia of chronic disease.
4. **Family history:** hemophilia, thalassemia, G6PD deficiency, others.
5. **Alcoholism:** tendency to have iron, folate, and vitamin B_{12} deficiencies as well as GI bleeds.

Steps in diagnosing the cause of anemia

1. **Complete blood count** with differential and RBC indices. First and foremost, the hemoglobin and hematocrit must be below normal. The mean corpuscular volume (MCV) tells you whether the anemia is microcytic (MCV < 80), normocytic (MCV = 80–100), or macrocytic (MCV > 100).
2. **Peripheral smear:** look for classic findings for an easy diagnosis.

SMEAR FINDING	USUAL CAUSE	SMEAR FINDING	USUAL CAUSE
Sickled cells	Sickle cell anemia	Teardrop-shaped RBCs (see figure)	Myelofibrosis
"Bite cells"	Hemolytic anemias	Rouleaux formation (see figure)	Multiple myeloma
Basophilic stippling	Lead poisoning	Parasites inside RBCs	Malaria, babesiosis

Myelofibrosis. Red cell anisocytosis and poikilocytosis with "tear-drop" forms (*arrows*) are shown. (From Hoffbrand AV, Pettit JE: Non-leukaemic myeloproliferative disorders. In Hoffbrand AV, Pettit JE (eds): Color Atlas of Clinical Hematology, 3rd ed. St. Louis, Mosby, 2000, pp 247–258, with permission.)

Multiple myeloma. Marked rouleaux formation (i.e., "stack of coins") is evident. (From Hoffbrand AV, Pettit JE: Myeloma and related conditions. In Hoffbrand AV, Pettit JE (eds): Color Atlas of Clinical Hematology, 3rd ed. St. Louis, Mosby, 2000, pp 233–246, with permission.)

(*Table continued on next page.*)

SMEAR FINDING	USUAL CAUSE	SMEAR FINDING	USUAL CAUSE
Heinz bodies	G6PD deficiency	Echinocytes/burr cells (see figure)	Uremia
Target cells (see figure)	Thalassemia, liver disease	Hypersegmented neutrophils	Folate/vitamin B_{12} deficiency
Howell-Jolly bodies	Asplenia/splenic dysfunction		
Iron inclusions in RBCs of bone marrow	Sideroblastic anemia	Schistocytes, helmet cells, fragmented RBCs	Intravascular hemolysis
Spherocytes, elliptocytes	Hereditary spherocytosis/elliptocytosis	Polychromasia →	Reticulocytosis (consider hemolysis)

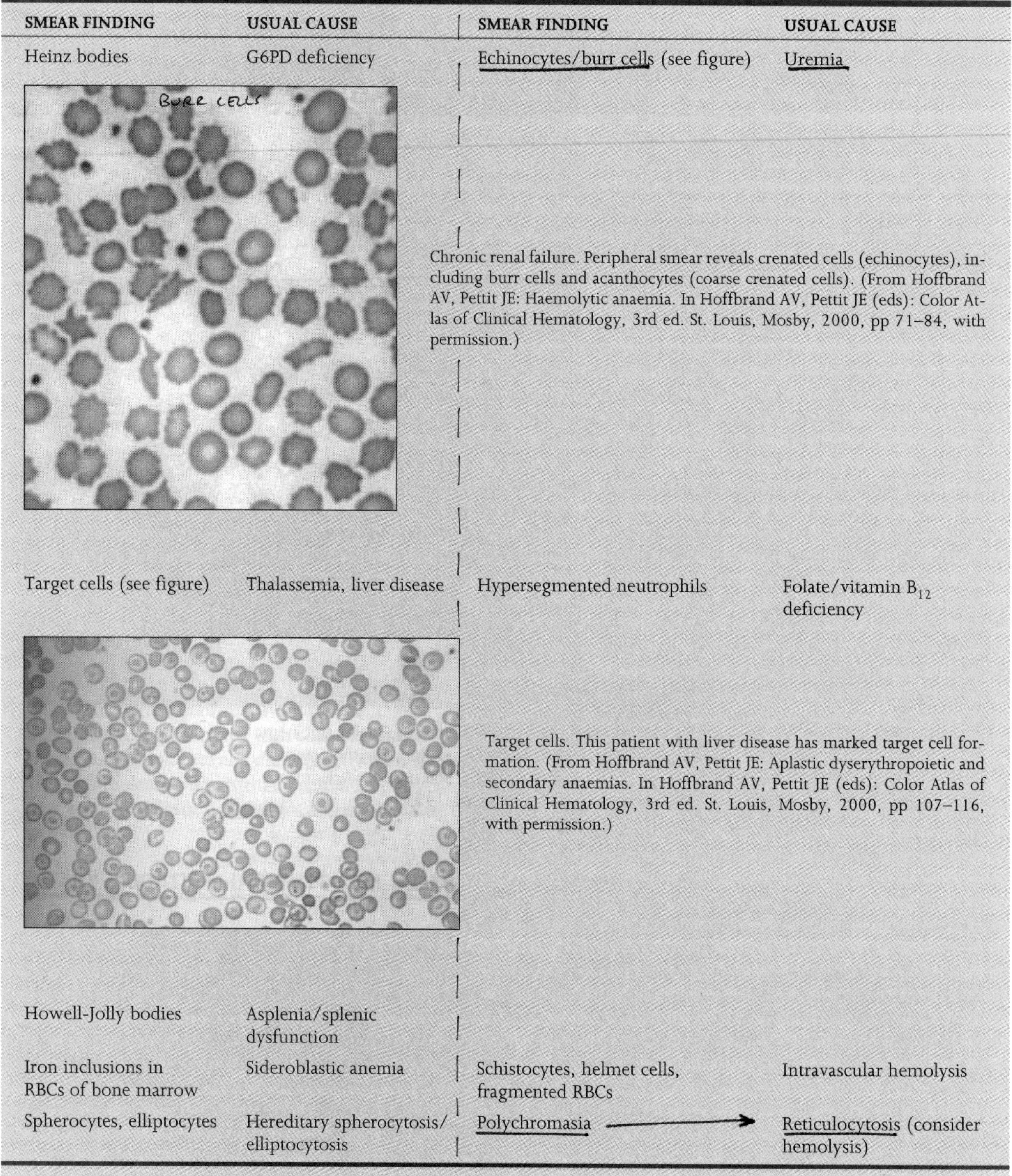

Chronic renal failure. Peripheral smear reveals crenated cells (echinocytes), including burr cells and acanthocytes (coarse crenated cells). (From Hoffbrand AV, Pettit JE: Haemolytic anaemia. In Hoffbrand AV, Pettit JE (eds): Color Atlas of Clinical Hematology, 3rd ed. St. Louis, Mosby, 2000, pp 71–84, with permission.)

Target cells. This patient with liver disease has marked target cell formation. (From Hoffbrand AV, Pettit JE: Aplastic dyserythropoietic and secondary anaemias. In Hoffbrand AV, Pettit JE (eds): Color Atlas of Clinical Hematology, 3rd ed. St. Louis, Mosby, 2000, pp 107–116, with permission.)

3. **Reticulocyte index (RI)** should be > 2% with anemia; otherwise, the marrow is not responding properly. If the index is very high, consider hemolysis as the cause (the marrow is responding properly and is not the problem).

With these three parameters, you can form a reasonable differential diagnosis if the cause is still uncertain.

MICROCYTIC	NORMOCYTIC	MACROCYTIC
Normal to elevated RI	*Normal to elevated RI*	*All have low RI*
Thalassemia/hemoglobinopathy	Acute blood loss	Folate deficiency
	Hemolytic (multiple causes)	Vitamin B_{12} defiency
	Medications (antibody-causing)	Medications (methotrexate, phenytoin)
Low RI	*Low RI*	Cirrhosis/liver disease
Iron deficiency	Cancer/dysplasia (e.g., myelophthisic)	
Sideroblastic	Anemia of chronic disease (some)	
Anemia of chronic disease (some)	Aplastic anemia	
Lead poisoning	Endocrine failure (thyroid, pituitary)	
	Renal failure	

Clues to presence of hemolytic anemia: elevated lactate dehydrogenase (LDH); elevated bilirubin (unconjugated as well as conjugated if the liver functions properly); jaundice; **low or absent haptoglobin** (seen with **intravascular** hemolysis); and positive urobilinogen, bilirubin, or hemoglobin in urine. Only conjugated bilirubin appears in the urine, and hemoglobin appears only when haptoglobin has been saturated, as in brisk intravascular hemolysis.

Microcytic anemias

1. **Iron deficiency anemia:** the most common cause of anemia in the U.S. Look for **low iron or ferritin level, elevated total iron-binding capacity (TIBC;** also known as **ferritin**), and **low TIBC saturation.** Rarely patients have a craving for ice or dirt (pica) or **Plummer-Vinson syndrome** (esophageal web producing dysphagia, iron deficiency anemia, and glossitis). Iron deficiency anemia is common in women of reproductive age because of menstrual irregularities. To treat iron deficiency anemia, correct the underlying cause, if possible, and treat with oral iron supplementation.

   ➤ **CASE SCENARIO:** A 22-year-old woman with menorrhagia presents with fatigue and has lab values consistent with iron deficiency anemia. How long should you treat her with iron? For roughly 3–6 months.

2. **Thalassemia** must be differentiated from iron deficiency. Iron levels are normal in thalassemia, and iron supplementation is contraindicated because it may cause iron overload. Look for **elevated hemoglobin A_2** (β-thalassemia only) or **hemoglobin F** (β-thalassemia only); target cells, nucleated RBCs, or diffuse basophilia on peripheral smears; x-ray of the skull showing "crew-cut" or "hair-on-end" appearance (see figure); splenomegaly; and family history. Thalassemia is more common in blacks, Mediterraneans, and Asians. No treatment is required for minor thalassemia; patients often are asymptomatic because they are accustomed to living at a lower level of hemoglobin. Thalassemia major is more dramatic and severe. Treat with transfusions as needed and iron chelation therapy to prevent hemochromatosis. Diagnosis is confirmed with hemoglobin electrophoresis.

   ➤ **CASE SCENARIO:** If a child is asymptomatic at birth and develops symptoms of anemia around 6 months of age, could he or she have thalassemia? Yes. There are four gene loci for the alpha chain and only two for the beta chain. Patients with alpha-thalassemia are symptomatic at birth or die in utero (due to fetal hydrops), but patients with beta-thalassemia (see figure) have no symptoms until they run out of fetal hemoglobin (usually around 6 months).

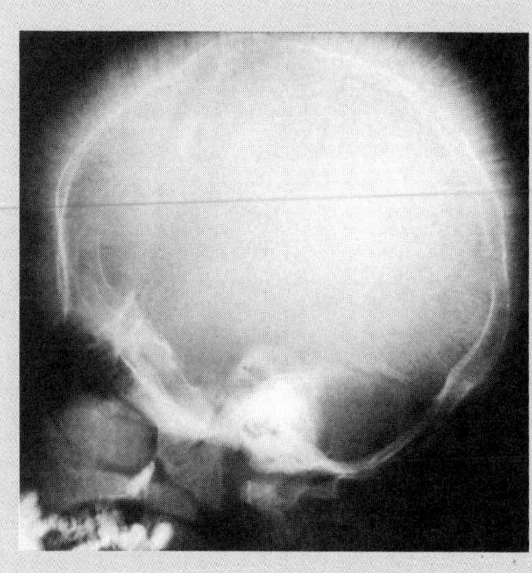

Beta-thalassemia major. Lateral skull radiograph shows typical "hair-on-end" appearance, with thinning of cortical bone and expansion of the marrow cavity. (From Hoffbrand AV, Pettit JE: Genetic disorders of haemoglobin. In Hoffbrand AV, Pettit JE (eds): Color Atlas of Clinical Hematology, 3rd ed. St. Louis, Mosby, 2000, pp 85–106, with permission.)

3. **Lead poisoning:** classically seen in children. With acute poisoning, look for vomiting, ***ataxia, colicky abdominal pain,*** irritability (aggression, behavioral regression), and ***encephalopathy, cerebral edema,*** or ***seizures.*** Usually poisoning is chronic. The history may include residence in an old or neglected building (paint chips and dust in old buildings may still contain lead) or residence near or family members who work at a lead-smelting or battery-recycling plant. Lab tests show ***basophilic RBC stippling*** and elevated free erythrocyte protoporphyrin. Screening is important (see pediatric section) to prevent neurologic damage. Order serum lead level if lead poisoning is suspected.

4. **Sideroblastic anemia:** increased or normal iron and ferritin/TIBC saturation (which distinguish it from iron deficiency), polychromatophilic stippling, and the classic "***ringed sideroblast***" in the bone marrow. Sideroblastic anemia may be related to myelodysplasia or future blood dyscrasia. Manage supportively. In rare cases, the anemia responds to ***pyridoxine.*** Do not give iron.

5. **Anemia of chronic disease** may be microcytic or normocytic. Look for diseases that cause chronic inflammation. Serum iron is low, but so is TIBC (thus, the % saturation may be near normal). *Serum ferritin is elevated because ferritin is an acute-phase reactant*. Treat the underlying disorder to correct the anemia. Do not give iron.

Normocytic anemias

1. **Acute blood loss:** immediately after blood loss, hemoglobin may be normal (takes a few hours to re-equilibrate). Look for pale cold skin, tachycardia, and hypotension. Transfuse if indicated, even with a normal hemoglobin in the appropriate acute setting.

2. **Autoimmune hemolytic anemia** has multiple etiologies: lupus (or medications that cause lupus, like ***procainamide, hydralazine,***and ***isoniazid***), drugs (classic is methyldopa, also penicillins/cephalosporins/sulfas and quinidine), leukemia/lymphoma or infection (classic is mycoplasma, also Epstein-Barr virus and syphilis). ***Coombs test*** is positive, may have spherocytes due to incomplete macrophage destruction.

3. **Spherocytosis (normochromic):** diagnosis based on blood-smear, family history (***autosomal dominant*** inheritance), splenomegaly, ***positive osmotic fragility test,*** and an increased mean corpuscular hemoglobin concentration (MCHC). Treatment often involves splenectomy. Spherocytes also may be seen in extravascular hemolysis, but the osmotic fragility test is normal.

4. **End-stage renal disease:** the kidney makes erythropoietin; give erythropoietin to correct the anemia.

5. **Aplastic anemia** is usually idiopathic but may be caused by chemotherapy or radiation, malignancy (especially leukemias), benzene, and medications (e.g., chloramphenicol, carbamazepine, phenylbutazone, sulfa drugs, zidovudine). Look for decreased white blood cells and platelets. Treat by stopping any possible causative medication. Patients may need antithymocyte globulin (ATG) or bone marrow transplant.

6. **Myelophthisic anemia** usually is due to myelodysplasia/myelofibrosis or malignant invasion and destruction of bone marrow (most common cause). Look for marked anisocytosis (different sizes), poikilocytosis (different shapes), nucleated RBCs, giant and/or bizarre-looking platelets, and teardrop-shaped RBCs on the peripheral smear. A bone marrow biopsy is usually done and may reveal no cells ("dry tap"due to fibrotic marrow in myelofibrosis) or malignant-looking cells.

7. **Glucose-6-phosphate dehydrogenase (G6PD) deficiency** is an X-linked recessive trait , thus is clinically seen in males. It is most common in blacks and Mediterraneans. Look for sudden hemolysis or anemia after expsoure to *fava beans* or certain drugs (*antimalarials*, salicylates, *sulfa drugs*) or after infection. Diagnosis is based on the RBC enzyme assay. Do not perform the assay immediately after hemolysis; you may get a false-negative result, because all of the older RBCs have been destroyed and the younger RBCs are not affected in many patients. Treat by avoiding precipitating foods and medications. Discontinue the triggering medication first.

Macrocytic anemias

1. **Folate deficiency** is classically seen in alcoholics and pregnant women. Rare causes include poor diet (e.g., tea and toast), methotrexate, prolonged therapy with trimethoprim/sulfamethoxazole, anticonvulsant therapy (especially phenytoin), and malabsorption. Check folate level (serum or RBC). Treat with oral folate.

2. **Vitamin B_{12} deficiency** is most commonly due to *pernicious anemia* (antiparietal cell antibodies) but also may be due to gastrectomy, terminal ileum resection, diet (strict vegan), chronic pancreatitis and *Diphyllobothrium latum* (fish tapeworm) infection. Look for *neurologic deficiencies* (loss of sensation or position sense, paresthesias, ataxia, spasticity, hyperreflexia, positive Babinski, dementia) and achlorhydria (no stomach acid secretion, elevated stomach pH). Check serum levels of vitamin B_{12}. A *Schilling test* usually determines the etiology.

   ➤ *CASE SCENARIO:* A 24-year-old woman with a history of hypothyroidism who eats a normal diet presents with tingling in her legs and macrocytic anemia with hypersegmented neutrophils. How should she be treated? With intramuscular vitamin B_{12} injections, usually given monthly. Oral supplements cannot be used, because the patient almost surely has pernicious anemia and cannot absorb oral supplements.

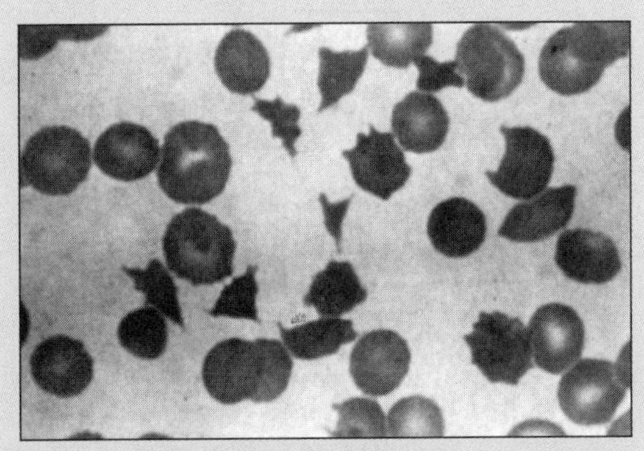

Peripheral blood film from a patient with thrombotic thrombocytpenic purpura. Fragmented cells are prominent. Platelets are decreased. This smear also could be seen in patients with disseminated intravascular coagulation, hemolytic uremic syndrome, malignant hypertension, prosthetic or pathologic heart valves, or large hemangiomas. (From Wood ME (ed): Hematology/Oncology Secrets, 2nd ed. Philadelphia, Hanley & Belfus, 1999, with permission.)

Other causes of anemia

1. **Mechanical heart valves** (hemolyze red blood cells).

2. **Hemolysis due to "microangiopathy"** (e.g., disseminated intravascular coagulation, thrombotic thrombocytopenic purpura [see figure], hemolytic uremic syndrome). Look for schistocytes and RBC fragments.

3. **Infections:** *Clostridium perfringens*, malaria, babesiosis.
4. **Hypersplenism**: all patients have splenomegaly; other common findings include low platelets and low white blood cell (WBC) count.

Transfusions. Different blood components have different indications:

1. **Whole blood:** used only for rapid, massive blood loss or exchange transfusions (poisoning, thrombotic thrombocytopenic purpura).
2. **Packed RBCs:** used instead of whole blood when the patient needs a transfusion.
3. **Washed RBCs:** free of traces of plasma, white blood cells, and platelets. Good for IgA deficiency and allergic or previously sensitized patients.
4. **Platelets:** given for symptomatic thrombocytopenia (usually $\leq$ 10,000/μl).
5. **Granulocytes:** rarely used for neutropenia with sepsis caused by chemotherapy.
6. **Fresh frozen plasma** (FFP): contains all clotting factors; used for bleeding diathesis when the patient cannot wait for vitamin K to take effect (e.g., disseminated intravascular coagulation, severe warfarin poisoning) or when vitamin K is not effective (liver failure).
7. **Cryoprecipitate:** contains fibrinogen and factor 8; used in hemophilia, von Willebrand disease, and disseminated intravascular coagulation.

> ➤ *CASE SCENARIO:* A 47-year-old man presents for a routine health visit. He is asymptomatic. A routine hemoglobin level is 6 mg/dl. How many units of blood should you transfuse? None. Transfusion should be based on clinical grounds. Treat the patient, not the lab value. There is no such thing as a "trigger value" for transfusion. An asymptomatic patient rarely needs a transfusion.

The most common cause of **blood transfusion reaction** is lab error. Type O negative blood can be used to avoid reactions when you cannot wait for blood typing or the blood bank does not have the patient's type. Types of transfusion reactions:

1. **Febrile reaction** (chills, fever, and headache/back pain) from antibodies to WBCs.
2. **Hemolytic reaction** (anxiety/discomfort, dyspnea, chest pain, shock, jaundice) from antibodies to RBCs.
3. **Allergic reaction** (urticaria, edema, dizziness, dyspnea/wheezing, anaphylaxis) from reaction to component in donor serum.
   - If the patient has associated oliguria, treat with IV fluids and diuresis (mannitol or furosemide). Massive transfusions may result in bleeding diathesis from dilutional thrombocytopenia and citrate (a calcium chelator found in transfused blood; calcium is required for proper coagulation). Look for oozing from puncture or IV sites. The patient also may have hyperkalemia.

> ➤ *CASE SCENARIO:* A 52-year-old man receives a transfusion for severe anemia due to a GI bleed. He develops chills, fever, and low back pain during the transfusion. What should you do? The first step is to stop the transfusion. Next, have the lab check to make sure that no error or blood mix-up occurred while you monitor the patient and his urine output.

Disseminated intravascular coagulation (DIC) most commonly is due to **pregnancy** or obstetric complications (50%), **malignancy** (33%), **sepsis,** or **trauma** (especially head trauma, prostate surgery, and snake bites). DIC usually manifests with bleeding diathesis. Look for the classic **oozing or bleeding from puncture or IV sites.** However, it also may be associated with thrombotic tendencies. Look for prolonged prothrombin time (PT), partial thromboplastin time (PTT), and bleeding time (BT); positive D-dimer test; increased fibrin degradation products; thrombocytopenia; decreased fibrin; decreased clotting factors; and schistocytes. Treat the underlying cause (e.g., evacuate the uterus, give antibiotics). Patients may need transfusions/FFP or, rarely, heparin (only if thrombosis occurs).

Eosinophilia may be idiopathic or caused by allergy, eczema, atopy, angioedema, drug reactions, parasitic infections, blood dyscrasias (especially lymphoma), Löffler syndrome (pulmonary eosinophilia), autoimmune diseases, IgA deficiency, and adrenal insufficiency.

Basophilia: think of allergies, neoplasm or blood dyscrasia.

Bleeding problems: the lupus anticoagulant may cause a prolonged PTT, but patients have a tendency toward thrombosis. Look for associated lupus, positive test for syphilis (Veneral Disease Research Laboratory or rapid plasmin reagin test), and/or history of miscarriages. Factor V Leyden, thrombin variant, protein C, protein S, and antithrombin III deficiencies also may cause an increased tendency toward thrombosis. Treat with anticoagulant therapy to prevent deep venous thrombosis and pulmonary embolism.

Clotting tests: use PT for extrinsic system (prolonged by warfarin), PTT for intrinsic system (prolonged by heparin), and bleeding time (BT) for platelet function.

DISEASE	PT	PTT	BT	PLATELET COUNT	RBC COUNT	OTHER
Von Willebrand disease	Normal	High	High	Normal	Normal	Autosominal dominant (look for family history)
Hemophilia A/B	Normal	High	Normal	Normal	Normal	X-linked recessive; A = low factor 8; B = low factor 9
DIC	High	High	High	Low	Normal/low	Appropriate history, factor 8 level low
Liver failure	High	High	Normal	Normal/low	Normal/low	Jaundice, normal level of factor 8; do not give vitamin K (ineffective)
Heparin	Normal	High	Normal	Normal/low	Normal	Watch for thrombocytopenia/ thrombosis
Warfarin	High	Normal	Normal	Normal	Normal	Vitamin K antagonist (factors 2, 7, 9, and 10)
ITP	Normal	Normal	High	Low	Normal	Watch for preceding URI
TTP	Normal	Normal	High	Low	Low	Hemolysis, CNS symptoms; treat with plasmapheresis; do not give platelets
Scurvy	Normal	Normal	Normal	Normal	Normal	Fingernail and gum hemorrhages, bone hemorrhages

PT = prothrombin time, PTT = partial thromboplastin time, BT = bleeding time, RBC = red blood cell, DIC = disseminated intravascular coagulation, URI = upper respiratory infection, ITP = idiopathic thrombocytpenic purpura, TTP = thrombotic thrombocytopenic purpura, CNS = central nervous system.

Thrombocytopenia may be caused by idiopathic thrombocytopenic purpura, thrombotic thrombocytopenic purpura (TTP), hemolytic uremic syndrome, disseminated intravascular coagulation, HIV infection, splenic sequestration, heparin (treat by first stopping heparin), other medications (especially quinidine and sulfa drugs), autoimmune disorders, and alcohol. Bleeding from thrombocytopenia is in the form of **petechiae, nose-bleeds,** and ***easy* bruising.** Do not give platelet transfusions to a patient with TTP or heparin-associated thrombocytopenia; this may cause thrombosis!

➤ **CASE SCENARIO:** A 72-year-old man who eats "hot dogs and soda" for every meal complains of bleeding gums and muscle pain. On exam, you notice petechiae and splinter hemorrhages under his fingernails. Platelets and coagulation studies are normal. The patient takes no medications. What does the patient have? Vitamin C deficiency (scurvy). Treat with oral vitamin C and diet counseling.

IMMUNOLOGY

HIV Infection and AIDS

Initial seroconversion may present as a mononucleosis-type syndrome (fever, malaise, pharyngitis, rash, lymphadenopathy). Keep in the back of your mind as a differential diagnosis for any sore throat or Epstein-Barr virus (EBV)-type presentation.

➤ ***CASE SCENARIO:*** How do you make the diagnosis of HIV infection? First order an enzyme-linked immunosorbent assay (ELISA); positive results should be confirmed with a Western blot test. Do all tests before you tell the patient anything!

➤ ***CASE SCENARIO:*** How long does it take for the HIV test to become positive once a person contracts the virus? Generally, it takes at least 1 month for antibodies to develop. If a patient presents because of specific recent risk-taking behavior and wants testing, you should retest the patient in 6 months if the initial test is negative.

Other HIV/AIDS CASE SCENARIOS:

- Once the diagnosis of HIVinfection is made, how often should you check the CD4 count? Every 6 months.
- When should you start antiretroviral therapy? When the CD4 count falls below 500/mm^3 (or sooner!).
- When should you start prophylaxis for *Pneumocystis carinii* pneumonia (PCP)? When the CD4 count is < 200/mm^3. What drug should you give for PCP prophylaxis? Trimethoprim-sulfamethoxazole (TMP-SMZ), dapsone, or pentamidine (2nd line agent).
- When should you start prophylaxis for *Mycobactrium avium* infection (MAI)? When the CD4 count is < 100/mm^3.
- What drug should you use for MAI prophylaxis? Azithromycin, clarithromycin, or rifabutin.
- Below what CD4 count is a person with HIV said to have AIDS even if he or she is asymptomatic? Below 200/mm^3.
- What is the only live vaccine given to HIV-positive patients? Measles, mumps, and rubella (MMR).
- What are the two classic malignancies in patients with AIDS? Kaposi sarcoma and non-Hodgkin lymphoma (especially primary CNS B-cell lymphomas).
- AIDS plus a positive India ink preparation of the cerebrospinal fluid indicates what infection? *Cryptococcus neoformans.*
- AIDS plus ring-enhancing lesions in the brain indicates which infection? Toxoplasma or cysticercosis (*Taenia solium*).
- What is the treatment of choice for cytomegalovirus (CMV) retinitis? Ganciclovir/valganciclovir (foscarnet and cidofovir are other choices).
- What two protozoal causes of diarrhea are fairly unique to patients with AIDS? *Cryptosporidium* and *Isospora* spp.
- Should HIV-positive mothers be allowed to breast feed? No. The virus can be transmitted through breast milk.

HIV sequelae include wasting syndrome (progressive weight loss), dementia, peripheral neuropathies, thrombocytopenia, and loss of delayed hypersensitivity (type IV) on skin testing (also known as anergy).

In any patient with AIDS and pneumonia, think of **PCP pneumonia** first (although community-acquired pneumonia is more common). Look for severe hypoxia with normal x-ray or **diffuse, bilateral interstitial infiltrates.** Usually the patient has a dry, nonproductive cough.

You may be able to detect PCP with silver stains (Wright-Giemsa, Giemsa, or methenamine silver) after induced sputum; if not, bronchoscopy with bronchoalveolar lavage and brush biopsy can be used to make the diagnosis. In the correct clinical setting, patients often are treated empirically without securing a diagnosis.

Any adult patient with **thrush** should raise suspicion of HIV, leukemia, or diabetes and any young adult who presents with **herpes zoster** should raise suspicion of HIV.

To prevent HIV transmission to infants, give zidovudine (AZT) to HIV-positive women during the last trimester of pregnancy. Give the infant AZT for 6 weeks after delivery. This protocol reduces the transmission rate from approximately 25% to 8%. The infant may have a positive HIV test for 6–12 months because of maternal antibodies. Use PCR to detect HIV directly. Recent studies indicate that cesarean section may reduce transmission.

Hypersensitivity Reactions

1. **Type I: anaphylactic.** Due to preformed IgE antibodies that cause release of vasoactive amines (e.g., histamine, leukotrienes) from mast cells and basophils. Examples are **anaphylaxis** (bee stings, food allergy [especially peanuts and shellfish], medications [especially penicillin and sulfa drugs], rubber glove allergy), **atopy, hay fever, urticaria,** allergic rhinitis, and some forms of asthma.
   - With chronic type I hypersensitivity (atopy, some forms of asthma, allergic rhinitis), look for **eosinophilia,** elevated IgE levels, family history, and seasonal exacerbations. Patients also may have allergic "shiners" (bilateral infrarorbital edema) and a transverse nasal crease (from frequent nose rubbing). Pale, bluish, edematous nasal turbinates with many eosinophils in clear, watery nasal secretions are also classic.
   - Treat acute reactions immediately by securing the airway, if needed. Laryngeal edema may prevent intubation, in which case a cricothyrotomy should be performed. Give **epinephrine.** Steroids are sometimes given for severe reactions (choose only if other options are not present).
   - Watch for **C1 esterase inhibitor (complement) deficiency** as a cause for hereditary angioedema. Patients have diffuse swelling of lips, eyelids, and possibly the airway, unrelated to any allergen exposure. The disorder is inheritied in an autosomal dominant pattern; look for family history. C4 complement levels are low. Treat acutely like anaphylaxis. Androgens are used for long-term treatment to increase liver production of C1 esterase inhibitor.
     - **CASE SCENARIO:** What drug should be avoided in patients with asthma and nasal polyps? Aspirin, which may precipitate a severe asthmatic attack.
     - **CASE SCENARIO:** What can be done if you suspect an allergy but are not sure of the trigger? Skin testing.
2. **Type II: cytotoxic.** Due to pre-formed IgG and IgM which react with antigen and cause secondary inflammation. Examples are **autoimmune hemolytic anemia** (classic causes are methyldopa or penicillin/sulfas) or other cytopenias caused by antibodies (e.g., ITP), **transfusion reactions,** erythroblastosis fetalis (Rh incompatibility), **Goodpasture syndrome** (watch for linear immunofluorescence on kidney biopsy), myasthenia gravis, Graves disease, pernicious anemia, pemphigus, and hyperacute transplant rejection (as soon as the anastomosis is made at transplant surgery, the transplanted organ deteriorates in front of your eyes)
   - **CASE SCENARIO:** What test can be used to screen for suspected antibody-mediated hemolytic anemia? The Coombs test.

3. **Type III: immune complex-mediated.** Due to antigen-antibody complexes that usually are deposited in blood vessels and cause an inflammatory response. Examples are **serum sickness, lupus** and other autoimmune disorders, chronic hepatitis, cryoglobulinemia, and glomerulonephritis.
4. **Type IV: cell-mediated (delayed).** Due to sensitized T lymphocytes that release inflammatory mediators. Examples include the **purified protein derivative (PPD) tuberculosis skin test, contact dermatitis** (especially poison ivy, nickel earrings, cosmetics, and topical medications), chronic transplant rejection, and **granulomatous diseases** (e.g., sarcoidosis).

INFECTIOUS DISEASE

Empirical therapy while awaiting culture and sensitivity results:

CONDITION	MAIN ORGANISM(S)	EMPIRICAL ANTIBIOTICS
Urinary tract infection	*Escherichia coli*	Trimethoprim-sulfamethoxazole, nitrofurantoin, amoxicillin, quinolones
Bronchitis	Virus, *Haemophilus influenzae, Moraxella* spp.	Amoxicillin, erythromycin
Pneumonia (classic)	*Streptococcus pneumoniae, H. influenzae*	Third-generation cephalosporin, azithromycin
Pneumonia (atypical)	*Mycoplasma, Chlamydia* spp.	Macrolide antibiotic, doxycycline
Osteomyelitis	*Staphylococcus aureus, Salmonella* spp.	Antistaphylococcal penicillin (e.g., dicloxacillin, methicillin); vancomycin
Cellulitis	Streptococci, staphylococci	Antistaphylococcal penicillin (covers both)
Meningitis (neonate)	Streptococci B, *E. coli, Listeria* spp.	Ampicillin + aminoglycoside, third-generation Cephalosporin
Meningitis (child/adult)	*S. pneumoniae, Neisseria meningitidis**	Third-generation cephalosporin or meropenem + vancomycin + dexamethasone
Sepsis	Gram-negative organisms, streptococci, staphylococci	Third-generation penicillin/cephalosporin + aminoglycoside, imipenem
Septic arthritis[t]	*S. aureus* Gonococci	Antistaphylococcal penicillin, vancomycin Ceftriaxone, fluoroquinolone, spectinomycin
Endocarditis	Staphylococci, streptococci	Antistaphylococcal penicillin (or vancomycin) + aminoglycoside

**H. influenzae* type b is no longer as common a cause of meningitis in children because of widespread vaccination. In a child with no history of immunization, *H. influenzae* is the most likely cause of meningitis.

[t]Think of staphylococci if the patient is monogamous or not sexually active. Think of gonorrhea for younger adults who are sexually active.

Empirical antibiotics of choice for different organisms:

ORGANISM*	ANTIBIOTIC	OTHER CHOICES
Streptococci A or B	Penicillin, cephazolin	Erythromycin
S. pneumoniae	Third-generation cephalosporin, fluoroquinolone	Fluoroquinolone (e.g., levofloxacin)
Enterococci	Penicillin or ampicillin +aminoglycoside	Vancomycin + aminoglycoside
Staphylococci	Antistaphylococcal penicillin (e.g. methicillin)	Vancomycin (MRSA)
Gonococci[t]	Ceftriaxone or fluoroquinolone	Spectinomycin
Meningococci	Penicillin/ampicillin	Cefotaxime, chloramphenicol

(Table continued on next page.)

ORGANISM*	ANTIBIOTIC	OTHER CHOICES
Haemophilus spp.	Second- or third-generation cephalosporin	Ampicillin
Pseudomonas spp.	Antipseudomonal penicillin + aminoglycoside	Aztreonam, imipenem
Bacteroides spp,	Metronidazole	Clindamycin
Mycoplasma spp,	Erythromycin, azithromycin	Doxycycline
Treponema pallidum	Penicillin	Doxycycline
Chlamydia spp.	Doxycycline, azithromycin	Erythromycin, fluoroquinolone
Lyme disease	Ceftriaxone, doxycycline	Erythromycin, amoxicillin

*Always use culture sensitivities to guide therapy once available.

ᵗWith genital infections, always treat for presumed *Chlamydia* coinfection with azithromycin or doxycycline.

Tuberculosis therapy:

CLINICAL SETTING/FINDINGS	TREATMENT
Exposed adult with negative PPD test	None
Exposed child < 5 years old with negative PPD test	Isoniazid (INH) for 3 mo
Prophylaxis for PPD conversion (negative to positive), no active disease	INH for 6–12 months
Acute pulmonary disease/positive culture	INH/rifampin/pyrazinamide for 2 mo, then INH/rifampin for 4 mo

PPD = purified protein derivative.

Important Tb points

1. If the patient is noncompliant, **directly observed therapy** (someone watches the patient take medications every day) is recommended.
2. Watch for **liver dysfunction** in patients on therapy.
3. Consider supplementation with **vitamin B_6** (pyridoxine) for patients on INH, or watch for signs of deficiency.
4. Multidrug resistant Tb is an increasing problem and requires the addition of streptomycin or ethambutol until sensitivities known.

Streptococcal and Staphylococcal Infections

Skin infections often occur after a break in the skin due to trauma, scabies, or insect bite. Watch for development of poststreptococcal glomerulonephritis.

1. **Impetigo:** maculopapules to vesicopustules or bullae to **honey-colored, crusted lesions.** Staphylococci are a more common cause than streptococci. Definitely think of staphylococci if a **furuncle** or **carbuncle** is present; if glomerulonephritis develops, think of streptococci. Impetigo is contagious: look for sick contacts. Treat empirically with antistaphylococcal penicillin (e.g., dicloxacillin) to cover both organisms.
2. **Erysipelas:** a superficial cellulitis that is red, shiny, swollen, and tender. It may be associated with vesicles or bullae, fever, and lymphadenopathy.

3. **Cellulitis:** involves subcutaneous tissues (deeper than erysipelas). Streptoccoci are the most common cause, but staphylococci also may be implicated. Treat empirically with antistaphylococcal penicillin or vancomycin to cover both. Other causes:
   - *Pseudomonas* spp. (diabetic patients with foot ulcers, burns, severe trauma): treat with broad-spectrum,"big-gun" antibiotics.
   - *Pastuerella multocida* (after dog/cat bites): treat with ampicillin.
   - *Vibrio vulnificus* (fishermen or other salt-water exposure): treat with tetracycline.
4. **Necrotizing fasciitis:** progression of cellulitis to necrosis and gangrene, crepitus, and systemic toxicity (tachycardia, fever, hypotension). Multiple organisms (aerobes and anaerobes) often are involved. Treat with intravenous fluids, debridement, and broad-spectrum, "big-gun" antibiotics.

Endometritis and **puerperal fever** usually result from streptococcal infection and cause postpartum fever and uterine tenderness. Treat with amoxicillin/ampicillin.

Streptococcus viridans: causes subacute endocarditis and dental caries (*Streptococcus mutans*).

Enterococcus faecalis: normal bowel flora; causes endocarditis, urinary tract infection, and sepsis.

Streptococcus pneumoniae: common cause of pneumonia, otitis media, meningitis, sinusitis, and sepsis.

Staphylococcus aureus is a common cause of abscess (especially in the breast after breast-feeding or in the skin after a furuncle), **endocarditis** (especially in drug users), **osteomyelitis** (most common cause), **septic arthritis,** food poisoning (preformed toxin), **toxic shock syndrome** (preformed toxin; classically a woman who leaves tampon in place too long and develops hypotension, fever, and rash that desquamates; see figure), scalded skin syndrome (preformed toxin, affects younger children who often start with impetigo, then desquamate), impetigo, cellulitis, wound infections, pneumonia (often forms lung abscess/empyema), and furuncle/carbuncle. Health care workers who are chronic nasal carriers may cause nosocomial infections; treat carriers with antibiotics. Treat patients with antistaphylococcal penicillin or vancomycin; abscesses require surgical drainage.

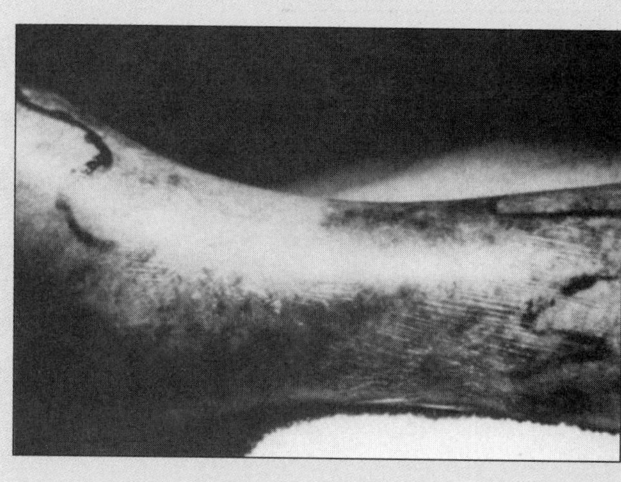

Skin desquamation secondary to toxic shock syndrome. (From Cunha BA: Infectious Disease Pearls. Philadelphia, Hanley & Belfus, 1999, with permission.)

Staphylococcus epidermidis: causes IV catheter infections, infections of prosthetic implants (heart valves, vascular grafts), and sepsis. Treat empirically with antistaphylococcal penicillin or vancomycin.

Staphylococcus saprophyticus: causes urinary tract infections.

Miscellaneous Infections

Endocarditis can either be **acute** (fulminant, most commonly caused by *S. aureus*) or **subacute** (insidious onset, most commonly caused by viridans streptococci). Look for general signs of infection (e.g., fever, tachycardia, malaise) plus **new-onset heart murmur,** embolic phenomena (stroke and other infarcts), **Osler nodes** (painful palpable nodules on tips of fingers), **Roth spots** (round retinal hemorrhages with white centers), **Janeway lesions** (nontender, erythematous lesions on palms and soles), **splinter hemorrhages** (small, asymptomatic linear hemorrhages under the nails) and septic shock (more dramatic with acute than subacute disease). The diagnosis is made by blood cultures, and empiric treatment is begun with wide-spectrum antibiotics (to cover strep and staph species) until culture results are known.

- People more likely to be affected include IV drug abusers (who classically develop right-sided valve lesions), patients with abnormal heart valves (prosthetic valves, rheumatic valvular disease, congenital heart defects) and postoperative patients (especially after genitourinary, gastrointestinal, or dental surgery; thus the need for prophylaxis in susceptible people).
  - ➤ **CASE SCENARIO:** If a patient has a secundum atrial septal defect (the more common type) or mitral valve prolapse, do you need to give endocarditis prophylaxis? No. The exception is patients with mitral valve prolapse who have an audible murmur (uncommon); such patients should receive prophylaxis.

Rabies usually is due to bites from bats, skunks, raccoons, or foxes in the U.S.(vaccination has eliminated dog rabies). The incubation period is usually around 1–2 months. The classic symptoms are hydrophobia and CNS signs (paralysis). After a bite, several steps should be taken:

1. **Local wound treatment.** Cleanse thoroughly with soap, and do not cauterize or suture the wound.
2. **Observe the animal.** If possible, capture and observe a dog or cat to see if it develops rabies. If a wild animal (bats, skunks, raccoons, foxes) is caught, it should be killed and tissue examined for rabies.
3. **Prophylaxis and vaccination** with rabies immune globulin and rabies vaccine:
   - If a captured or killed animal has rabies, definitely give prophylaxis and vaccinate.
   - If a wild animal (bats, skunks, raccoons, and foxes only) bites and escapes, give prophylaxis and vaccine.
   - If a dog or cat bites and escapes, do not give prophylaxis or vaccine unless the animal acted strangely and/or bit the patient without provocation and rabies is prevalent in the area (very rare).
   - Do not give prophylaxis or vaccine for bites by a rabbit or rodent (rats, mice, squirrels, chipmunks).

Syphilis screen: 1. VDRL / RPR 2. MHA-TP

Syphilis: screen with Venereal Disease Research Laboratory (VDRL) or rapid plasmin reagin (RPR) test. If the result is positive, confirm with the fluorescent treponemal antibody, absorbed test (FTA-ABS) or the microhemagglutination-*Treponema pallidum* test (MHA-TP). *T. pallidum* can be seen with darkfield microscopy but not with Gram stain. Screen all pregnant women with VDRL/RPR. Treat with penicillin; use erythromycin in penicillin-allergic patients. Three stages are listed below:

1. **Primary:** look for painless chancre (typically appears as a superficial ulcer with indurated, raised edges and a yellow base) that resolves on its own within 8 weeks.
2. **Secondary:** roughly 6 weeks to 18 months after infection. Look for condyloma lata, maculopapular rash (especially involving the palms of the hands and soles of the feet), and lymphadenopathy (see figure). Between secondary and tertiary stages is the **latent phase,** in which the disease is quiet and asymptomatic.

latent phase

3. **Tertiary:** occurs years after initial infection. Look for **gummas** (granulomas in many different organs), neurologic symptoms and signs (neurosyphilis, Argyll Robertson pupil, dementia, paresis, tabes dorsalis, Charcot joints), and/or thoracic aortic aneurysms. See gynecology section for other sexually transmissable diseases.

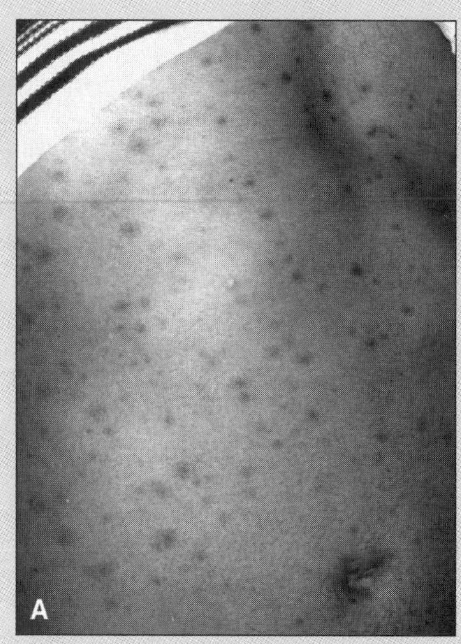

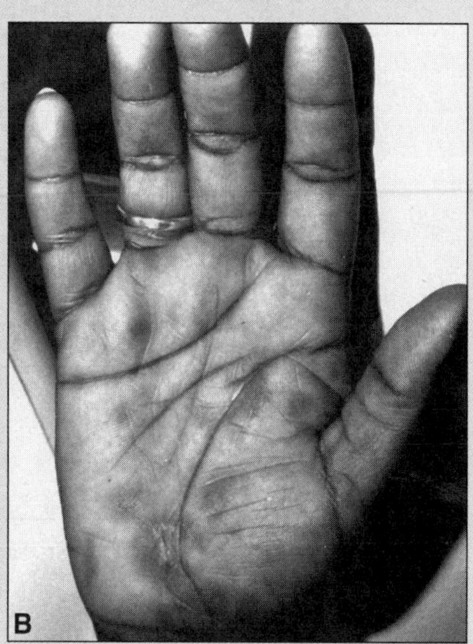

Syphiloderm of secondary syphilis. **A,** Hyperpigmented macules of secondary syphilis. The patient initially presented with a genital ulcer that was treated as chancroid. Note the strong similarity of these lesiosn to pityriasis rosea. **B,** Characteristic papulosquamous lesions of secondary syphilis on the palm. (From Fitzpatrick FE, Aeling JL: Dermatology Secrets. Philadelphia, Hanley & Belfus, 1996, with permission.)

➤ ***CASE SCENARIO:*** What is the classic disease that can cause a false-positive result on the VDRL or RPR test? Lupus erythematosus.

Classic case scenarios and word associations

- Elderly person with community-acquired, typical pneumonia: *S. pneumoniae.*
- Child with community-acquired, typical pneumonia: *H. influenzae.*
- Lung infection in a patient with cystic fibrosis: *Pseudomonas* spp., *S. aureus.*
- Atypical pneumonia in a college student: *Mycoplasma* spp. (positive cold-agglutinin titer), *Chlamydia* spp.
- Lung infection in a child younger than 1 year: respiratory syncytial virus (RSV).
- Lung infection in a person with AIDS: *Pneumocystis carinii.*
- Patient stuck with a thorn or gardening: *Sporothrix schenkii* (see figure). Treat with ketoconazole. it's a fungus
- Aplastic crisis in sickle cell disease/other hemoglobinopathy: parvovirus B19.
- Sepsis after splenectomy (or autosplenectomy in sickle cell disease): *S. pneumoniae, H. influenzae, N. meningitidis* (encapsulated organisms).

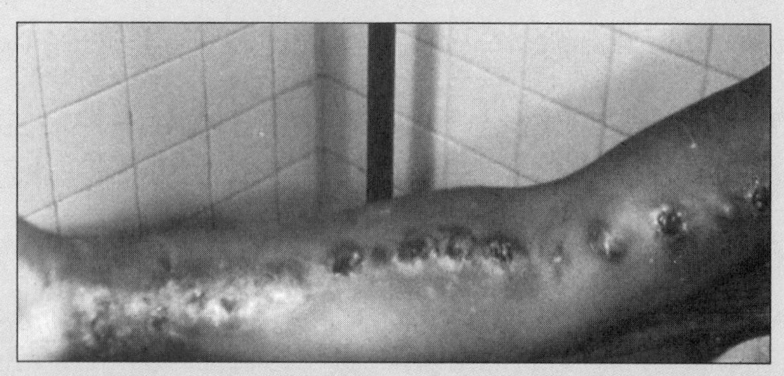

Sporotrichosis. *Sporothrix schenckii* is a dimorphic fungus that classically spreads via the lymphatics and can lead to lesion development in a linear manner along the lymphatic drainage pathway of the limb, as shown. (From du Vivier A: Tropical infections of the skin. In Atlas of Clinical Dermatology, 3rd ed. New York, Churchill Livingstone, 2002, pp 343–365, with permission.)

- Pneumonia in the southwest (California, Arizona): *Coccidioides imitis*. Treat with fluconazole or amphotericin B if severe.
- Pneumonia after cave exploring (or exposure to bird droppings) in Ohio and Mississippi River valleys: *Histoplasma capsulatum*.
- Pneumonia after being around a parrot or exotic bird: *Chlamydia psittaci*.
- Fungus ball or hemoptysis after tuberculosis cavitary disease: *Aspergillus* spp.
- Pneumonia in a patient with silicosis: tuberculosis.
- Diarrhea after hiking or drinking from a stream: *Giardia lamblia*.
- Pregnant women with cats: *Toxoplasma gondii*.
- Vitamin B_{12} deficiency and abdominal symptoms: *Diphyllobothrium latum*.
- Seizures with ring-enhancing brain lesion on CT: *Taenia solium* (cysticercosis) or Toxoplasmosis.
- Bladder cancer (squamous cell) in Middle East and Africa: *Schistosoma hematobium*.
- Worm infection in infants: *Enterobius* spp. (positive tape test, perianal itching).
- Fever, muscle pain, eosinophilia, and periorbital edema after eating raw meat: *Trichinella spiralis* (trichinosis).
- Gastroenteritis in young children: rotavirus.
- Food poisoning after eating reheated rice: *Bacillus cereus*.
- Food poisoning after eating raw seafood: *Vibrio parahemolyticus*.
- Diarrhea after traveling to Mexico: *E. coli* (Montezuma's revenge).
- Diarrhea after antibiotics: *Clostridium difficile* (treat with metronidazole or vancomycin).
- Infant paralyzed after eating honey: *Clostridium botulinum* (toxin blocks acetylcholine release).
- Genital lesions in children in the absence of sexual abuse or activity: Molluscum contagiosum virus.
- Cellulitis from cat or dog bites: *Pasteurella multocida* (some physicians treat cat and dog bites with prophylactic ampicillin).
- Slaughterhouse worker with fever: *Brucella* spp.
- Pneumonia after being in a hotel or near air conditioner or water tower: *Legionella pneumophila* (treat with azithromycin).
- Burn wound infection with blue-green color: *Pseudomonas* spp. (*S. aureus* also is common but is not associated with a blue-green color).

Staining hints: gram-positive organisms are blue/purple, and gram-negative organisms are red (as seen on a slide).

- Gram-positive cocci in chains = streptococci.
- Gram-positive cocci in clusters = staphylococci.
- Gram-positive cocci in pairs (diplococci) = *S. pneumoniae*.
- Gram-negative coccobacilli (small rods) = *Hemophilus* spp.
- Gram-negative diplococci = *Neisseria* spp. (urethritis, septic arthritis, meningitis) or *Moraxella* spp. (lungs, sinusitis).
- Gram-negative rod that is plump and has thick capsule ("mucoid" appearance) = *Klebsiella* spp.
- Gram-positive rods that form spores = *Clostridium*, *Bacillus* spp. (food poisoning from reheated rice).
- Pseudohyphae = *Candida* spp.
- Acid-fast organisms = *Mycobacterium*, *Nocardia* spp.

- Gram-positive with sulfur granules = *Actinomyces* spp. (pelvic inflammatory disease in women who use intrauterine devices; rare cause of neck mass or cervical adenitis).
- Silver-staining = *Pneumocystis carinii* and cat-scratch disease
- Positive India ink preparation (with thick capsule) = *Cryptococcus* spp. (see figure)

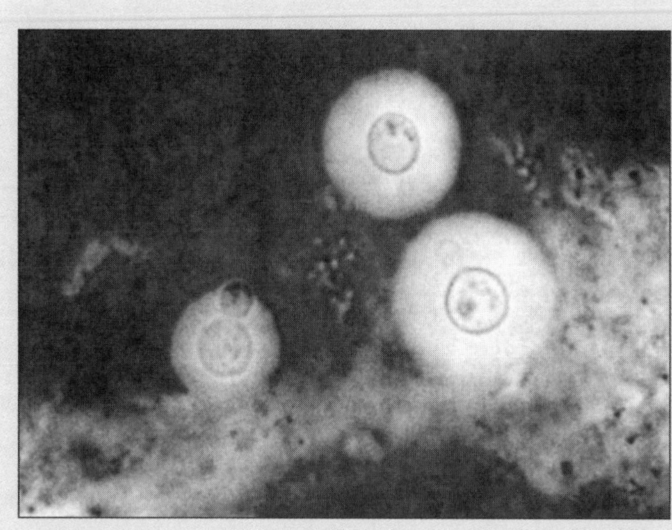

Positive India ink preparation of the cerebrospinal fluid in a patient with cryptococcal meningitis. Note the rounding of the yeast, which is classically budding. (From Cunha BA: Infectious Disease Pearls. Philadelphia, Hanley & Belfus, 1999, with permission.)

- Spirochete = *Treponema, Leptospira* spp. (both seen only on darkfield microscopy), *Borrelia* spp. (seen with regular light microscope).

NEPHROLOGY

Acute Renal Failure

Look for a progressive rise in **creatinine** and **blood urea nitrogen (BUN),** metabolic acidosis, **hyperkalemia,** and hypervolemia (pulmonary rales, elevated jugular venous pressure, dilutional hyponatremia, peripheral edema). Three categories to think about:

1. **Prerenal** (most common): hypovolemia (dehydration, hemorrhage), cardiac/"pump" failure, renovascular hypertension. Look for **BUN:creatinine ratio > 15 or 20.** Patients have signs of hypovolemia (e.g., tachycardia, weak pulse) or congestive heart failure. Give intravenous fluids and/or blood (if needed) for hypovolemia, diuretics (e.g., furosemide) for failure. Other causes are sepsis (treat the sepsis and give IV fluids) and liver failure (hepatorenal syndrome; treat supportively).

   ➤ **CASE SCENARIO:** A 45-year-old man has a massive heart attack and develops renal failure. How may the two conditions be related? If the massive heart attack caused heart failure (not uncommon), it would prevent adequate perfusion of the kidneys and cause prerenal kidney failure. Digitalis/dobutamine and diuretics may reverse the renal failure by optimizing cardiac function.

2. **Postrenal:** the classic cause is **benign prostatic hypertrophy (BPH).** Watch for a man over 50 with symptoms of BPH (hesitancy, dribbling) and anuria; hydronephrosis is seen bilaterally on ultrasound. Treat with catheterization (suprapubic catheterization, if needed) to relieve the obstruction and prevent further renal damage. Then consider surgery (transurethral resection of the prostate [TURP]).

   ➤ **CASE SCENARIO:** A patient has urolithiasis and acute renal failure with no history of kidney disease. How did the stone cause renal failure? It probably did not—unless the patient had bilateral stones or a bladder neck stone. A unilateral ureteral stone does not usually cause failure, because the other kidney, *if normal,* picks up the slack.

3. **Renal: acute tubular necrosis** is the most common type. Examples of renal causes:
   - **IV contrast:** be careful in patients with diabetes and/or renal disease, as you may precipitate renal failure. Consider pre-hydrating patient with IV fluids if contrast is needed.
   - **Lupus erythematosus:** look for malar rash, arthritis, and other typical features. Renal failure is a major cause of morbidity and mortality in patients with lupus.
   - **Toxins/medications:** chronic NSAID use can cause **papillary necrosis** or acute tubular necrosis. Other implicated drugs include cyclosporine, **aminoglycosides,** and methicillin.
   - **Goodpasture syndrome:** due to antiglomerular basement membrane antibodies (**linear immunofluorescence pattern** on renal biopsy), which also react with the lungs. Look for a young man with hemoptysis, dyspnea, and renal failure. Treat with steroids and/or cyclophosphamide.
   - **Wegener granulomatosis** also has lung and kidney involvement. Look for **sinonasal involvement** (bloody nose, nasal perforation, sinusitis) or hemoptysis and pleurisy as presenting symptoms. Patients have positive **antineutrophilic cytoplasmic antibody (ANCA)** titer. Treat with cyclophosphamide.
   - **Glomerulonephritis:** prototype is poststreptococcal disease; usually seen in children with a history of upper respiratory infection or streptococcal infection 1–3 weeks earlier. They present with edema, hypervolemia, hypertension, and hematuria/oliguria. **RBC casts** on urinalysis clinch the diagnosis. Treat supportively.

     ➤ *CASE SCENARIO:* A 22-year-old man comes into the emergency room with nausea and muscle pain after running a marathon in hot weather. His creatinine and BUN are very high, but he has no history of renal failure. What is the cause of renal failure? What lab value goes with this condition? Rhabdomyolysis, which can result from strenuous exercise (e.g., marathon), alcohol, burns or muscle trauma, heat stroke, or neuroleptic malignant syndrome. Muscle breaks down and plugs up the renal filtration system. Look for very high levels of **creatine phosphokinase (CPK)** or **creatine kinase (CK).** Patients also may have myoglobinuria. Treat with hydration and diuretics.

In all cases of acute renal failure, **dialysis** may be required. Indications for dialysis include uremic encephalopathy, **pericarditis,** severe metabolic acidosis (roughly, pH < 7.25), heart failure, and **hyperkalemia** severe enough to cause an arrhythmia.

Chronic Renal Failure

Basically, any of the disorders that cause acute renal failure can cause chronic renal failure (CRF) if the insult is severe or prolonged. Most cases of CRF are due to **diabetes** (number-one cause) or **hypertension** (many patients have both). Another fairly common cause is polycystic kidney disease. Look for multiple cysts in the kidney, family history (usually **autosomal dominant;** the autosomal recessive form presents in children), hypertension, hematuria, palpable renal masses, berry aneurysms in the circle of Willis, and cysts in the liver.

Metabolic derangements due to CRF

1. Azotemia (high BUN/creatinine levels)
2. Metabolic acidosis
3. Hyperkalemia
4. Fluid retention (can cause hypertension, edema, heart failure, and pulmonary edema)
5. Hypocalcemia/hyperphosphatemia (impaired vitamin D production; bone loss leads to renal osteodystrophy)
6. Anemia due to lack of erythropoietin (synthetic erythropoietin may be given to correct the disorder)
7. Anorexia, nausea, and vomiting (from build-up of toxins)
8. CNS disturbances (mental status changes and even convulsions or coma from toxin build-up)

9. Bleeding (due to disordered platelet function)
10. Uremic pericarditis (**friction rub** may be heard on physical exam)
11. Skin pigmentation and pruritus (skin turns yellowish brown and itches due to metabolic byproducts)
12. Increased susceptibility to infection (due to impaired cellular immunity)

Treatment: regular dialysis, water-soluble vitamins (removed during dialysis), phosphate restriction and phosphate binders (calcium carbonate), erythropoietin, and control of hypertension. The only cure is renal transplant.

Urinary Tract Infection

Urinary tract infections (UTIs) in adults are much more common in women (by a 10–20:1 ratio). Most are caused by *Escherichia coli*; other enteric organisms also may be implicated. Look for urinary **urgency, dysuria, suprapubic or low back pain,** and low-grade fever. The gold standard for diagnosis is urine culture. At the least, get a mid-stream sample; a catheterized sample or suprapubic tap is best (though rarely indicated in uncomplicated cases). Urinalysis shows white blood cells, bacteria, positive **leukocyte esterase,** and/or positive **nitrite.** Treat with trimethoprim/ sulfamethoxazole, amoxicillin, nitrofurantoin, or first-generation cephalosporin for 5–10 days.

- Some women get recurrent UTIs related to sexual activity and can be given antibiotics to take after intercourse.
- Conditions that promote urinary stasis (enlarged prostate, pregnancy, stones, neurogenic bladder, vesicoureteral reflux) or bacterial colonization (indwelling catheter, fecal incontinence, surgical instrumentation) predispose to UTI. They also predispose to ascending UTI (pyelonephritis) and bacteremia/sepsis.
- Pyelonephritis (see figure) is also usually due to *E. coli.* The hallmark on physical exam is **costovertebral angle tenderness** with high fevers and shaking chills. Get blood and urine cultures. Most patients should be admitted to the hospital for inpatient treatment with intravenous antibiotics. If the patient does not improve within 48–72 hours, consider a CT scan to look for a renal abscess, which may need surgical drainage.

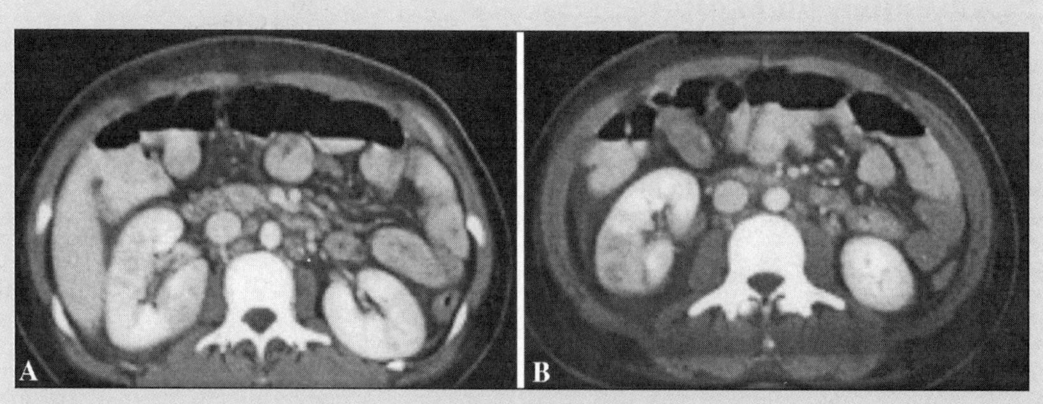

A and **B**, Pyelonephritis. The right kidney is swollen, and there are multiple wedge-shaped areas of decreased parenchymal enhancement. (From Katz DS, Math KR, Groskin SA (eds): Radiology Secrets. Philadelphia, Hanley & Belfus, 1998, p 187, with permission.)

➤ **CASE SCENARIO:** An asymptomatic 40-year old quadriplegic man with an indwelling urinary catheter has 3+ bacteria and 1+ WBCs in his urine on a routine urinalysis. Should you treat him? No. Asymptomatic bacteriuria is not treated, especially in chronically catheterized patients, who develop colonization and almost always have bacteria in the urine.

- ➤ ***CASE SCENARIO:*** On a routine urinalysis, a pregnant woman has 3+ bacteria on a mid-stream urine sample. She is asymptomatic and afebrile. Should you treat her? Yes. Asymptomatic bacteriuria has a high risk of progression to pyelonephritis in pregnancy. Use amoxicillin.

Other Conditions

Nephrotic syndrome: proteinuria (> 3.5 gm/day), hypoalbuminemia, edema (the classic example is morning periorbital edema), and hyperlipidemia/lipiduria. In children, nephrotic syndrome usually is due to ***minimal change disease*** (see loss of podocyte foot processes on electron microscopy), which is often postinfectious. Measure a 24-hour urine protein to clinch the diagnosis. Treat with steroids. Causes in adults include diabetes, hepatitis B, amyloidosis, lupus, and drugs (gold, penicillamine, captopril).

Nephritic syndrome: oliguria, azotemia (rising BUN/creatinine), hypertension, and hematuria. Some proteinuria may be present, but not in the nephrotic range. Nephritic syndrome classically is due to post-streptococcal glomerulonephritis. Patients classically have ***RBC casts*** (a sign of glomerulonephritis).

ONCOLOGY

Blood dyscrasias:

TYPE	AGE	WHAT TO LOOK FOR IN CASE DESCRIPTION/BUZZ WORDS
Acute lymphoblastic leukemia (ALL)	Children (peak at 3–5 yr)	Pancytopenia (bleeding, fever, anemia), radiation therapy, Down syndrome
Acute myelogenous leukemia (AML)	> 30 yr	Pancytopenia (bleeding, fever, anemia), Auer rods, disseminated intravascular coagulation
Chronic myelogenous leukemia (CML)	30–50 yr	WBC count > 50,000, Philadelphia chromosome, blast crisis, splenomegaly
Chronic lymphocytic leukemia (CLL)	> 50 yr	Male gender, lymphadenopathy, lymphocytosis, infections, smudge cells, splenomegaly
Hairy cell leukemia	Adults	Blood smear with hair-like projections, splenomegaly
Mycosis fungoides/ Sézary syndrome	> 50 yr	Plaque-like, itchy skin rash that does not improve with treatment, blood smear with cerebriform nuclei ("butt cells"), Pautrier abscesses in epidermis (see figure)

Mycosis fungoides-Sézary syndrome. Abnormal cells in the peripheral blood with characteristic cerebriform nuclei and scant cytoplasm (i.e., "butt" cells) are classic. (From Hoffbrand AV, Pettit JE: Chronic lymphoid leukaemias. In Hoffbrand AV, Pettit JE (eds): Color Atlas of Clinical Hematology, 3rd ed. St. Louis, Mosby, 2000, pp 177–190, with permission.)

(Table continued on next page.)

TYPE	AGE	WHAT TO LOOK FOR IN CASE DESCRIPTION/BUZZ WORDS
Burkitt lymphoma	Children	Associated with Epstein-Barr virus (in Africa)
CNS B-cell lymphoma	Adults	HIV/AIDS
T-cell leukemia	Adults	HTLV-1 is one cause.
Hodgkin disease	15–34 yr	Reed-Sternberg cells, cervical lymhadenopathy, night sweats
Non-Hodgkin lymphoma	Any age	Small follicular type has best prognosis, large diffuse type has worst; primary tumor may be located in GI tract
Myelodysplasia/ myelofibrosis	> 50 yr	Anemia, teardrop cells, "dry tap" on bone marrow biopsy, high mean corpuscular volume and red cell distribution index; associated with CML
Multiple myeloma	> 40 yr	Bence-Jones protein (IgG = 50%, IgA = 25%), osteolytic lesions, high calcium level (see figure)
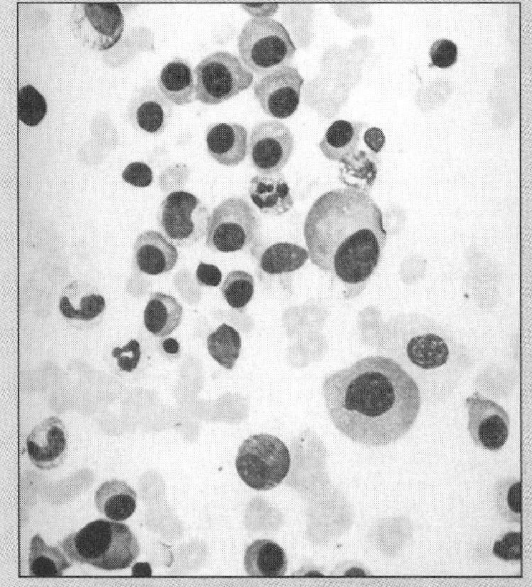		Multiple myeloma. The majority of cells seen in the bone marrow are atypical plasma cells. (From Hoffbrand AV, Pettit JE: Myeloma and related conditions. In Hoffbrand AV, Pettit JE (eds): Color Atlas of Clinical Hematology, 3rd ed. St. Louis, Mosby, 2000, pp 233–246, with permission.)
Waldenstrom disease	> 40 yr	Hyperviscosity, IgM spike, cold agglutinins (Raynaud phenomenon with cold sensitivity)
Polycythemia vera	> 40 yr	High hemoglobin, pruritus (after hot bath/shower). Use phlebotomy
Primary thrombo-cythemia	> 50 yr	Platelet count usually > 1,000,000/µl; patients may have bleeding or thrombosis

Cancer statistics:

OVERALL HIGHEST INCIDENCE		OVERALL HIGHEST MORTALITY RATE	
MALE	**FEMALE**	**MALE**	**FEMALE**
1. Prostate	1. Breast	1. Lung	1. Lung
2. Lung	2. Lung	2. Prostate	2. Breast
3. Colon	3. Colon	3. Colon	3. Colon

In children and younger adults, **leukemia** is the most common malignancy. Remember, however, that ***age*** has the most signifigant impact on the incidence and mortality of cancer (number one risk factor, but not modifiable so rarely talked about). In the U.S., the incidence of cancer roughly doubles every 5 years after age 25; therefore, cancer most commonly affects older adults. **Smoking** is the most significant modifiable risk factor.

- **CASE SCENARIO:** What is the most common malignancy seen in the liver? Metastatic disease! Do not be fooled into saying that hepatocellular carcinoma is the most common malignancy of the liver if metastatic cancer is a choice. Do not assume that the question refers to a primary tumor unless it specifically says so.
- **CASE SCENARIO:** A 73-year-old man with known stage IV prostate cancer presents with local spinal pain and acute onset of hyperreflexia and muscle weakness in the lower extremities. What should you do first? What factor is most closely linked to final outcome? Metastases to the spine can cause cord compression (local spinal pain, reflex changes, weakness, sensory loss, paralysis). This scenario is an emergency. The first step is to start high-dose corticosteroids; then order an MRI. The next step is is treat with radiation. Surgical decompression is used if radiation fails or the tumor is known not to be radiosensitive. The final outcome is most closely linked to pretreatment function. Do not wait to give steroids.

Genetic predisposition to cancer:

DISEASE/SYNDROME	INHERITANCE	TYPE OF CANCER (IN ORDER OF MOST LIKELY)/OTHER INFORMATION
Retinoblastoma	Autosomal dominant	Retinoblastoma, osteogenic sarcoma (later in life)
MEN, type I	Autosomal dominant	Parathyroid, pituitary, pancreas (islet cell tumors)
MEN, type IIa	Autosomal dominant	Thyroid (medullary cancer), parathyroid, pheochromocytoma
MEN, type IIb	Autosomal dominant	Thyroid (medullary cancer), pheochromocytoma, mucosal neuromas
Familial polyposis coli	Autosomal dominant	Hundreds of colon polyps that *always* result in colon cancer
Gardner syndrome	Autosomal dominant	Familial polyposis plus osteomas and soft tissue tumors
Turcot syndrome	Autosomal dominant	Familial polyposis plus central nervous system tumors
Peutz-Jeghers syndrome	Autosomal dominant	Look for perioral freckles (see figure) and multiple noncancerous GI polyps; increased incidence of noncolon cancer (stomach, breast, ovaries); no increased risk of colon cancer
Neurofibromatosis, type 1	Autosomal dominant	Mulitple neurofibromas, café-au-lait spots; increased number of pheochromocytomas, bone cysts, Wilms tumor, leukemia, gliomas
Neurofibromatosis, type 2	Autosomal dominant	Bilateral acoustic schwannomas, meningiomas

Peutz-Jeghers syndrome. Round, pigmented macules occur around the mouth and particularly on the lower lips. (From du Vivier A: Developmental disorders of the skin. In du Vivier A (ed): Atlas of Clinical Dermatology, 3rd ed. New York, Churchill-Livingstone, 2002, pp 439–488, with permission.)

(Table continued on next page.)

DISEASE/SYNDROME	INHERITANCE	TYPE OF CANCER (IN ORDER OF MOST LIKELY)/OTHER INFORMATION
Tuberous sclerosis (see figure)	Autosomal dominant	Adenoma sebaceum, seizures, mental retardation, glial nodules in brain; increased renal angiomyolipomas, and cardiac rhabdomyomas.
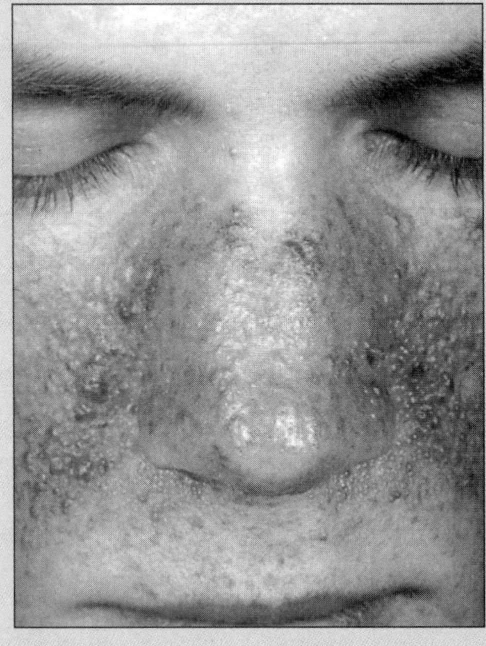		Adenoma sebaceum in tuberous sclerosis. Also known as angiofibromas, these lesions are small red or yellow tumors that typically first appear in childhood and occur symmetrically around the nose, chin, cheeks, and/or forehead. (From du Vivier A: Developmental disorders of the skin. In du Vivier A (ed): Atlas of Clinical Dermatology, 3rd ed. New York, Churchill-Livingstone, 2002, pp 439–488, with permission.)
Von Hippel-Lindau disease	Autosomal dominant	Hemangioblastomas in cerebellum, renal cell cancer; cysts in liver and/or kidney
Xeroderma pigmentosa	Autosomal recessive	Skin cancer
Albinism	Autosomal recessive	Skin cancer
Down syndrome	Trisomy 21	Leukemia

MEN = multiple endocrine neoplasia.

Other diseases associated with an increased incidence of cancer are immunodeficiency syndromes, Bloom syndrome, and Fanconi anemia. Breast, ovarian, and colon cancer are well known to have familial tendencies (as well as some other types of cancers), but rarely can a Mendelian inheritance pattern be shown (e.g., BRCA1 gene for breast cancer)

Alterable risk factors for development of cancer:

CANCER TYPE	AVOIDABLE RISK FACTOR(S) TO REDUCE INCIDENCE (GREATEST IMPACT LISTED FIRST)
Lung	Smoking, asbestos (also nickel, radon, coal, arsenic, chromium, uranium)
Mesothelioma	Asbestos
Leukemia	Chemotherapy, radiotherapy, other immunosuppressive drugs, benzene
Bladder	Smoking, aniline dyes (rubber and dye industry), schistosomiasis (in immigrants)
Skin	Ultraviolet light exposure, coal tar, arsenic
Liver	Alcohol, vinyl chloride (liver angiosarcomas), aflatoxins
Oral cavity	Smoking, alcohol

(Table continued on next page.)

CANCER TYPE	AVOIDABLE RISK FACTOR(S) TO REDUCE INCIDENCE (GREATEST IMPACT LISTED FIRST)
Pharynx/larynx	Smoking, alcohol
Esophagus	Smoking, alcohol
Pancreas	Smoking
Renal cell	Smoking
Stomach	Alcohol, nitrosamines/nitrites (from smoked meats/fish)
Clear cell cancer	Patient's mother should avoid diethylstilbesterol (DES) during pregnancy
Colorectal	High-fat, low-fiber diet
Breast	High-fat, low-fiber diet
Cervical	Smoking, sex, high parity
Thyroid	Childhood head, neck, or chest irradiation
Endometrial	Unopposed estrogen stimulation, obesity
All cancer	Smoking (alcohol is probably second)

Lung Cancer

Lung cancer is the number-one cause of overall cancer mortality in the U.S. The incidence is rising in women because of increased smoking. Look for **change in a chronic cough in a smoker**—the more pack years of tobacco use, the more suspicious you should be. Patients also may present with hemoptysis, pneumonia, and/or weight loss. Chest x-ray (CXR) may show pleural effusion; put a needle in the fluid and examine for malignant cells. After CXR, get a CT scan and tissue biopsy to confirm the diagnosis and define the histologic type. Non-small-cell cancer may be treated with surgery if the cancer remains within lung parenchyma. Small-cell cancer is treated with chemotherapy only; early metastases make surgery inappropriate.

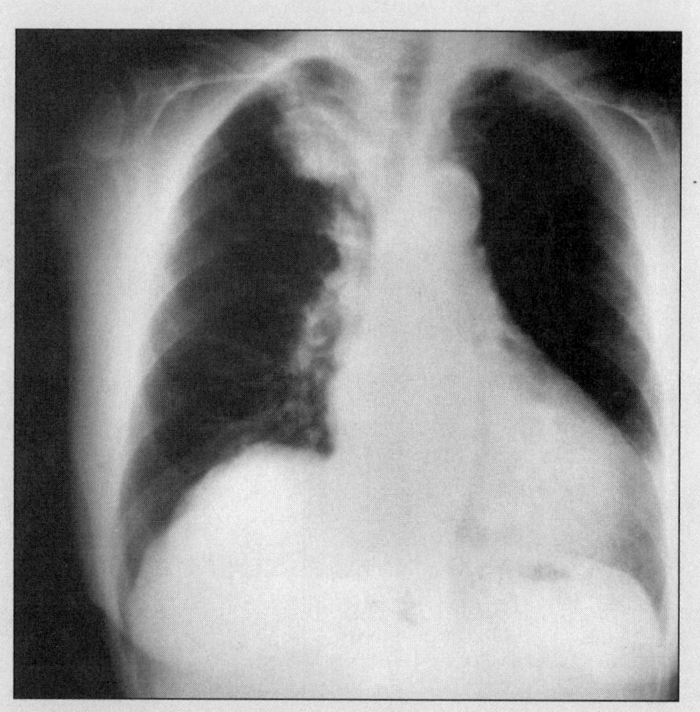

Right apical lung mass, also known as a Pancoast tumor. (From Sahn SA, Heffner JE: Critical Care Pearls, 2nd ed. Philadelphia, Hanley & Belfus, 1998, with permission.)

Weird (and tested) consequences of lung cancer

1. **Horner syndrome:** due to invasion of cervical sympathetic chain by an apical (Pancoast) tumor (see figure). Look for unilateral **ptosis, miosis,** and **anhidrosis** (no sweating).
2. **Diaphragm paralysis:** due to phrenic nerve involvement.
3. **Hoarseness:** due to recurrent laryngeal nerve involvement.
4. **Superior vena cava syndrome:** due to compression of superior vena cava with impaired venous drainage.

Look for edema and plethora (redness) of the neck and face and CNS symptoms (headache, visual symptoms, altered mental status).

5. **Cushing syndrome:** due to production of adrenocorticotropic hormone (ACTH) by a small-cell carcinoma.
6. **Syndrome of inappropriate antidiuretic hormone** (SIADH): due to ADH production by a small-cell carcinoma.
7. **Hypercalcemia:** due to bone metastases or production of parathyroid hormone by a squamous-cell carcinoma.
8. **Eaton-Lambert syndrome:** myasthenia gravis-like disease due to lung cancer that spares the ocular muscles. The muscles become stronger with repetitive stimulation (opposite of myasthenia gravis).

Solitary pulmonary nodule on chest x-ray (CXR). The first step is to compare the current x-ray with previous chest x-rays. If the nodule has remained the same size for > 2 years, it is generally not cancer. If no old films are available and the patient is older than 35 or has a smoking history, order a CT scan. If the CT scan is not definitive, do a biopsy of the nodule (via bronchoscopy or transthoracic biopsy, if possible) for a tissue diagnosis. If the patient is younger than 35 or has no smoking history, the cause is most likely infection (tuberculosis or fungi), hamartoma, or collagen vascular disease. Such patients can often undergo observation and follow-up with repeat CT or CXR.

Breast Cancer

Roughly 1 in 8–10 women will develop breast cancer in their lifetime.

Risk factors for breast cancer

1. History of breast cancer (biggest risk factor)
2. Family history in first-degree relatives
3. Age (breast cancer is rare before age 30; the incidence increases with age)
4. Early menarche, late menopause, and late first pregnancy or nulliparity (more menstrual cycles = higher risk)
5. Atypical hyperplasia of the breast
6. Radiation exposure before age 30

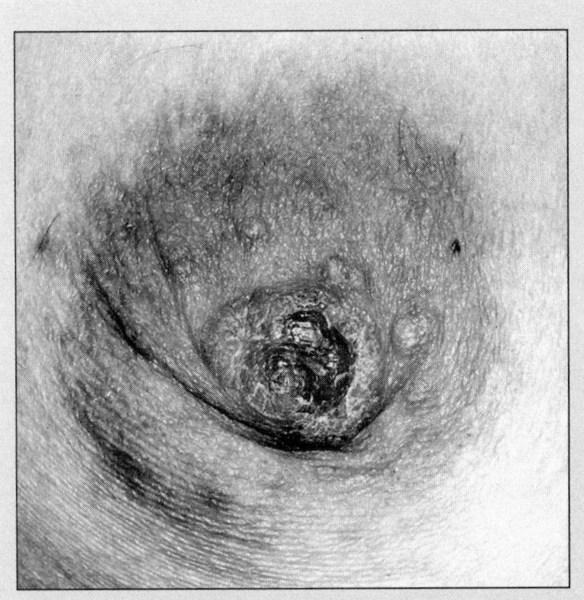

Paget disease of the nipple. (From James EC, Corry RJ, Perry FJ: Principles of Basic Surgical Practice. Philadelphia, Hanley & Belfus, 1987, with permission.]

The debate about breast cancer and birth control pills and estrogen replacement continues. A woman with a history of breast cancer should not receive estrogen (although this controversy is unlikely to appear on the boards).

Signs and symptoms that should make you think that a breast mass is cancer until proved otherwise: fixation of breast mass to the chest wall or overlying skin, satellite nodules or ulcers on the skin, lymphedema (also called **peau d'orange**), matted or fixed axillary lymph nodes, inflammatory skin changes (red, hot skin with enlargement of the breast due to inflammatory cancer of the breast), prolonged unilateral, scaling erosion of the nipple with or without discharge (may be Paget disease of the nipple; see figure), microcalcifications on mammography, and *any new breast mass in a postmenopausal woman.*

The **conservative approach** is best on the boards. In women over 35, when in doubt, consider biopsy of a palpable breast mass, especially if the woman has any risk factors. If the question does not want you to biopsy the mass, it will give clues that the mass is not a cancer (such as bilateral, lumpy breasts that become symptomatic with every menses and have no dominant mass or age < 30 years old).

In **women under 30,** breast cancer is extremely rare. With a discrete breast mass in this age group, think of **fibroadenoma.** Observe the mass over a few menstrual cycles before considering biopsy. Fibroadenomas are usually round, rubbery-feeling, and freely movable.

The **most common histologic type** of breast cancer is invasive ductal carcinoma.

In patients with a **palpable breast mass,** the decision to do a biopsy is a clinical one. A benign mammogram should not deter you from doing a biopsy. Furthermore, a lesion that is detected on mammography and looks suspicious should be biopsied, even if not palpable (needle localization biopsy).

Mammograms in women under 35 are rarely helpful (breast tissue is too dense to see cancer), unless the mammogram is ordered to have a baseline before removal of a breast mass.

Tamoxifen (or other endocrine therapy) generally improves survival if a breast cancer is estrogen receptor-positive—and even more so if the tumor is also progesterone receptor-positive.

Mastectomy vs. breast-conserving surgery plus radiation: considered equal in efficacy. In either, do an axillary node dissection (or a sentinel node dissection) to determine spread to the nodes. If nodes are positive, give chemotherapy.

Prostate Cancer

Risk factors

1. **Age** (not seen in men < 40; the incidence increases with age; 60% of men > 80 have prostate cancer)
2. **Race:** black > white > Asian.

Patients present late, because early prostate cancer is asymptomatic. Look for BPH-like symptoms (hesitancy, dysuria, frequency) with hematuria and/or elevated prostate-specific antigen (PSA) or acid phosphatase. Acid phosphatase is elevated only when the cancer has broken through the capsule; for this reason, it was replaced with the more sensitive PSA as a screening tool. Look for prostate irregularities (nodules) on rectal exam. Patients may present with **back pain from vertebral metastases** (osteoblastic, not lytic lesions).

Treatment: local prostate cancer is treated with surgery (prostatectomy) or radiation. With metastases, patients have several options for hormonal therapy: orchiectomy, gonadotropin-releasing hormone agonist (**leuprolide**), androgen-receptor antagonist (flutamide), estrogen (diethylstilbesterol), and others (e.g., cyproterone). Standard chemotherapy rarely helps; radiation therapy is also used for pain due to bone metastases.

Colorectal Cancer

Risk factors

1. **Age** (incidence begins to increase after age 40; peak incidence at 60–75 years)
2. **Family history** (especially with familial polyposis and Gardner, Turcot, or Lynch syndrome)
3. **Inflammatory bowel disease** (ulcerative colitis > Crohn disease, but both increase risk)

4. **Low-fiber, high-fat diet** (weak evidence)

Presentation: patients may present with asymptomatic blood in stool (visible streaks of blood or guaiac-positive stool), **anemia** with right-sided colon cancer, and **change in stool caliber** ("pencil stool") or frequency (alternating constipation and frequency) with left-sided colon cancer. As with any cancer, look for weight loss.

Occult blood in the stool of a person > 40 years old should be considered colon cancer until proved otherwise. To rule out colon cancer, do either a flexible sigmoidoscopy and barium enema *or* a total colonoscopy. If you see any lesions with a flexible sigmoidoscope or barium enema, you need to do a total colonoscopy with removal and histologic examination of all polyps or lesions. For this reason, many physicians now start with colonoscopy.

Carcinoembryonic antigen (CEA) is often elevated with colon cancer, and a preoperative level is usually measured. After surgery to remove the tumor, CEA should return to normal levels. Periodic monitoring of CEA after surgery helps to detect recurrence before it is clinically apparent. CEA is *not* generally used as a screening tool for colon cancer; it is used only to follow known cancer.

Treatment is primarily surgical, with resection of involved bowel. Adjuvant chemotherapy is sometimes used (e.g., 5-fluorouracil and levamisole or leucovorin).

Metastases frequently go to the liver; if the metastasis is solitary, surgical resection may be attempted. With metastases elsewhere, chemotherapy or local ablative treatments (e.g., radiofrequency ablation, chemoembolization) are the only option, and prognosis is poor.

Colon cancer is a common cause of a **large bowel obstruction** in adults.

Pancreatic Cancer

The **classic presentation** for adenocarcinoma (most common type of pancreatic cancer; see figure) is a smoker in the 40–80-year-old range who has **weight loss and jaundice.** Patients may have epigastric pain, migratory thrombophlebitis (**Trousseau syndrome,** which also may be seen with other visceral cancers), or a palpable, nontender gallbladder (**Courvoisier sign**). Pancreatic cancer is more common in men than women, blacks than whites, and diabetics than nondiabetics. Surgery (Whipple procedure) is rarely curative, and prognosis is dismal.

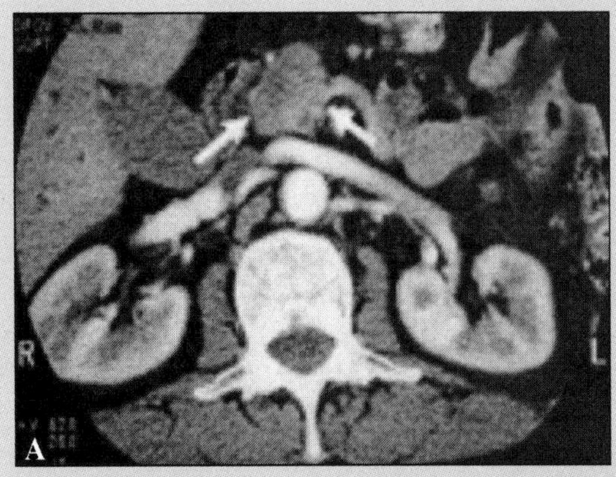

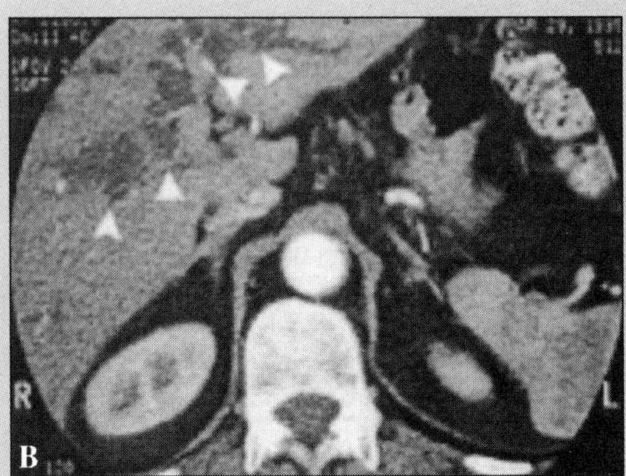

Small pancreatic head cancer (**A,** *arrows*) with resultant biliary dilatation (**B,** *arrowheads*). (From Katz DS, Math KR, Groskin SA (eds): Radiology Secrets. Philadelphia, Hanley & Belfus, 1998, p 128, with permission.)

Islet cell tumors

#1 1. **Insulinoma** (beta cell tumor): most common islet cell tumor. Look for two-thirds of ***Whipple's triad***: hypoglycemia (glucose < 50 mg/dl) and CNS symptoms due to hypoglycemia (confusion, stupor, loss of consciousness). As the good doctor, you provide the third part of Whipple's triad: give glucose to relieve symptoms. About 90% of insulinomas are benign; the cure is resection (if possible).

2. **Gastrinoma:** ***Zollinger-Ellison syndrome*** is gastrinoma plus acid hypersecretion and peptic ulcers (gastrin causes acid secretion). Peptic ulcers are often ***multiple and resistant to therapy;*** they may be found in unusual locations (distal duodenum or jejunum). More than half are malignant.

3. **Glucagonoma** (alpha cell tumor): hyperglycemia with high glucagon level and ***migratory necrotizing skin erythema.***

Ovarian Cancer

Presentation: ovarian cancer usually presents late with weight loss, pelvic mass, ***ascites*** and/or bowel obstruction in a post-menopausal woman. Any ***ovarian enlargement in a postmenopausal woman is cancer until proved otherwise.*** In women of reproductive age, most ovarian enlargements are benign. Ultrasound is a good first test to evaluate an ovarian lesion. Treatment consists of debulking surgery and chemotherapy; the prognosis is usually poor. Most ovarian cancers arise from the ovarian epithelium.
#1 ***Serous cystadenocarcinoma*** is the most common type; ***psammoma bodies*** often are seen on histopathologic exam.

Germ cell and stromal tumors make good questions:

1. **Teratoma/dermoid cyst:** look for a description of the tumor to include skin, hair, and/or teeth (which may show up on x-ray).
2. **Sertoli-Leydig cell tumor:** causes virilization (hirsutism, receding hairline, deepening voice, clitoromegaly)
3. **Granulosa/theca cell tumor:** causes feminization and precocious puberty

Meigs syndrome: ovarian fibroma, ascites, and right hydrothorax. TRIAD

Krukenberg tumor: stomach cancer with metastases to the ovaries.

Cervical Cancer

Pap smears decrease the incidence and mortality of invasive cervical cancer. Give every female patient a Pap smear if she is due, even if she presents with an unrelated complaint.

Follow any dysplastic Pap smear with colposcopy, directed biopsies, and endocervical curettage. If the Pap smear shows microinvasive cancer, proceed to conization. Invasive cervical cancer begins in the transformation zone and usually presents with vaginal bleeding or discharge (postcoital bleeding, intermenstrual spotting, or abnormal menstrual bleeding). Women with invasive cancer require surgery and/or radiation.

Risk factors for cervical cancer

1. **Age** < 20 years old at first coitus, pregnancy, or marriage
2. **Multiple sexual partners** (role of ***human papillomavirus*** and possibly herpes virus) or sexual relations with a promiscuous person
3. **Smoking**

4. **Low socioeconomic status**
5. **High parity** (which protects against endometrial and breast cancer)

Uterine Cancer

Presentation: ***Postmenopausal vaginal or uterine bleeding is cancer until proved otherwise,*** and endometrial cancer is the most common type to present in this fashion (fourth most common cancer in women). Any woman with unexplained gynecologic bleeding that persists needs a Pap smear, endocervical curettage, and endometrial biopsy.

Risk factors for endometrial cancer

1. **Obesity**
2. **Nulliparity**
3. **Late menopause**
4. **Diabetes**
5. **Hypertension**
6. **Gallbladder disease**
7. **Chronic, unopposed estrogen stimulation.** Examples include ***polycystic ovary*** (i.e. Stein-Levinthal) ***syndrome,*** estrogen-secreting neoplasm (e.g., granulosa/theca cell tumor), and estrogen replacement therapy (only if taken without progesterone).

Most uterine cancers are *adenocarcinomas* and spread by direct extension. The usual treatment includes surgery and radiation.

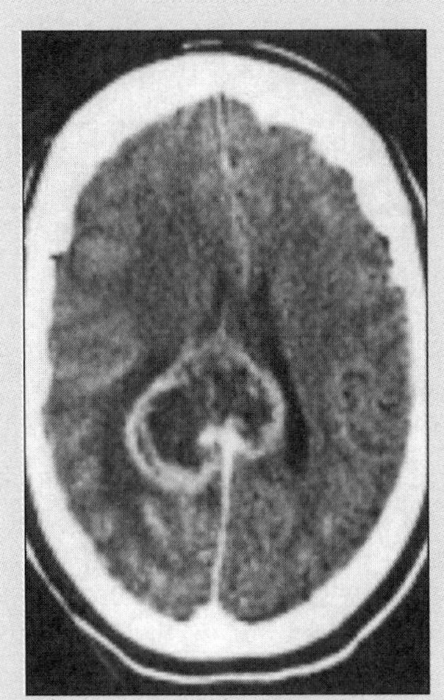

Contrast-enhanced CT image of a butterfly glioma. This tumor has grown from the right side to the left, crossing through the splenium of the corpus callosum. (From Katz DS, Math KR, Groskin SA (eds): Radiology Secrets. Philadelphia, Hanley & Belfus, 1998, p 352, with permission.)

Miscellaneous Neoplasms

Brain tumors: in adults, two-thirds of primary tumors are *supratentorial;* metastatic disease is as common as primary tumors. Look for new-onset seizures, neurologic deficits, or signs of intracranial hypertension (headache, blurred vision, ***papilledema,*** nausea, and projectile vomiting). The most common type is a glioma (most are intraparenchymal astrocytomas, with little or no calcification; see figure), followed by meningioma (often calcified and located external to the brain substance). Treatment is surgical removal, which may be followed by radiation and chemotherapy, depending on the tumor.

➤ **CASE SCENARIO:** A 24-year-old obese woman has headaches, papilledema, and vomiting with negative CT/MRI scans. What tumor does she have? Pseudotumor cerebri (not a neoplasm). Lumbar puncture reveals high pressure with no other abnormalities. Weight loss may help. Repeat lumbar punctures may be needed to lower intracranial pressure and prevent optic nerve damage and vision problems.

➤ **CASE SCENARIO:** A 9-year-old boy presents with visual disturbances, headaches, and vomiting. A skull x-ray shows calcification in the region of the sella turcica. What tumor does the child probably have? A craniopharyngioma (remnant of Rathke pouch), which is often heavily calcified.

Testicular cancer: most common solid malignancy in adult men < 30 years old. The main risk factor is cryptorchidism. Transillumination and ultrasound help to distinguish **hydrocele** (which is fluid-filled and transilluminates) from cancer (which is solid). The most common type is **seminoma** (radiosensitive).

Pituitary tumors: look for **bitemporal hemianopsia;** order an MRI if it is present. The most common type is **prolactinoma** (high prolactin levels with galactorrhea and menstrual/sexual dysfunction). Other types may cause hyperthyroidism or Cushing disease.

> ➤ ***CASE SCENARIO:*** A 34-year-old schizophrenic man taking haloperidol presents with galactorrhea, decreased libido, and an elevated prolactin level. Why? Because of the haloperidol, a dopamine antagonist. Dopamine inhibits prolactin production.

Nasopharyngeal carcinoma: most common in Asians; remember association with **Epstein-Barr virus.**

Esophageal cancer (see figure): classically associated with weight loss, possible anemia, and complaints that "my food is sticking," which progress to dysphagia for liquids in chronic smokers and drinkers over age 40 due to squamous cell carcinoma. However, adenocarcinoma is now more common than squamous cell carcinoma, and this is due to GERD/Barrett metaplasia, so tobacco and alcohol are not significant risk factors. Esophageal cancer typically presents late, because early disease is asymptomatic.

> ➤ ***CASE SCENARIO:*** In a 52-year-old man with severe heartburn, endoscopy reveals Barrett metaplasia in the distal esophagus. He begins taking omeprazole and feels better. What kind of follow-up does he need for the Barrett's? Periodic upper endoscopy with biopsies to make sure that he does not develop adenocarcinoma.

Obstructing carcinoma of the lower esophagus. (From James EC, Corry RJ, Perry FJ: Basic Principles of Surgical Practice. Philadelphia, Hanley & Belfus, 1987, p 215, with permission.)

Thyroid cancer: patients present with a nodule in the thyroid gland. Be suspicious for cancer in any of the following scenarios: **"cold nodule" on nuclear medicine scan,** male sex, history of **childhood irradiation,** nodule described as "stony hard," recent or rapid enlargement, and increased **calcitonin** level (which indicates medullary thyroid cancer, classically in patients with multiple endocrine neoplasia [MEN] type II). To evaluate a thyroid nodule, order thyroid function tests. Thyroid-stimulating hormone is the best screening test; "toxic" or functional nodules are unlikely to be cancer. Then order a nuclear scan ("cold" nodule or area of decreased uptake is more suspicious than a nodule with normal or increased uptake). The next step is ultrasound, fine-needle aspiration, or open biopsy.

Bladder cancer: look for **persistent, painless hematuria.** The patient is often a **smoker** or worked in the rubber/dye industry (aniline dye exposure). Cystoscopy is usually done first to evaluate a potential bladder cancer, after screening with CT scan with contrast or intravenous pyelogram.

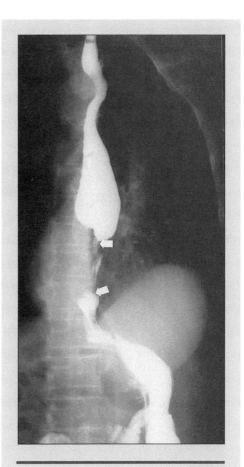

Liver tumors: hepatocellular carcinoma is caused by alcohol, hepatitis (B or C), hemochromatosis and essentially anything else that causes cirrhosis. **Alpha-fetoprotein** is often elevated and can be measured postoperatively to detect recurrences. Patients have one of the above histories and present with weight loss, right upper quadrant pain, and an enlarged liver. Surgery is usually the only hope for cure; prognosis is poor.

Other tumors of the liver

- **Hemangioma:** most common primary tumor of the liver; benign and generally left alone, but surgery may be done if the patient is symptomatic.
- **Hepatic adenoma:** appears most commonly in **women of reproductive age taking birth control pills.** Stop the pills! The tumor may regress; if not, surgical resection often is performed.
- **Cholangiosarcoma:** 50% of patients have inflammatory bowel disease (usually **ulcerative colitis**). Liver flukes (*Clonorchis* spp.) increase the risk in immigrants.
- **Angiosarcoma:** look for exposure to industrial vinyl chloride.
- **Hepatoblastoma:** the main primary liver tumor in children.

Adrenal tumors may be functional and cause primary hyperaldosteronism (Conn syndrome) or hyperadrenalism (Cushing syndrome). The tumor also can be a pheochromocytoma (see figure); look for intermittent, severe hypertension with mental status changes, headaches, and diaphoresis. Check 24-hour urine catecholamine product levels (e.g., metanephrines, vanillylmandelic acid, homovanillic acid).

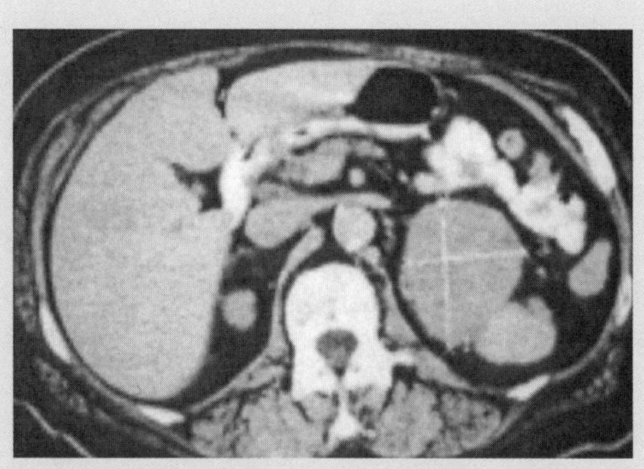

A 71-year-old woman with a left adrenal pheochromocytoma (between the the x signs). (Photo courtesy of Dr. Steven Perlmutter.) (From Katz DS, Math KR, Groskin SA (eds): Radiology Secrets. Philadelphia, Hanley & Belfus, 1998, p 207, with permission.)

Stomach cancer: risk factors are Japanese ethnicity, increasing age, smoking, and ingestion of smoked meat. *Helicobacter pylori* infection also has been implicated. A **Krukenberg tumor** is stomach cancer (or other GI malignancy) with ovarian metastases. A **Virchow node** is a left supraclavicular node enlargement due to visceral cancer spread (classically stomach cancer). If a gastric ulcer is seen on upper GI barium series or endoscopy, perform a biopsy to exclude malignancy.

Carcinoid tumors: the most common location is the small bowel, but carcinoid is also the most common appendiceal tumor. Carcinoid syndrome consists of **episodic cutaneous flushing, abdominal cramps, diarrhea,** and **right-sided heart valve damage** from serotonin and other secreted substances. Urinary levels of **5-hydroxyindoleacetic acid** (**5-HIAA,** a serotonin breakdown product) are increased.

> ➤ CASE SCENARIO: A patient has intermittent flushing, diarrhea, cramps, and increased urinary 5-HIAA. Is the GI carcinoid benign or malignant? Malignant, because the liver breaks down serotonin and other vasoactive secreted substances to make the tumor asymptomatic. However, when carcinoid metastasizes to the liver and vasoactive products reach the systemic circulation, symptoms begin.

Kaposi sarcoma: most common in HIV-positive patients. Kaposi sarcoma is a vascular skin tumor that starts out as a papule or plaque, commonly on the upper body or in the oral cavity. The classic description is a **rash that does not respond to multiple treatments.** Associated with human herpesvirus 8 infection.

Skin cancer: ultraviolet light increases the risk of basal cell, squamous cell, and melanoma skin cancer. The ***ABCDs of melanoma*** should make you suspicious of malignancy. Biopsy any lesion with any of these characteristics: **a**symmetry, **b**orders (irregular), **c**olor (change in color or multiple colors), and **d**iameter (the bigger the lesion, the more likely that it is malignant). Know the classic appearance of basal cell cancer: ***pearly and umbilicated with telangiectasias.*** Basal cell cancer is extremely common but almost never metastasizes. Metastasis is uncommon in squamous cell cancer but common in melanoma.

> ➤ CASE SCENARIO: A 54-year-old woman reports that a mole on her back has changed in appearance and now itches. You note asymmetry, irregular borders, and multiple colors. What kind of biopsy should you perform—punch, excisional, needle, or shave? Excisional biopsy.

You should cut out the entire lesion. New-onset itching in a mole that never itched before is a classic sign of melanoma.

Oral cancer is typically due to smoking or chewing tobacco and ethanol. Also look for poor oral hygiene. The lesion often starts as **leukoplakia** (white-colored plaque-like lesion), which must be differentiated from oral hairy leukoplakia, an Epstein-Barr virus-associated disease that affects HIV-infected patients. Leukoplakia is rarely cancerous at presentation and often regresses if the person quits tobacco and alcohol use. **Erythroplakia** (red-colored plaque-like lesion) is more worrisome; if it is present, consider a biopsy.

Histiocytosis: CD1-positive histiocytes are the malignant cell. Look for **Birbeck granules** (cytoplasmic inclusion bodies that look like tennis rackets).

Patients with cancer, like all other patients, have the **right to refuse any treatment.** However, watch for and treat **depression,** even in terminal patients.

> **CASE SCENARIO:** A 54-year-old man was diagnosed with pancreatic cancer and told of his odds for survival. He refuses all treatment, "even for a sore throat." The patient mentions insomnia, lack of appetite, and loss of interest in his hobbies. He mentions that the world would "probably be better off without me" and starts crying. He hands you an advance directive that states that he refuses any type of medical treatment whatsoever under any circumstances. What should you do with his advance directive? Tell him that you refuse to honor it until his depression has been treated and offer the patient antidepressants and counseling.

Tumor markers:

MARKER	CANCER(S)
Alpha fetoprotein	Liver, testicular (yolk sac tumor)
Carcinoembryonic antigen (CEA)	Colon, pancreas, other GI tumors
Prostate-specific antigen (PSA)	Prostate (early)
Acid phosphatase	Prostate (only with extension outside the capsule)
Human chorionic gonadotropin (HCG)	Hydatiform moles, choriocarcinoma
CA-125	Ovary
CA 19–9	Pancreas

PULMONOLOGY

Asthma

FEV1/FVC

High-yield pearls

CAUSES OF WHEEZING: ASTHMA, BRONCHIOLITIS, FB, CF

- Usually presents during childhood.
- The "atopic triad" is classic: **wheezing, eczema,** and **seasonal rhinitis.** If one parent has asthma, the child has a 25% risk; if both parents have asthma, the child's risk is 50%.
- Do not forget other causes of wheezing, such as bronchiolitis, foreign body, and cystic fibrosis.
- The best way to make the diagnosis is with spirometry and pulmonary function tests. A decreased ratio of forced expiratory volume in 1 second (FEV_1) to forced vital capacity (FVC) that should reverse (at least partially) with bronchodilators.

> **CASE SCENARIO:** What class of medications should be avoided in patients with asthma or chronic obstructive pulmonary disease? Beta blockers, which block the beta-2 receptors that are needed to open the airways.

- ➤ **CASE SCENARIO:** What infection should you suspect when wheezing occurs in children less than 2 years old? Respiratory syncytial virus or bronchiolitis. Look for coexisting fever.
- ➤ **CASE SCENARIO:** What should you suspect in a young child with unilateral wheezing of acute onset and no prior history of symptoms? Foreign body inhalation.
- ➤ **CASE SCENARIO:** A child has symptoms of wheezing only during gym class and soccer practice. What test should you use to confirm a suspicion of asthma? Have the child exercise immediately before performing spirometry (exercise challenge or provocation). The child's trigger is probably exercise.

Management issues

- Avoid any known triggers, and ask the patient's parents to stop smoking.
- In one-half of children with asthma, the symptoms resolve by early adulthood. No symptoms = no treatment.
- The first-line agent for maintenance therapy and acute attacks is a beta-2 agonist. Use as needed for mild symptoms or before triggers, such as exercise. Use regularly for moderate-to-severe asthma.
- Use inhaled steroids if the child does not respond to beta-2 agonists or has frequent attacks ($>$ 2/week). Children that need hospitalization because asthma does not respond to emegency treatment also commonly receive IV steroids for their delayed effect.

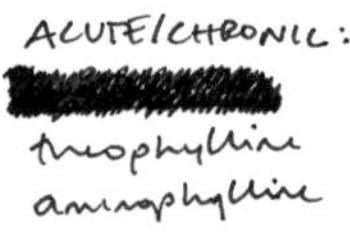

- Cromolyn and zafirlukast are alternatives or additional agents for prophylaxis, not acute attacks. Phosphodiesterase inhibitors (theophylline, aminophylline) are older, second-line agents that can be used in acute or chronic settings when other agents fail.
- Follow children with frequent exacerbations with peak flow measurements. The child should have a peak flow meter at home, and the parents should call the physician when values start to drop so that early treatment can be initiated.
  - ➤ **CASE SCENARIO:** A child in the emergency department with a severe asthma attack is no longer hyperventilating and her carbon dioxide level is now normal. The patient seems calm and sleepy. What should you do? Check arterial blood gas immediately. The patient may be crashing and require intubation. Fatigue alone is sufficient reason to intubate an asthmatic patient.

Emphysema/Chronic Obstructive Pulmonary Disease

High-yield pearls

- The cause is almost always smoking.
- In chronic obstructive pulmonary disease (COPD), the FEV_1/FEV ratio is less than normal ($<$ 0.75–0.80), whereas in restrictive lung disease, the FEV_1/FEV is often normal. **FEV_1 may be equal in both conditions, but the ratio of FEV_1 to FEV is different.**
- Treat with bronchodilators, usually beta-2 agonists or anticholinergics (e.g., ipratropium). Consider steroids for acute exacerbations and antibiotics for signs of infection (change in sputum color or amount).
- Remember pneumococcal and annual influenza vaccines.
- Long-term oxygen therapy reduces mortality and should be used when oxygen saturation is ≤ 90% (or partial arterial oxygen tension [PaO_2] is $<$ 60) while the patient is breathing room air.
- Consider pulmonary rehabilitation (supervised exercise), if given the option, for its long-term benefit.
  - ➤ **CASE SCENARIO:** What is the best way to reduce mortality in a patient with emphysema? Stop smoking.

> ➤ **CASE SCENARIO:** A 72-year-old man with severe emphysema comes to the emergency department because of a stubbed toe. Oxygen level = 50 mmHg, carbon dioxide level = 50 mmHg. He denies respiratory complaints and says that his toe hurts. Should you admit the patient and intubate him? No. Treat the patient, not the lab value. Remember that a patient with chronic COPD may normally live at higher carbon dioxide and lower oxygen levels. If the patient is asymptomatic and talking to you calmly, the lab value should not make you panic (also: did you accidentally get venous blood on this one?).

> ➤ **CASE SCENARIO:** What should you suspect in a patient with chronic bronchitis who has a "change" in his chronic cough but no other symptoms of infection? Lung cancer.

As a rough rule of thumb, you should **prepare to intubate** any patient whose carbon dioxide is > 50 mmHg or whose oxygen is < 50 mmHg, especially if the pH in either situation is < 7.30 while the patient is breathing room air (this is a guideline—treat the patient, not the lab). Usually, unless the patient is crashing rapidly, a trial of oxygen by nasal cannula is given first. If this approach fails or the patient becomes too tired (using accessory muscles is a good clue to the work of breathing), consider intubation.

Miscellaneous Conditions

Certain clues point to the cause of a **single pulmonary nodule:**

- Immigrant: think of tuberculosis, and do a skin test.
- Southwest United States: think of *Coccidioides immitis.*
- Cave explorer, exposure to bird droppings, or Ohio/Mississippi River valleys (Midwest): think of histoplasmosis.
- Smoker over the age of 50: think of lung cancer; do bronchoscopy and biopsy.
- Person under 40 with none of the above: think of hamartoma

> ➤ **CASE SCENARIO:** What is the first step you should take if a patient has a single pulmonary nodule on a chest x-ray? Check for old chest x-rays. If the lesion has not changed in 2 years, it is very likely to be benign.

Although a baseline chest x-ray (CXR) is standard preoperative evaluation for patients over 60 or patients with known pulmonary or cardiovascular disease, when to order pulmonary function tests is not as clear. Overall, the best indicator of possible postoperative pulmonary complications is preoperative pulmonary function. Aggressive pulmonary toileting, incentive spirometry, minimal narcotics, and early ambulation help to minimize or prevent postoperative pulmonary complications.

> ➤ **CASE SCENARIO:** What is the best way to reduce postoperative pulmonary complications in a smoker? Stop smoking preoperatively.

Note: The most common cause of a postoperative fever in the first 24 hours is **atelectasis.**

Adult respiratory distress syndrome (ARDS): acute lung injury that results in **noncardiogenic pulmonary edema,** respiratory distress, and **hypoxemia.** Common causes are sepsis, major trauma, pancreatitis, shock, near drowning, and drug overdose. Look for ARDS to develop within 24–48 hours of the initial insult. Classic patients have mottled or cyanotic skin, intercostal retractions, rales or rhonchi, and **no improvement in hypoxia with oxygen administration.** X-rays show pulmonary edema with normal cardiac silhouette (no congestive heart failure). Treat with intubation, mechanical ventilation with high percentage of oxygen, and positive end-expiratory pressure (PEEP), while addressing the underlying cause if possible.

Pneumonia usually is diagnosed on the basis of clinical findings plus elevated white blood cell count and CXR abnormalities. On physical exam, try to differentiate between typical (*Streptococcus pneumoniae*) and atypical (other organisms) community-acquired pneumonia, although the distinction is not always clear:

	TYPICAL PNEUMONIA	ATYPICAL PNEUMONIA
Prodrome	Short (< 2 days)	Long (> 3 days): headache, malaise, aches
Fever	High (> 102°F)	Low (< 102°F)
Age	> 40 yr	< 40 yr
CXR	One distinct lobe involved	Diffuse or multilobe involvement
Organism	*S. pneumoniae*	Many (*Haemophilus influenzae*, *Mycoplasma* or *Chlamydia* spp.)
Medications*	Third-generation cephalosporin or broad-spectrum fluoroquinolone	Azithromycin

*Avoid the temption to pull out the "big-gun" antibiotics (with a very wide spectrum) unless the patient is crashing or unstable.

Clinical clues that should suggest certain organisms:

HISTORY	THINK OF THESE BUGS
College student	*Mycoplasma* spp. (cold agglutinins) or *Chlamydia* spp.
Alcoholic	*Klebsiella* spp. ("currant jelly" sputum), *Staphylococcus aureus*, other enteric organisms (aspiration)
Cystic fibrosis	*Pseudomonas* spp. or *S. aureus*
Immigrant or silicosis	Tuberculosis
Chronic obstructive pulmonary disease	*Haemophilus influenzae*, *Moraxella* spp.
Patient with Tb and pulmonary cavitation	*Aspergillus* spp.
Exposure to air conditioner	*Legionella* spp.
HIV/AIDS	*Pneumocystis carinii* or cytomegalovirus (with koilocytosis)
Exposure to bird droppings	*Chlamydia psittaci* or *Histoplasma capsulatum*
Child < 1 year old	Respiratory syncytial virus
Child 2–5 years old	Parainfluenza (croup) or epiglottitis (less common)

➤ ***CASE SCENARIO:*** A young child has recurrent pneumonia in the right middle lobe, with no other signs of immune deficiency. What should you suspect? Foreign body aspiration. Remember that a foreign body is most likely to go down the right bronchus. Congenital malformation in the affected lung segment is another possibility.

Pleural effusion: if you do not know the cause, always consider thoracentesis and examine the fluid by doing a Gram stain, culture (including tuberculosis), cell count with differential, cytology, glucose level (low in infection), and protein level (high in infection). A pleural effusion can be normal in the setting of pneumonia, but watch for possible progression to an empyema (infected, loculated pleural fluid), which requires chest tube drainage (see figure).

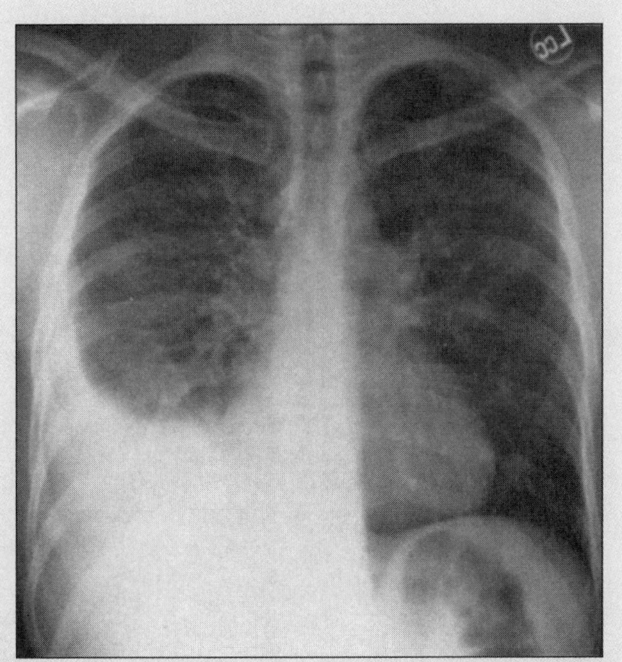

Pleural effusion. (From Sahn SA. Heffner JE: Pulmonary Pearls II. Philadelphia, Hanley & Belfus, 1995, with permission.

RHEUMATOLOGY

Arthritis: a large majority of cases are due to osteoarthritis (OA). When in doubt, or if you suspect something other than OA, aspirate fluid from the affected joint for examination. Examine the fluid for cell count and differential, glucose, bacteria (Gram stain and culture), and crystals.

	OA	RA	GOUT	PSEUDOGOUT	SEPTIC ARTHRITIS
Usual age/sex	Older adults	Females 20–45	Older males	Older adults	Any age
Classic joints	DIP, PIP, hip, knee	PIP, MCP, wrist	Big toe	Knees, elbows	Knee
Joint fluid WBC	< 2,000	> 2,000	> 2,000	> 2,000	> 50,000
% Neutrophils	< 25%	> 50%	> 50%	> 50%	> 75%

OA = osteoarthritis, RA = rheumatoid arthritis, DIP = distal interphalangeal, PIP = proximal interphalangeal, MCP = metacarpophalangeal, WBC = white blood cells.

➤ *CASE SCENARIO:* A 50-year-old man presents with an acutely painful, hot, swollen, stiff right knee with no history of trauma or musculoskeletal problems. What should you do next? Arthrocentesis and joint fluid examination.

Other key differences/points

1. **Osteoarthritis (OA):** little evidence of inflammation on exam (no hot, red, tender joints as seen in most other rheumatologic/arthritic disorders). Classic signs and symptoms include **Heberden nodes** at the distal interphalangeal (DIP) joint and **Bouchard nodes** at the proximal interphalangeal (PIP) joint; worsening symptoms in the evening or after use; and bony spurs. The incidence increases with age. Treat with weight reduction and as-needed NSAIDs or acetaminophen.

2. **Rheumatoid arthritis (RA):** positive rheumatoid factor (RF) clinches the diagnosis, although children with RA are often RF-negative. Look for systemic symptoms (fever, malaise, subcutaneous nodules [see figure], pericarditis/pleural effusion, uveitis), prolonged morning stiffness, **swan neck** and **boutonnière** deformities. The buzz word is **pannus** (articular cartilage looks like granulation tissue due to chronic inflammation). Treated with NSAIDs (for symptom relief only; they do not halt disease progression like other agents), hydroxychloroquine, etanercept, and corticosteroids (for bad flare-ups), among others.

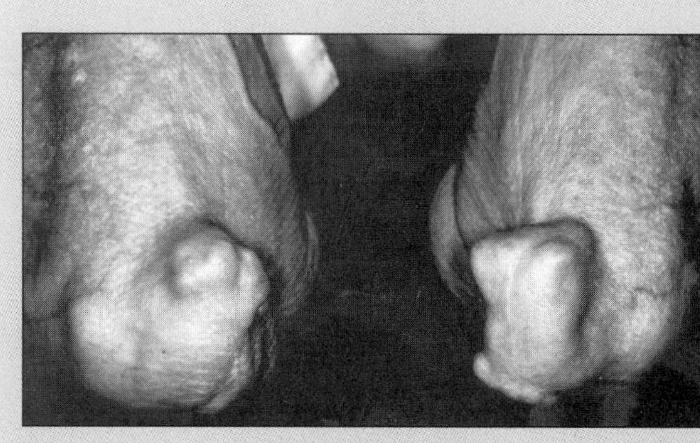

Unusually large dermal and subcutaneous rheumatoid nodules in a patient with severe rheumatoid arthritis. (From Fitzpatrick JE, Aeling JL: Dermatology Secrets. Philadelphia, Hanley & Belfus, 1999, with permission.)

3. **Gout:** classically starts with **podagra** (gout in the big toe). Look for **tophi** (subcutaneous uric acid deposits, punched out lesions on bone x-ray) and **needle-shaped crystals** (often inside leukocytes) with **negative birefringence.** Gout is more common in men than in women. Patients should avoid alcohol, which may precipitate an attack. Colchicine or NSAIDs (not aspirin, which causes decreased excretion of uric acid by the kidney) are used for acute attacks. For maintenance therapy, high fluid intake, alkalinization of the urine, and **allopurinol** may be used.

   ➤ **CASE SCENARIO:** A 58-year-old obese man presents with acute onset of pain, redness, and swelling in the big toe. Joint aspiration reveals needle-shaped crystals with negative birefringence. Should you use low-dose or high-dose allopurinol? Neither. Allopurinol and probenicid should not be given for acute attacks, because they make matters worse. They are maintenance agents that should be used once the acute attack has resolved.

4. **Pseudogout: rhomboid-shaped** calcium pyrophosphate dihydrate crystals with **weakly positive birefringence.** Mnemonic: **p**seudogout = **p**yrophosphate and **p**ositive birefringence. Treat with NSAIDs or colchicine.

5. **Septic arthritis:** synovial fluid shows bacteria on Gram stain. *Staphylococcus aureus* is the most common organism, except in sexually active young adults (in whom the most common organism is *Neisseria gonorrhoeae*). Do blood cultures in addition to joint cultures, because the organism usually reaches the joint via the hematogenous route. Do urethral swabs and cultures in appropriate patients.

Other causes of arthritis

1. **Psoriasis:** in the presence of classic skin lesions, always consider psoriatic arthritis. The disease usually affects hands and feet. The arthritis resembles RA, but rheumatoid factor is negative. Treat with NSAIDs or steroids (for severe cases).

2. **Lupus erythematosus or inflammatory bowel disease:** look for other symptoms of the primary disease.

3. **Ankylosing spondylitis:** remember the association with **HLA-B27.** Most often a 20–40-year-old man with a positive family history presents with back pain and morning stiffness. The patient may

assume a bent-over posture. Sacroiliac joints are primarily affected, and x-rays may show a **"bamboo spine."** Watch for other autoimmune symptoms, such as fever, elevated sedimentation rate, anemia, and **uveitis.** Treatment is exercise and NSAIDs.

4. **Reiter syndrome:** also associated with **HLA-B27.** The classic triad of symptoms is urethritis (due to chlamydial infection), conjunctivitis, and arthritis (the patient "***can't pee, can't see, and can't climb a tree***"). Reiter syndrome also may follow enteric bacterial infections. Superficial oral and penile ulcers may occur. Diagnose and treat the sexually transmitted disease, if present; also treat the patient's sexual partners. Use NSAIDs for arthritis.
5. **Hemophilia:** recurrent hemarthroses can cause a debilitating arthritis. Treat with acetaminophen; avoid antiplatelet agents.
6. **Lyme disease:** look for tick bite, ***erythema chronicum migrans*** (see figure), and migratory arthritis later. Treat with doxycycline, ceftriaxone or amoxicillin (best agent for pregnant women).
7. **Rheumatic fever:** look for previous streptococcal pharyngitis. ***Migratory polyarthritis*** is one of the major Jones criteria.
8. **Sickle cell disease:** patients frequently have arthralgias and ***avascular necrosis*** of the humeral or femoral head, which can lead to severe arthritic changes and deformities.
9. **Trauma**
10. **Childhood orthopedic problem:** slipped capital femoral epiphysis, congenital hip dysplasia, and Legg-Calvé-Perthes disease may cause arthritis as an adult. Use history (age of onset) and x-ray to figure out which disease the patient had (see Pediatric Orthopedics section).

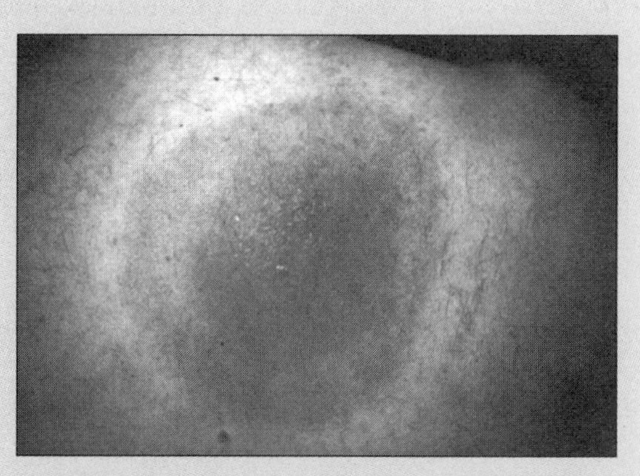

Erythematous, annular rash known as erythema (chronicum) migrans, which is characteristic of Lyme disease. (From Cunha BA: Infectious Disease Pearls. Philadelphia, Hanley & Belfus, 1999, with permission.)

11. **Charcot joint:** most commonly seen in ***diabetics;*** also seen in other neuropathies. 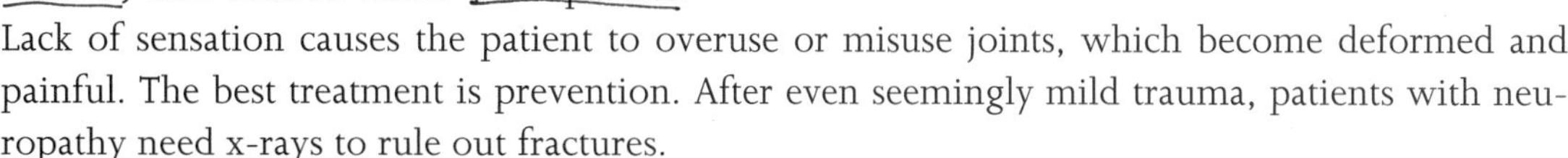Lack of sensation causes the patient to overuse or misuse joints, which become deformed and painful. The best treatment is prevention. After even seemingly mild trauma, patients with neuropathy need x-rays to rule out fractures.
12. 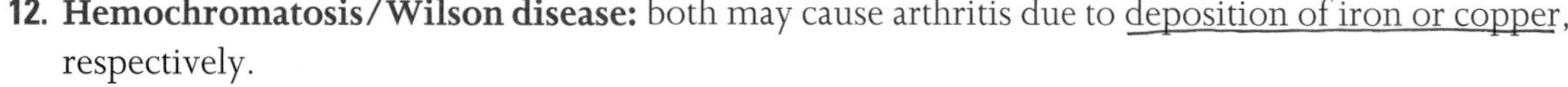**Hemochromatosis/Wilson disease:** both may cause arthritis due to deposition of iron or copper, respectively.

Autoimmune diseases affect women of reproductive age unless otherwise specified. For board purposes, classic disease findings differentiate one condition from the other. Almost all have systemic signs of inflammation (elevated sedimentation rate/C-reactive protein, fever, anemia of chronic disease, fatigue, weight loss).

1. **Lupus erythematosus:** malar rash, discoid rash, photosensitivity, kidney damage, arthritis, pericarditis or pleuritis, positive ***antinuclear antibody (ANA),*** positive ***anti-Smith antibody,*** positive syphilis test (Veneral Disease Research Laboratory, rapid plasma reagin), positive lupus anticoagulant, thrombocytopenia, leukopenia, anemia, pancytopenia, neurologic disturbances (depression, psychosis, seizures), and oral ulcers may be presenting symptoms. Use ANA titer as a screening test; confirm with the anti-Smith antibody test. Treat with NSAIDs, hydroxychloroquine, and corticosteroids.
2. **Scleroderma/progressive systemic sclerosis:** look for **CREST** symptoms (calcinosis, Raynaud phenomenon, esophageal dysmotility, sclerodactyly, telangiectasias), ***heartburn,*** and mask-like,

leathery facies. The screening test is the ANA assay; confirmatory tests are **anticentromere antibody** (for CREST) and **antitopoisomerase** (for scleroderma). Steroids may help.

3. **Sjögren syndrome:** dry eyes (**keratoconjunctivitis sicca**) and dry mouth (xerostomia); often associated with other autoimmune disease. Treat with eye drops and good oral hygiene.
4. **Dermatomyositis:** polymyositis (see below) plus skin involvement (**heliotrope rash around the eyes with associated periorbital edema** is classic). Patients classically have difficulty in rising out of a chair or climbing steps becasue the disease affects proximal muscles. Muscle enzymes (i.e. creatine kinase or creatine phosphokinase) are elevated, and electromyography is irregular. Muscle biopsy establishes the diagnosis. Patients have an increased incidence of **malignancy.**
5. **Polyarteritis nodosa:** remember the association with **hepatitis B** infection and cryoglobulinemia. Patients present with fever, abdominal pain, weight loss, renal disturbances, and/or peripheral neuropathies. Lab abnormalities include high sedimentation rate, leukocytosis, anemia, and hematuria/proteinuria. Vasculitis involves medium-sized vessels. Biopsy is the gold standard for diagnosis.
6. **Wegener granulomatosis:** resembles Goodpasture syndrome, but instead of anti-glomerular antibodies, look for positive **antineutrophilic cytoplasmic antibody *(ANCA)*** titer. Also look for **sinonasal involvement** (nose bleeds, nasal perforation), which is not seen in Goodpasture syndrome, as well as involvement of lungs (hemoptysis, dyspnea) and kidneys (hematuria, acute renal failure). Treat with cyclophosphamide.
7. **Kawasaki syndrome:** typically affects **children less than 5 years old** and is more common in Japanese children and girls. Patients present with truncal rash, high fever (lasting > 5 days), conjunctival infection, cervical lymphadenopathy, **"strawberry" tongue,** late **skin desquamation** of palms and soles, and/or arthritis. Patients can develop coronary vessel vasculitis and subsequent **aneurysms,** which may thrombose and cause a myocardial infarction. You should consider Kawasaki disease in any child who has a myocardial infarction. Treat during the acute stage with aspirin (one of the few times to use aspirin in children) and IV immunoglobulins to reduce the risk of coronary aneurysm.
8. **Takayasu arteritis:** tends to affect Asian women between 15 and 30 years of age. It is also called "**pulseless disease**" because you may not be able to feel the patient's pulse or get a blood pressure measurement on one side. Vasculitis affects the aortic arch and the branches that arise from it; carotid involvement may cause neurologic signs or stroke. Heart failure is not uncommon. An angiogram shows characteristic lesions. Treat with steroids and/or cyclophosphamide.
9. **Behçet syndrome:** the classic patient is a man in his 20s with **painful oral and genital ulcers.** May also have uveitis, arthritis and other skin lesions (especially erythema nodosum). Steroids may help.

Fibromyalgia vs. polymyositis vs. polymyalgia rheumatica:

	FIBROMYALGIA	POLYMYOSITIS	POLYMYALGIA RHEUMATICA
Classic age/sex	Young adult woman	40–60 y.o. woman	Woman > 50 y.o.
Location	Various	Proximal muscles	Pectoral and pelvic girdles, neck
ESR	Normal	Elevated	Markedly elevated (often > 100)
Muscle biopsy/EMG	Normal	Abnormal	Normal
Classic findings	Anxiety, stress, insomnia; point tenderness over affected muscles; negative work-up	Elevated CPK; abnormal EMG and biopsy; greater risk of cancer	Temporal arteritis; great response to steroids, very high ESR; elderly patient
Treatment	SSRIs, NSAIDs, rest	Steroids	Steroids

ESR = erythrocyte sedimentation rate, CPK = creatine phosphokinase, EMG = electromyography, SSRIs = serotonin-specific reuptake inhibitors, NSAIDs = nonsteroidal anti-inflammatory drugs.

> ➤ **CASE SCENARIO:** A 65-year-old woman presents with unilateral scalp tenderness, fatigue, and muscular weakness. Her sedimentation rate is markedly elevated. She mentions that she is having trouble seeing out of her right eye. What should you do next? Start steroids immediately. Do not wait to confirm the diagnosis of temporal arteritis with a biopsy, because the patient may go blind while you are waiting for the biopsy results.

Paget disease: a disease of bone in which bone is broken down and regenerated, often simultaneously. The disease is seen in patients **> 40 years old,** more commonly in men, and often is discovered in an asymptomatic patient on an x-ray. Classic signs include pelvic and skull involvement; watch for a patient who has had to buy larger-sized hats. Patient may have bone pain, arthritis, or nerve deafness. **Alkaline phosphatase** is markedly elevated in the presence of **normal calcium and phosphorus levels.** Patients have an increased risk of osteosarcoma in affected bones. Treat with NSAIDs for symptom relief, possibly a bisphosphonate (e.g., etidronate) for severe disease.

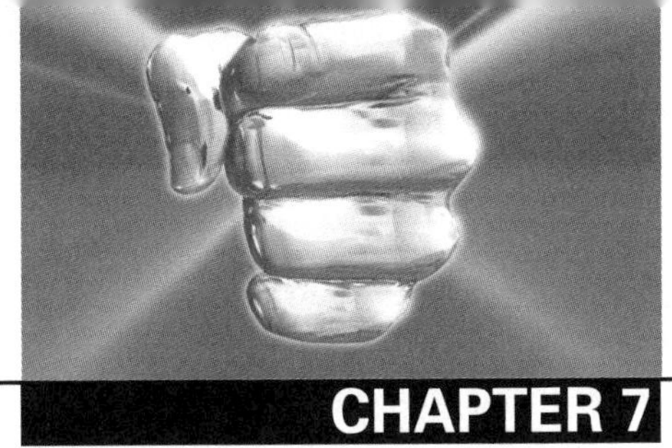

CHAPTER 7

Other Important Topics

DERMATOLOGY

Common terms used to describe skin findings:

1. Macule: a flat spot < 1 cm (nonpalpable, but visible). Example: freckles.
2. Patch: same as macule but > 1 cm. Example: port-wine birthmarks.
3. Papule: solid, elevated lesion < 1 cm (palpable). Examples: wart, acne, lichen planus.
4. Plaque: same as papule but > 1 cm and flat-topped. Example: psoriasis.
5. Nodule: a palpable, solid lesion > 1 cm and not flat-topped. Examples: small lipoma, erythema nodosum.
6. Vesicle: elevated, circumscribed lesion < 5 mm containing fluid (small blister). Examples: chickenpox, genital herpes.
7. Bulla: same as vesicle but > 5 mm (large blister). Examples: contact dermatitis, pemphigus.
8. Wheal: itchy, transiently edematous area. Example:allergic reaction.

Vitiligo: depigmentation of unknown etiology (see figure); associated with other autoimmune conditions, such as **pernicious anemia** and hypothyroidism. Patients may have antibodies to melanin.

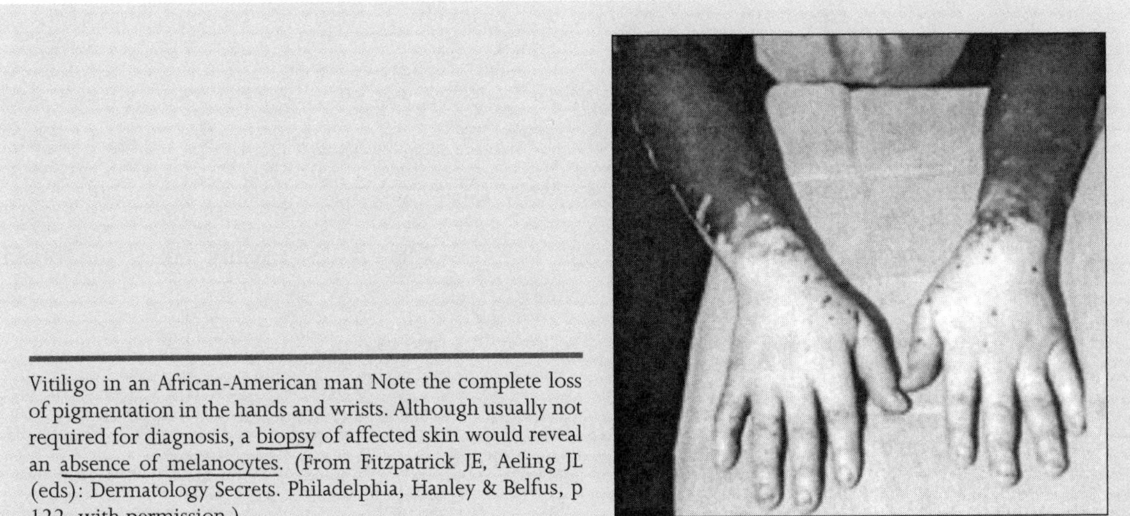

Vitiligo in an African-American man Note the complete loss of pigmentation in the hands and wrists. Although usually not required for diagnosis, a biopsy of affected skin would reveal an absence of melanocytes. (From Fitzpatrick JE, Aeling JL (eds): Dermatology Secrets. Philadelphia, Hanley & Belfus, p 122, with permission.)

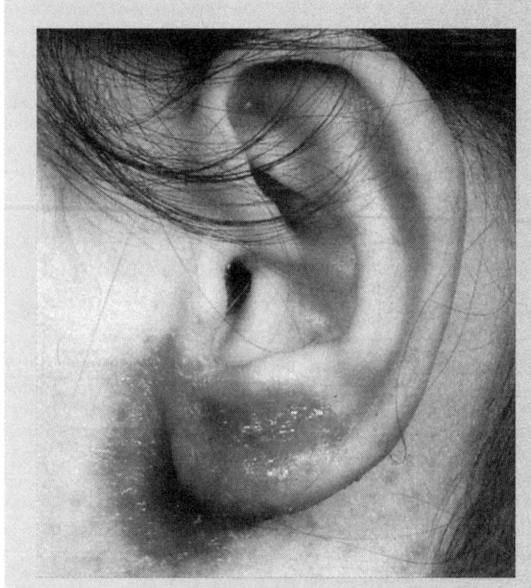

Nickel dermatitis, the most common form of contact dermatitis in women, from nickel earrings. In this case, secondary infection was also present. Jean studs, zippers, spectacle frames, and jewelry are other potential causes of nickel dermatitis. (From du Vivier A: Disorders of pigment and of pigmented skin. In du Vivier A (ed): Atlas of Clinical Dermatology, 3rd ed. New York, Churchill Livingstone, 2002, pp 649–666, with permission.)

Pruritus: may be a clue to a diagnosis of **obstructive biliary disease** (classically primary biliary cirrhosis), **uremia, polycythemia rubra vera** (classically after a warm shower or bath), contact or **atopic dermatitis,** scabies, and lichen planus.

Contact dermatitis: often due to a type IV hypersensitivity reaction; also may be due to irritating or toxic substance. Look for question to mention new exposure to a classic offending agent (e.g., poison ivy, nickel earrings, deodorant). The rash is well circumscribed and found only in the area of exposure (see figure). The skin is **red and itchy** and often has **vesicles** and **bullae.** Avoidance of the agent is required. Patch testing can be done, if needed, to determine the antigen.

Atopic dermatitis: look for family and personal history of **allergies** (e.g., hay fever) or **asthma.** This is a chronic condition that begins in the first year of life with **red, itchy, weeping skin** on the head and upper extremities and sometimes around the diaper area. The major problem is pruritis and resultant scratching, which leads to skin breaks and possible bacterial infection. Treatment involves avoidance of drying soaps and the use of **antihistamines** and **topical steroids.**

Seborrheic dermatitis: causes the common conditions known as cradle cap and **dandruff** as well as **blepharitis** (eyelid inflammation). Look for scaling skin on the scalp and eyelids. Treat with dandruff shampoo (i.e., selenium sulfide).

Fungal skin infections, dermatophyte infections, and **ringworm,** depending on the location, are defined as:

1. **Tinea corporis** (body/trunk): look for **red, ring-shaped lesions** that have **raised borders** and tend to **clear centrally while they expand peripherally.**
2. **Tinea pedis** (athlete's foot): look for **macerated, scaling web spaces between the toes that often itch** and associated thickened, distorted toenails (**onychomycosis**). Good foot hygiene is part of the treatment.
3. **Tinea unguium** (nails; also known as onychomycosis): **thickened, distorted nails** with debris under the nail edges.
4. **Tinea capitis** (scalp): mainly affects children (highly contagious), who have scaly patches of hair loss and may have an inflamed, boggy granuloma of the scalp (known as a **kerion**). On the boards you may be shown a picture of this finding. The condition usually resolves with antifungal treatment (not a tumor).
5. **Tinea cruris** (jock itch): more common in obese males; usually seen in the **crural folds of the upper, inner thighs**.

Most of these infections are due to **Trichophyton species.**

- Diagnosis of any of these infections can be confirmed by scraping the lesion and using a potassium hydroxide (KOH) preparation to visualize the fungus or by doing a culture.
- Oral agents (e.g., **terbinafine, fluconazole**) must be used to treat tinea capitis and onychomycosis; the others can be treated with topical antifungals (imidazoles such as miconazole, clotrimazole, ketoconazole), or oral agents.
- In tinea capitis, if the hair **fluoresces under the Wood's lamp, Microsporum sp.** is the cause; if the hair does *not* fluoresce, the probable cause is **Trichophyton sp.**

Candidiasis: thrush (creamy white patches on the tongue or buccal mucosa that can be scraped off) may be seen in normal children, and candidal vulvovaginitis is seen in normal women, especially during pregnancy or after taking antibiotics. However, at other times and in different patients, candidal infections may be a sign of **diabetes** or **immunodeficiency.** For example, thrush in an adult man should raise the possibility of **HIV/AIDS.** Treat with local/topical nystatin or imidazoles (e.g., miconazole, clotrimazole); oral therapy (nystatin or ketoconazole) is used for extensive or resistant disease.

Tinea versicolor: *Pityrosporum* infection that presents most commonly in young adults with **multiple patches of various size and color (brown, tan, and white) on the torso.** Often the lesions become noticeable in the summer because the affected areas *fail to tan* and look white. Diagnose from lesion scrapings (KOH preparation). Treat with selenium sulfide shampoo or topical imidazoles.

Scabies: caused by the mite ***Sarcoptes scabei,*** which tunnels into the skin and leaves **visible "burrows"** on the skin, classically in the **finger web spaces** and **flexor surface of the wrists.** Watch for severe pruritus and itching, which can lead to secondary bacterial infection. Diagnosis is made by scraping the mite out of a burrow and seeing it under a microscope. Remember to treat *all* contacts (e.g., the whole family).

> ➤ **CASE SCENARIO:** What is the preferred treatment for scabies? **Permethrin** cream applied to the whole body. Do not use lindane unless permethrin is not a choice. Lindane used to be the treatment of choice but can cause neurotoxicity, especially in young children.

Lice (pediculosis): lice can infect the head (*Pediculus capitis;* common in school children), body (*Pediculus corporis;* unusual in people with good hygiene), or pubic area (*Phthirus pubis,* also known as "crabs"; transmitted sexually). Infected areas tend to itch, and diagnosis is made by **seeing the lice on hair shafts.** Treat with **permethrin** cream (preferred over lindane due to lindane's neurotoxicity) and decontaminate sources of reinfection. Wash and sterilize combs, hats, bed sheets, and clothing.

Warts: caused by **human papillomavirus (HPV)**. Warts are infectious and most commonly seen in older children, often on the hands. Treatments are multiple and include salicylic acid, liquid nitrogen, curettage, and others. Genital warts are also caused by HPV; types 16 and 18 are associated with cervical cancer.

Molluscum contagiosum: a **poxvirus** infection that is common in children but also may be transmitted sexually. A child who has genital molluscum may or may not have contracted the disease from sexual contact; autoinnoculation is possible. Do not automatically assume child abuse, although it must be ruled out. The diagnosis is made by the characteristic appearance of the lesions (**skin-colored, smooth, waxy papules with a central depression** [umbilicated] that are roughly 0.5 cm) or by looking at the contents of the lesion, which include cells with characteristic **inclusion bodies.** Molluscum contagiosum usually is treated with freezing or curettage.

Acne: know the medical description of acne: **comedones (whiteheads/blackheads), papules, pustules, inflamed nodules,** and **superficial pus-filled cysts** with possible inflammatory skin changes. ***Propionibacterium acnes*** is thought to be partially involved in pathogenesis as is blockage of pilosebaceous glands. Acne has *not* been proved to be related to food, but if the patient makes such a relation, you can try discontinuance of the presumably offending food. Acne is not related to exercise, sex, or masturbation, but cosmetics may aggravate it. Treatment options are multiple. Start with **topical benzoyl peroxide;** then try **topical clindamycin,** oral tetracycline, or oral erythromycin (for *P. acnes* eradication). The next step is to try topical tretinoin. The last resort is **oral isotretinoin.** Isotretinoin is highly effective but **teratogenic** and can cause **dry skin and mucosae, muscle and joint pain,** and **abnormal liver function tests.**

Rosacea: looks like acne but starts in middle age. Look for ***rhinophyma*** (bulbous red nose) and coexisting blepharitis. Treat with topical metronidazole or oral tetracycline. The pathogenesis is unknown, but it is not related to diet.

Hirsutism: most commonly idiopathic, but look for other signs of **virilization** (deepening voice, clitoromegaly, frontal balding) to represent an androgen-secreting ovarian tumor. Other causes include

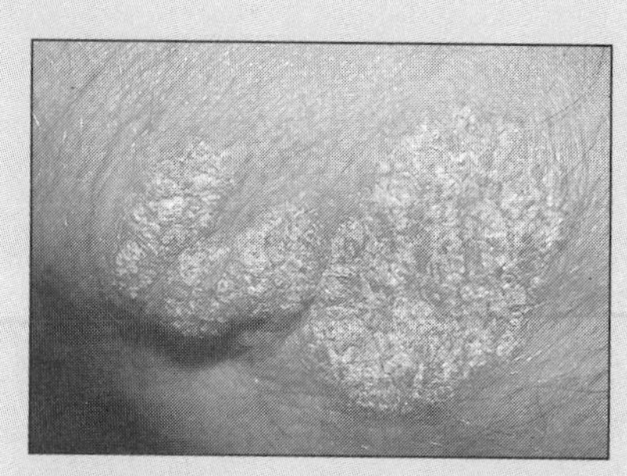

Psoriasis. Elbow involvement of psoriasis vulgaris, demonstrating typical well-demarcated, red plaques with silvery scale. (From Fitzpatrick JE, Aeling JL: Dermatology Secrets. Philadelphia, Hanley & Belfus, 1998, with permission.)

corticosteroid administration, Cushing syndrome, Stein-Leventhal syndrome (polycystic ovary disease), and drugs (**minoxidil** and **phenytoin**).

Baldness: watch for exotic causes of irregular, patchy baldness, such as **trichotillomania,** a psychiatric disorder in which patients pull out their own hair, and **alopecia areata,** which is idiopathic and associated with antimicrosomal and other autoantibodies. Alopecia areata also is seen in patients with lupus or syphilis and after chemotherapy. Male-pattern baldness is benign and considered to be a genetic disorder that requires androgens to be expressed.

Psoriasis: Classic lesions are **dry, not pruritic, well-circumscribed, silvery, scaling papules and plaques** found on the **extensor surfaces of the elbows and knees** (see figure) or the **scalp.** The family history is often positive. Psoriasis occurs mostly in whites with onset in early adulthood. Patients may have **pitting of the nails** and an arthritis that resembles rheumatoid arthritis but is rheumatoid factor-negative. Diagnosis made by appearance, but biopsy can be used if there is doubt. Treatment is complex (shouldn't be asked about in detail on USMLE) but involves exposure to **ultraviolet light** (e.g., sunlight), lubricants, topical corticosteroids, and keratolytics (coal tar, salicylic acid, anthralin).

Pityriasis rosea: usually seen in adults. Look for a "**herald patch**" (scaly, slightly erythematous, ring-shaped or oval patch classically seen on the trunk), followed 1 week later by many similar lesions that tend to **itch.** Look for lesions on the back with a long axis that **parallels the Langerhan's skin cleavage lines,** typically in a "**Christmas tree**" pattern. The disease usually remits spontaneously in 1 month. Syphilis is in the differential diagnosis. Treat with reassurance, as rash generally goes away within a few months.

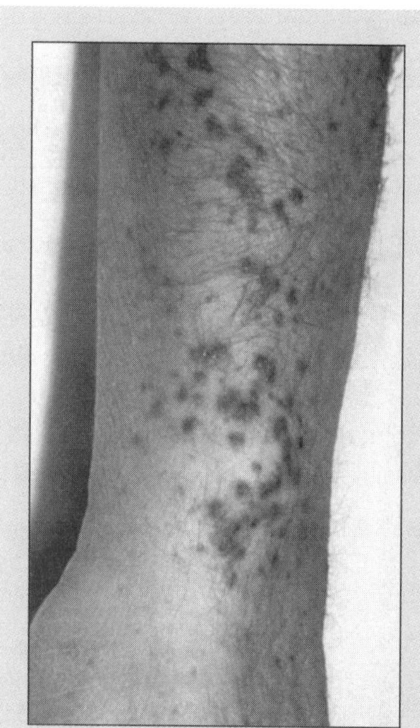

Drug reaction resulting in palpable purpura due to vasculitis. This type of rash is also classically seen in Henoch-Schonlein purpura, meningococcal meningitis/sepsis, and other autoimmune/vasculitis disorders. (From Silver RM, Smith EA: Rheumatology Pearls. Philadelphia, Hanley & Belfus, 1997, with permission.)

Lichen planus: look for oral mucosal lesions (**patches of fine white lines and dots**) and the **4 Ps:** **p**ruritic, **p**urple, **p**olygonal **p**apules, classically on the **wrists** and/or **ankles.** The condition is usually self-limiting and goes away within a few years and only symptomatic treatment (i.e. relieve itching) is typically needed.

Drug reactions and skin (see figure): penicillin, cephalosporins, and sulfa drugs commonly cause rashes; tetracyclines and phenothiazines commonly cause **photosensitivity.**

Erythema multiforme: look for classic **target** (also known as **iris**) lesions. This condition is usually caused by drugs or infections (e.g., herpes virus). The severe form, which may be fatal, is known as Stevens-Johnson syndrome (eye and oral mucosal involvement); treat supportively. (See figure on next page.)

Erythema nodosum: inflammation of the subcutaneous tissue and skin, classically over the shins (pretibial). Tender, red nodules are present. Look for exotic diseases such as **sarcoidosis, coccidiomycosis,** and **ulcerative colitis** to be the cause, although more commonly the cause is unknown or due to a streptococcal infection.

Pemphigus vulgaris: an autoimmune disease of middle-aged and elderly people that presents with **multiple bullae,** starting in the **oral mucosa** and spreading to the skin of the rest of the body, with subsequent sloughing of the blisters that leaves raw, denuded skin. Biopsy can be stained for antibody and shows a **lacelike or fishnet immunofluorescence pattern** (versus a **linear pattern in bullous pemphigoid,** a similar but milder condition). Treat with corticosteroids to prevent death from skin infection or fluid losses.

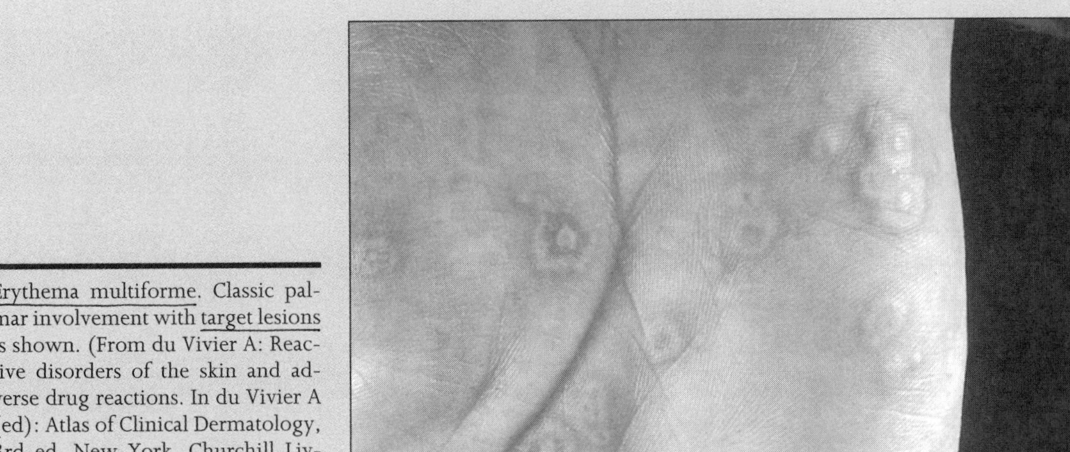

Erythema multiforme. Classic palmar involvement with target lesions is shown. (From du Vivier A: Reactive disorders of the skin and adverse drug reactions. In du Vivier A (ed): Atlas of Clinical Dermatology, 3rd ed. New York, Churchill Livingstone, 2002, pp 367–416, with permission.)

Dermatitis herpetiformis: should alert you to the presence of **gluten-sensitivity** (i.e. **celiac disease**). Look for diarrhea and weight loss. The skin has **IgA deposits** even in unaffected areas. Patients present with intensely **pruritic vesicles, papules, and wheals on the extensor aspects of the elbows and knees,** possibly on the face and neck. Treat with gluten-free diet.

Decubitus ulcers (bedsore or pressure sore): due to prolonged pressure against the skin. Cleanliness and dryness help to prevent this condition, and periodic skin inspection makes sure that you catch the problem early. When missed, the lesions can ulcerate down to the bone and become infected, possibly leading to sepsis and death. Treat major skin breaks with aggressive surgical debridement; use antibiotics if the patient has signs of infection.

- **CASE SCENARIO:** What is the best way to prevent bedsores? Periodic turning of paralyzed, bedridden, or debilitated patients (those at highest risk). Special air mattresses also change areas of pressure continuously and can help in prevention.
- **CASE SCENARIO:** What are the two classic causes for new onset of excessive perspiration? Hyperthyroidism and pheochromocytoma (if intermittent). Also consider hypoglycemia.

Moles: common and benign, but malignant transformation is possible. Excise any mole (or do a biopsy if the lesion is very large) if it **enlarges suddenly, develops irregular borders, darkens or becomes inflamed, changes color** (even if only one small area of the mole changes color), **begins to bleed, begins to itch,** or **becomes painful.** Dysplastic nevus syndrome is a genetic condition with multiple dysplastic-appearing nevi (usually > 100). Also look for a family history of melanoma. Treat with careful follow-up and excision/biopsy of any suspicious-looking lesions as well as sun avoidance and sunscreen use.

Keratoacanthoma: mainly important because it mimics skin cancer (especially squamous cell cancer). Look for a flesh-colored lesion with a central crater that contains keratinous material, classically on the face. The best way to differentiate it from cancer is that a keratoacanthoma has a **very rapid onset and grows to its full size in 1 or 2 months** (which almost never happens with squamous cell cancer). The lesion involutes spontaneously in a few months and requires no treatment. If you are unsure, the best step is a biopsy; but choose observation if the history is classic.

Keloid: an overgrowth of scar tissue after an injury, most frequently seen in **blacks.** The lesion usually is slightly pink and classically found on the upper back, chest, and deltoid area. Also look for keloids to develop after ear piercing. Do not treat or excise the lesion; you may make it worse.

Basal cell skin cancer: begins as a shiny papule and slowly enlarges and develops an **umbilicated center,** which later may **ulcerate,** with **peripheral telangiectasias** (see figure). Almost never metastasizes. As with all

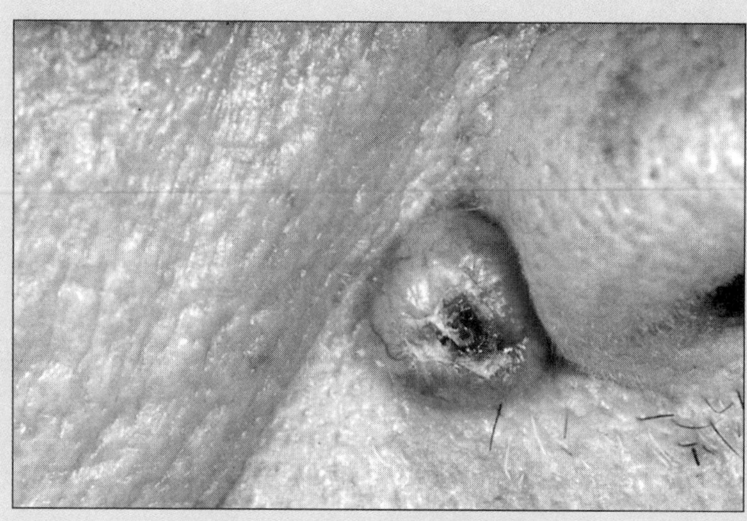

Basal cell carcinoma, the most common skin cancer of the face, adjacent to the nose. There is a pearly papule or nodule with classic central ulceration and peripheral telangiectasias. Typically, the lesion is painless but bleeds, forms a scab, and fails to heal. (From du Vivier A: Differential diagnosis. In du Vivier A (ed): Atlas of Clinical Dermatology, 3rd ed. New York, Churchill Livingstone, 2002, pp 693–724, with permission.)

skin cancer, ***sunlight exposure*** increases the risk and it is more common in light-skinned people. Treat with excision. Biopsy any suspicious skin lesion in elderly patients.

Squamous cell cancer: look for preexisting ***actinic keratoses*** (hard, sharp, red, often scaly lesions in sun-exposed areas) or burn scars to become nodular, warty, or ulcerated. Do a biopsy if this happens. Squamous cell cancer in situ is known as ***Bowen disease.***

Malignant melanoma: ***superficial spreading melanoma*** (see figure), which tends to stay superficial, has the best prognosis and ***nodular melanoma*** the worst, because it tends to grow downward (i.e. vertical spread) first. Although uncommon in blacks, melanoma tends to be of the ***acrolentiginous*** type; look for black dots on the ***palms*** or ***soles*** or ***under the fingernail*** (i.e. subungual). Treat with surgery; if surgery fails, the prognosis is poor.

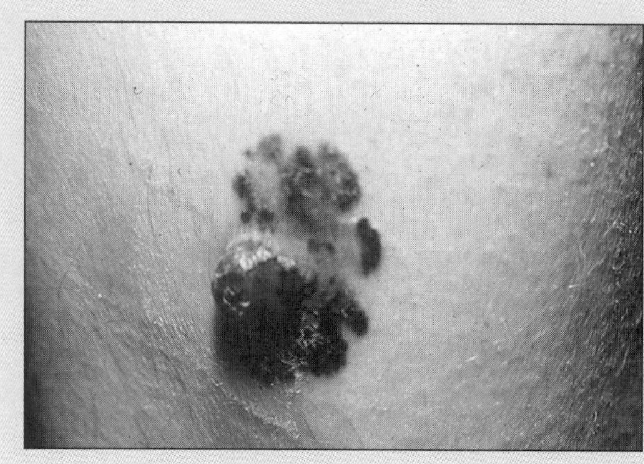

Superficial spreading malignant melanoma that has developed a nodular melanoma. (From Fitzpatrick JE, Aeling JL: Dermatology Secrets. Philadelphia, Hanley & Belfus, 1996, with permission.)

➤ ***CASE SCENARIO:*** What characteristic of the primary lesion is most closely related to prognosis in melanoma? The depth of vertical invasion.

Kaposi sarcoma: classically seen in patients with AIDS. Look for classic mucosal lesions (e.g., inside the mouth) or an expanding, strange rash or skin lesion that does not respond to multiple treatments.

Paget disease of the nipple: watch out for a ***unilateral red, oozing/crusting nipple*** in an adult woman. You must rule out an underlying breast adenocarcinoma with extension to the skin.

➤ ***CASE SCENARIO:*** What is the classic nutritional cause of stomatitis? Deficiencies of B-complex vitamins (riboflavin, niacin, pyridoxine). Vitamin C deficiency also may cause stomatitis.

NEUROLOGY

Delirium and Dementia

	DELIRIUM	DEMENTIA
Onset	Acute and dramatic	Chronic and insidious
Common causes	Illness, toxin, withdrawal	Alzheimer disease, multi-infarct dementia, HIV/AIDS
Reversible	Usually	Usually not
Attention	Poor	Usually unaffected
Arousal level	Fluctuates	Normal

Both may be associated with **hallucinations, illusions, delusions, orientation difficulties** (unawareness of time, place, or person), and "**sundowning**" (worsening symptoms at night). Memory impairment is usually global in delirium, whereas **remote memory is spared** in early dementia.

- Watch for "**pseudodementia**" in the elderly, a manifestation of depression that is reversible with treatment.
- Treatable causes of dementia include vitamin B_{12} deficiency, endocrine disorders (especially thyroid and parathyroid disorders), uremia, syphilis, brain tumors, and normal pressure hydrocephalus. Treatment of Parkinson syndrome also may improve dementia.
- Watch for thiamine deficiency in alcoholics as the cause of delirium (***Wernicke encephalopathy***). The classic presentation includes **ataxia, ophthalmoplegia, nystagmus,** and **confusion.** If untreated, the delirium may progress to **Korsakoff syndrome,** which involves **anterograde amnesia** (inability to form new memories) and **confabulation** and usually is irreversible. Give thiamine before glucose in an alcoholic to prevent precipitating Wernicke encephalopathy.

Headaches

Tension headaches: most common headache cause. Look for long history of headaches and **stress,** plus a feeling of tightness or stiffness, usually frontal or occipital and bilateral. Treat with stress reduction and acetaminophen or NSAID.

Cluster headaches: unilateral, severe, tender and occur in clusters. **Oxygen** may abort an attack acutely.

Migraine headaches: look for ***aura, photophobia, nausea and vomiting,*** and positive family history. Patients may occasionally have neurologic symptoms during attack. Migraines usually begin between ages 10 and 30 years. Treat or prevent with antimigraine medication (e.g., **sumatriptan**).

Tumor/mass: look for progressive neurologic symptoms, **papilledema,** intracranial hypertension (classically with nausea and vomiting, which may be projectile), mental status changes, and headaches every day that are classically **worse in the morning.** CT or MRI with contrast should be ordered.

Pseudotumor cerebri: may mimic tumor or mass because it also causes intracranial hypertension, papilledema, and daily headaches that are classically worse in the morning and also may be accompanied by nausea and vomiting. Pseudotumor cerebri is typically found in **young, obese women,** and the CT/MRI scans are negative. Lumbar puncture reveals markedly **elevated opening pressure** with no other abnormalities. Patients may have permanent vision loss without treatment. Treatment is supportive; **weight loss** usually helps. If not repeat lumbar punctures or a shunt may be needed. Large doses of vitamin A, tetracyclines, and withdrawal from corticosteroids are possible causes.

Meningitis: look for fever, Brudzinski and Kernig signs, CSF findings (see table in later part of this section).

Subarachnoid hemorrhage: often described as the "worst headache" of the patient's life; may be due to congenital berry aneurysm rupture or trauma. Look for grossly bloody cerebrospinal fluid, though the diagnosis should be made with a noncontrast CT, *not* lumbar puncture. Treat supportively and try to diagnose an aneurysm if no history of trauma (i.e. order cerebral angiogram).

Extracranial causes: eye pain (optic neuritis, eyestrain from refractive errors, iritis, glaucoma), middle ear pain (otitis media, mastoiditis), sinus pain (sinusitis), oral cavity pain (toothache), herpes zoster infection with cranial nerve involvement, and nonspecific causes (malaise from any illness).

Cranial Nerves

Olfactory (CN 1): rarely important clinically. **Kallman syndrome** is anosmia plus hypogonadism due to deficiency of gonadotropin-releasing hormone.

Optic (CN 2), oculomotor (CN 3), trochlear (CN 4), and abducens (CN 6): see Ophthalmology section.

Trigeminal (CN 5): innervates **muscles of mastication** and **facial sensation** (including the afferent limb of the corneal reflex). The classic disorder is **trigeminal neuralgia** (tic douloureux), an idiopathic disorder that causes **unilateral shooting facial pain in older adults** that is often triggered by minor activity (e.g., brushing teeth). It is best treated with **antiepilepsy medications** (e.g., gabapentin, carbamazepine).

Facial (CN 7): innervates **muscles of facial expression, taste in the anterior two-thirds of the tongue,** skin of the external ear, lacrimal and salivary glands (except parotid gland), and **stapedius muscle** (thus CN 7 lesions may cause hyperacusis). See Ear, Nose, and Throat Surgery section.

> ➤ **CASE SCENARIO:** How can you tell the difference between an upper motor neuron (UMN) and lower motor neuron (LMN) facial nerve lesion using only physical examination? With an UMN, the forehead is *not* involved on the affected side due to dual UMN innervation. With a LMN, the forehead is involved on the affected side.

Vestibulocochlear (CN 8): important for hearing and balance. Lesions cause **deafness, tinnitus,** and/or **vertigo.** See Ear, Nose, and Throat Surgery section.

Glossopharyngeal (CN 9): innervates pharyngeal muscles and mucous membranes (afferent limb of gag reflex), parotid gland, taste in posterior third of the tongue, skin of the external ear, and carotid body/sinus. Look for **loss of gag reflex** and loss of taste in posterior third of tongue.

Vagus (CN 10): innervates muscles of palate, pharynx, larynx (efferent limb of gag reflex), taste buds in the base of the tongue, abdominal viscera, and skin of the external ear. Look for **hoarseness, dysphagia,** and **loss of gag or cough reflex.** Think of aortic aneurysms or tumors (especially Pancoast lung tumors).

Spinal accessory (CN 11): innervates sternocleidomastoid and trapezius muscles. Patients with lesion have **difficulty in turning their head to the side opposite the lesion** and **ipsilateral shoulder droop.**

Hypoglossal (CN 12): innervates muscles of the tongue. Lesions produce **deviation of a protruded tongue to the affected side.**

Seizures

Six main types of seizures are likely to be tested on the boards:

1. **Simple partial (local, focal) seizures** may be motor (e.g,. Jacksonian march), sensory (e.g., hallucinations) or "psychic" (cognitive or affective symptoms). The key point is that **consciousness is not impaired.** Treat with phenytoin, valproate, or carbamazepine.
2. **Complex partial (psychomotor) seizures:** any simple partial seizure followed by **impairment of consciousness.** Patients perform purposeless movements and may become aggressive if restraint is attempted. People who get in fights or kill other people, however, are not having a seizure! The first-line agents are phenytoin, valproate and carbamazepine.
3. **Absence (petit mal) seizures:** start **before the age of 20.** They are brief (duration of 10–30 seconds), generalized seizures of which the main manifestation is a **loss of consciousness,** often with **eye or muscle flutterings.** The classic description is a child in a classroom who stares off into space in the middle of a sentence, then 20 seconds later resumes the sentence where he or she left off. The child is having a seizure—*not* daydreaming. There is **no postictal state** (important differential point). The first-line agents are ethosuximide and valproate.
4. **Tonic clonic (grand mal) seizures:** the classic seizures that may have an **aura; tonic muscle contraction is followed by clonic contractions,** usually lasting 2–5 minutes. **Incontinence** (urine and/or feces) often is an associated symptom, and the postictal state is characterized by **drowsiness, confusion, headache,** and muscle soreness. Treat with phenytoin, valproate or carbamazepine.
5. **Febrile seizures:** between the ages of 6 months and 5 years, children may have a seizure due to fever. The seizure is usually of the tonic-clonic, generalized type, and no specific seizure treatment is required. Treat the underlying cause of the fever, if possible, and give **acetaminophen.** Such children do *not* have epilepsy, and the chances of developing it are only slightly higher than in the general population. Make sure that the child does not have meningitis, tumor, or any other serious cause of seizure. The question should give clues in the case description if you are expected to pursue the work-up of a serious condition.
6. **Secondary seizure disorder:** due to a **mass** (tumor, hemorrhage), **metabolic disorder** (hypoglycemia, hypoxia, phenylketonuria), **toxins** (lead, cocaine, carbon monoxide poisoning), **drug withdrawal** (alcohol, barbiturates, benzodiazepines, too rapid a withdrawal from anticonvulsants), **cerebral edema** (severe hypertension, eclampsia), **CNS infections** (meningitis, encephalitis, toxoplasmosis [see figure]), **trauma,** or **stroke.** Treat the underlying disorder. Use diazepam and/or phenytoin acutely to control seizures.

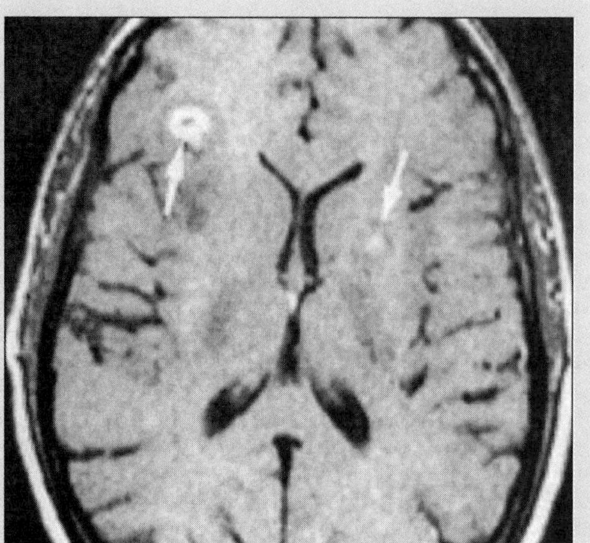

Toxoplasmosis in an immunosuppressed patient. Lesions on contrast-enhanced MRI may be eitehr ring-enhancing (*left arrow*) or nodular (*right arrow*). (From Katz DS, Math KR, Groskin SA (eds); Radiology Secrets. Philadelphia, Hanley & Belfus, 1998, p 369, with permission.)

Important points

1. **For all seizures,** secure the airway and, if possible, roll the patient onto his or her side to prevent aspiration.

2. **Cysticercosis** is due to infection with the larval form of *Taenia solium,* the pork tapeworm. This infection is seen most commonly in patients with ***AIDS*** and in ***immigrants*** (most common cause of seizures in South America). CT often reveals calcified and/or "ring-enhancing" lesions. Treat with niclosamide or praziquantel.
3. Remember **hypertension** as a cause of ***seizures*** or convulsions, ***headache, confusion,*** and/or ***mental status changes.***

Status epilepticus: when any type of seizure follows one after the other with ***no intervening periods of consciousness.*** Status epilepticus may occur spontaneously or result from too rapid a withdrawal of anticonvulsants. Treat with IV diazepam or lorazepam and phenytoin. Remember to protect the airway and intubate, if necessary.

> ➤ ***CASE SCENARIO:*** What is the most important point to remember when treating younger women with epilepsy? Anticonvulsants are teratogenic. Women need counseling about the risks of pregnancy. Do a pregnancy test before starting an anticonvulsant.

Cerebrovascular Disease

Cerebrovascular disease (stroke, cerebrovascular accident) is the most common cause of neurologic disability in the U.S. and the ***third leading cause of death.*** Watch for classic causes: ischemia due to atherosclerosis (by far the most common), atrial fibrillation with resultant clot formation and emboli to the brain, and septic emboli from endocarditis.

Treatment for acute stroke in evolution is supportive (e.g., airway protection, oxygen, intravenous fluids). Heparin is controversial and should be avoided for board purposes. The vascular surgery section discusses the role of carotid endarterectomy (CEA), which is not done emergently.

> ➤ ***CASE SCENARIO:*** What is the first test performed for suspected acute stroke? Noncontrast CT scan to rule out hemorrhagic stroke (see figure).

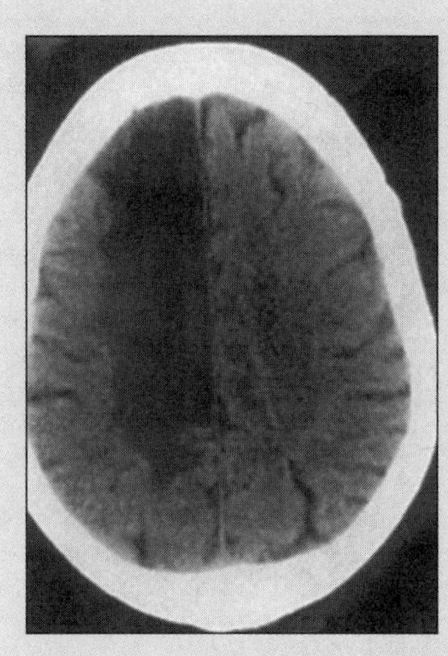

Noncontrast CT scan of the brain showing a well-established ischemic stroke in the territory of the anterior cerebral artery. (From Rolak LA: Neurology Secrets, 2nd ed. Philadelphia, Hanley & Belfus, 1998, with permission.)

> ➤ ***CASE SCENARIO:*** A patient has clinical symptoms of a stroke that started 2 hours ago, but the CT is negative. What does the patient have? A stroke or a transient ischemic attack (only time will tell which). Remember that the CT can be negative in the first 24–36 hours.

> ➤ ***CASE SCENARIO:*** A patient has symptoms of an acute stroke, and the CT scan reveals no hemorrhage. What is the best acute treatment? Aspirin and supportive therapy. Thrombolysis requires that the patient meet strict criteria and carries a risk of hemorrhage.

Transient ischemic attack (TIA): focal neurologic deficit that lasts seconds to hours (usually lasts less than 2–3 minutes), then resolves spontaneously; often a precursor to a stroke. The classic symptoms are ipsilateral blindness (**amaurosis fugax**) and/or unilateral hemiplegia, hemiparesis, weakness, or clumsiness. Order a carotid duplex ultrasound scan or magnetic resonance angiography (MRA) to look for stenosis. Heparin is somewhat controversial; avoid for boards purposes. The best choice for therapy is aspirin and antiplatelet medications or elective CEA (with carotid stenosis > 70%).

Localizing a stroke or other CNS lesion:

SYMPTOM/SIGN	THINK OF THIS AREA
Decreased or no reflexes/fasciculations	Lower motor neuron lesion (or possibly a muscle problem)
Hyperreflexia	Upper motor neuron lesion (cord or brain)
Apathy/inattention/uninhibited/labile affect	Frontal lobes
Broca (motor) aphasia	Dominant frontal lobe*
Wernicke (sensory) aphasia	Dominant temporal lobe*
Memory impairment, aggression, hypersexuality	Temporal lobes
Inability to read, write, name, or do math	Dominant parietal lobe*
Ignoring one side of the body/difficulty in dressing	Nondominant parietal lobe*
Visual hallucinations or illusions	Occipital lobes
Cranial nerves 3 and 4	Midbrain
Cranial nerves 5, 6, 7, and 8	Pons
Cranial nerves 9, 10, 11, and 12	Medulla
Ataxia, dysarthria, nystagmus, intention tremor, dysmetria, scanning speech	Cerebellum
Resting tremor, chorea	Basal ganglia
Hemiballismus	Subthalamic nuclei

*The left side is dominant in > 95% of population (99% of right-handed people and 60–70% of left-handed people).

Movement Disorders

Huntington disease: autosomal dominant condition usually beginning between 35 and 50 years of age. Look for **choreiform movements** (irregular, spasmodic, involuntary movements of the limbs or facial muscles) and **progressive intellectual deterioration, dementia,** or **psychiatric disturbances. Atrophy of the caudate nucleus** may be seen on CT/MRI. Treatment is supportive; antipsychotics may help.

Parkinson disease: classic tetrad of **slowness or poverty of movement; muscular rigidity** ("lead pipe" or "cogwheel"); **resting tremor** ("pill-rolling" tremor that disappears with movement and sleep); and **postural instability** (shuffling gait and festination). Patients also may have dementia and depression. The mean age of onset is around 60. The cause is a loss of dopaminergic neurons, especially in the **substantia nigra;** therefore, dopamine is decreased in the basal ganglia.

Drug therapy aims to increase dopamine and includes **levodopa** (given with **carbidopa**), bromocriptine or pergolide, monoamine oxidase-B inhibitors (selegiline), amantidine, anticholinergics (trihexyphenidyl, benztropine), and antihistamines (diphenhydramine).

> ➤ **CASE SCENARIO:** A 27-year-old man treated with haloperidol develops slowness of movement and muscular rigidity (Parkinsonism). What should you do? Treat with anticholinergics (benztropine, trihexyphenidyl) or antihistamines (diphenhydramine).

Note: Besides Parkinson disease, a resting tremor may be due to hyperthyroidism, anxiety, drug withdrawal or intoxication, or a benign (essential) hereditary tremor. Benign hereditary tremors usually are autosomal dominant. Look for a family history, and use beta blockers to reduce the tremor. Also watch for Wilson disease (hepatolenticular degeneration) as a cause of tremor. **Asterixis** (outstretched hands flap slowly and involuntarily) occurs in patients with liver and kidney failure.

Cerebellar disorders: typically cause an **intention tremor** (tremor only during attempted voluntary movement; goes away at rest). In children, think of **brain tumor** (cerebellar astrocytoma, medulloblastomas), hydrocephalus (enlarging head in child younger than 6 months, may be related to Arnold-Chiari or Dandy-Walker syndrome or prior meningitis), Friedreich ataxia, or ataxia-telangiectasia (the diagnosis is in the name). **Friedreich ataxia,** an autosomal recessive disorder, starts between 5 and 15 years of age. Look for cardiomyopathy. In adults, think of **alcoholism,** tumor, ischemia/hemorrhage, or multiple sclerosis.

Amyotrophic lateral sclerosis (ALS; also known as Lou Gehrig's disease): an idiopathic degeneration of both upper motor neurons (UMNs) and lower motor neurons (LMNs). ALS is more common in men. The mean age at onset is 55 years. The key is to notice a **combination of UMN lesion signs** (spasticity, hyperreflexia, positive Babinski sign) and **LMN lesion signs** (fasciculations, atrophy, flaccidity). Treatment is supportive. Fifty percent of patients die within 3 years of onset.

Miscellaneous Topics

Know the **classic cerebrospinal fluid (CSF) findings** in different conditions. Remember: do not perform a lumbar puncture in patients with acute head trauma or signs of intracranial hypertension until you have a CT/MRI. You may cause the patient's death (from uncal herniation).

CONDITION	CELLS/μL*	GLUCOSE (mg/dL)	PROTEIN (mg/dL)	PRESSURE (mmHg)
Normal CSF	0–3 (L)	50–100	20–45	100–200
Bacterial meningitis	≥ 1000 (PMN)	≤ 50	About 100	> 200
Viral/aseptic meningitis	≥ 100 (L)	Normal	Normal/slightly increased	Normal/slightly increased
Pseudotumor cerebri	Normal	Normal	Normal	≥ 200
Guillain-Barre syndrome	0–100 (L)	Normal	≥ 100	Normal
Cerebral hemorrhage[t]	"Bloody" (RBC)	Normal	> 45	> 200
Multiple sclerosis	Normal/slightly increased (L)	Normal	Normal/slightly increased	Normal

*Main cell type is put in parenthesis after the number (L = lymphocytes, PMN = neutrophils, RBC = red blood cells).

[t]Think of subarachnoid hemorrhage, but also may occur after an intracerebral bleed.

Note: With multiple sclerosis, look for **oligoclonal bands** on electrophoresis of the CSF, due to increased IgG production, and an increased level of **myelin basic protein** during active demyelination.

> **CASE SCENARIO:** A 32-year-old man with AIDS presents with gradual onset of lethargy, photophobia, low-grade fever, and headaches. Lumbar puncture reveals low glucose, high protein, and a high white blood cell count, which is due predominantly to high lymphocytes. What two types of meningitis should you consider? Tuberculous and fungal meningitis. Watch for a **positive India ink preparation** for cryptococcal meningitis.

Multiple sclerosis: look for insidious onset of neurologic symptoms in **women aged 20–40** years with **exacerbations and remissions.** Common presentations include paresthesias or numbness, weakness or clumsiness, **visual disturbances** (decreased vision and pain due to optic neuritis; diplopia due to cranial nerve involvement), gait disturbances, incontinence or urgency, and vertigo. Also look for emotional lability or other mental status changes. Internuclear ophthalmoplegia and scanning speech are classic symptoms, and patients may have a **positive Babinski sign. MRI** with and without contrast is the most sensitive diagnostic tool to show demyelination plaques. Also look for **increased IgG/oligoclonal bands** and **myelin basic protein** in the cerebrospinal fluid. Treatment is not highly effective but includes corticosteroids, interferons and other immune system modulators.

Guillain-Barré syndrome: look for a history of mild infection or immunization roughly **1 week before the onset of symmetric, distal lower extremity weakness or paralysis** and **loss of deep tendon reflexes** in affected areas. Sensory disturbances (e.g., paresthesias) are mild or absent. As the ascending paralysis/weakness progresses in more severe cases, respiratory paralysis may occur; watch the patient carefully. Usually spirometry is used to follow inspiratory ability. Intubation may be required. Diagnosis is made by a combination of clinical symptoms, cerebrospinal fluid analysis (usually normal except for markedly increased protein), and nerve conduction velocities (slowed). Disease usually stops spontaneously. **Plasmapheresis** may reduce the severity and duration of disease. Do not use steroids; you may make the patient worse.

Electromyography (EMG): measures the electrical (contractile) properties of muscle. Lower motor neuron lesions are associated with **fasciculations/fibrillations at rest.** With disease in the muscle itself, there is little electrical activity at rest (which is normal), but amplitude is decreased with contraction of the muscle.

Syncope: the most common cause is **vasovagal** (e.g., after stress or fear). Other possibilities include cardiac events (especially arrhythmias; order an EKG) and neurologic disorders (especially seizures; consider CT/MRI of head only if other neurologic symptoms are present).

> ➤ **CASE SCENARIO:** A patient passes out. Should you worry about a stroke? Syncope is uncommon in the setting of stroke; if it occurs, it is usually due to a lesion in the posterior circulation (vertebrobasilar system).

For delirious or unconscious patients in the emergency department with no history of trauma, first think of **hypoglycemia** (treat with glucose), **opioid overdose** (treat with naloxone), and **thiamine deficiency** (treat with thiamine before giving glucose in a suspected alcoholic). Other common causes are alcohol, illicit drugs, prescription medications, diabetic ketoacidosis, stroke, and epilepsy/postictal state.

Important causes of peripheral neuropathies

1. **Metabolic disorders:** diabetes (autonomic and sensory neuropathy), uremia, hypothyroidism.
2. **Nutritional disorders:** deficiencies of vitamin B_{12}, B_6 (look for a history of isoniazid use), thiamine ("dry" beriberi), or vitamin E.
3. **Toxins/medications:** lead or other heavy metals, isoniazid, vincristine, ethambutol (optic neuritis). In patients with lead poisoning, the classic symptom is **wrist drop** or **foot drop;** look for coexisting CNS and abdominal symptoms.
4. **Postinfection, immunization, autoimmune disorders:** Guillain-Barré, systemic lupus erythematosus, polyarteritis nodosa, scleroderma, sarcoidosis, amyloidosis.
5. **Trauma:** carpal tunnel syndrome (median nerve entrapped at the wrist), pressure paralysis (radial nerve palsy in alcoholics), or fractures. Carpal tunnel syndrome usually is due to repetitive physical activity but may be a presentation of acromegaly or hypothyroidism; look for a positive **Tinel** or **Phalen sign.**
6. **Infection:** Lyme disease, diphtheria, HIV, tick bite, leprosy.

➤ **CASE SCENARIO:** What is the hallmark effect of peripheral neuropathies and demyelinating diseases on nerve conduction velocity? Nerve conduction velocity is slowed.

Myasthenia gravis (MG): autoimmune disease that destroys acetylcholine receptors. MG usually presents in **women aged 20–40 years.** Look for **ptosis, diplopia,** and general muscle fatigability, especially **toward the end of the day.** The diagnosis can be made with the Tensilon test: muscle weakness improves after injection of **edrophonium** (Tensilon), a short-acting anticholinesterase. Watch for an associated **thymoma;** most patients with MG improve after removal of the thymus (thymectomy considered part of standard treatment). Most patients have antibodies to acetylcholine receptors in the serum. Treat with long-acting anticholinesterase (**pyridostigmine,** neostigmine); **plasmapheresis** can help in the setting of an acute crisis.

Eaton-Lambert syndrome (ELS): paraneoplastic syndrome classically seen with **small cell lung cancer.** ELS also is associated with muscle weakness but **spares the extraocular muscles,** whereas in MG involvement of extraocular muscles is almost always a prominent feature. ELS also has a different mechanism of disease (impaired release of acetylcholine from nerves).

➤ **CASE SCENARIO:** How can you tell the difference between MG and ELS by using repetitive muscle stimulation? In patients with MG fatigue *increases* with stimulation, whereas in patients with ELS fatigue *decreases* with stimulation.

Important points

1. Do not forget organophosphate poisoning as a cause for myasthenic-like muscle weakness. It usually results from agricultural exposure. Look for parasympathomimetic effects (e.g., miosis, excessive bronchial secretions, urinary urgency, diarrhea). Treatment includes **atropine** and **pralidoxime.**
2. **Aminoglycosides** in high doses may cause myasthenic-like muscular weakness and prolong the effects of muscular blockade in anesthesia.

➤ **CASE SCENARIO:** What conditions may occur in a patient with a port-wine stain over the right side of the face in the distribution of the first and second divisions of the trigeminal nerve? Seizures and glaucoma, as part of the **Sturge-Weber syndrome.**

GENETICS

Questions may ask you to give **genetic counseling** to a parent and/or to predict the likelihood of having a second affected child after the first is born with a disease. It is assumed that you know the inheritance pattern of the disease.

Autosomal dominant: look for an affected mother or father who passes the disease to 50% of offspring.

- von Willebrand disease
- Neurofibromatosis: café-au-lait spots, profuse peripheral nerve tumors, acoustic schwannoma
- Multiple endocrine neoplasia (MEN) I and II syndromes
- Achondroplasia (diagnosis from picture of the patient)
- Marfan syndrome: tall height, arachnodactyly, mitral valve prolapse, aortic dissection, lens dislocation
- Huntington disease
- Familial hypercholesterolemia: look for xanthomas and early coronary artery disease, markedly elevated cholesterol
- Familial polyposis coli
- Adult polycystic kidney disease
- Hereditary spherocytosis (see figure)

- Tuberous sclerosis: ***facial angiofibromas*** (i.e., ***adenoma sebaceum***), ***seizures, mental retardation*** (i.e., classic triad: "zits, fits, and nitwits"), CNS hamartomas, cardiac rhabdomyomas, renal angiomyolipomas, and hypopigmented skin macules
- Myotonic dystrophy: muscle weakness with ***inability to release grip***, balding, cataracts, mental and mental retardation
  - ***CASE SCENARIO:*** A 45-year-old man is diagnosed with adult polycystic kidney disease. His wife has no kidney disease and no family history of kidney disease. He wants to know the likelihood that his two children may have the disease. What do you tell him? Each child has roughly a 50% chance of having the disease.

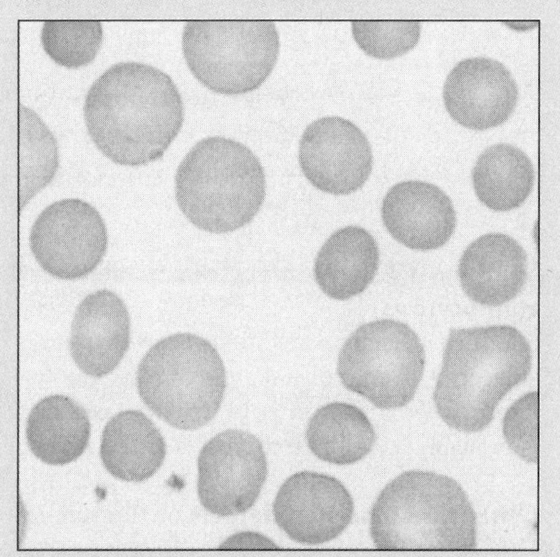

Hereditary spherocytosis. Smaller spherocytes are noted among larger polychromatic red cells. Note also the lack of normal central pallor in the spherocytes. Patients often improve after splenectomy. (From Hoffbrand AV, Pettit JE: Haemolytic anemia. In Color Atlas of Clinical Hematology, 3rd ed. New York, Churchill Livingstone, 2000, pp 71–84, with permission.)

Autosomal recessive: look for family history and unaffected parents who pass the disease to 25% of children.

- Sphingolipidoses (e.g., Tay-Sachs disease, Gaucher disease; the exception is Fabry disease, which is X-linked)
- Mucopolysaccharidoses (e.g., Hurler disease; the exception is Hunter disease, which is X-linked)
- Glycogen storage diseases (e.g., Pompe disease, McArdle disease)
- Cystic fibrosis
- Galactosemia: look for congenital cataracts, neonatal sepsis; avoid galactose- and lactose-containing foods
- Amino acid disorders (e.g., phenylketonuria, alkaptonuria)
- Sickle cell disease
- Childhood or infantile polycystic kidney disease
- Wilson disease
- Hemochromatosis (usually)
- Adrenogenital syndrome (e.g., 21-hydroxylase deficiency)
  - ***CASE SCENARIO:*** An asymptomatic couple has a child with phenylketonuria. What is the chance that their next child will have it? 25%.

X-linked recessive: look for affected fathers who pass the gene only to their daughters (who become carriers but do not get disease) and carrier mothers (family history in male relatives) who pass the disease to their sons.

- Hemophilia
- G6PD deficiency
- Fabry disease
- Hunter disease
- Lesch-Nyhan syndrome: hypoxanthine-guanine phosphoribosyltransferase (HPRT enzyme) deficiency. Look for mental retardation and **self-mutilation** (patients may bite off their own fingers).

- Duchenne muscular dystrophy
- Wiscott-Aldrich syndrome
- Bruton agammaglobulinemia
- Fragile X syndrome: second most common cause of mental retardation in males (after Down syndrome). Patients have large testes.

> ➤ ***CASE SCENARIO:*** A healthy man had a father with hemophilia. He wants to know the likelihood that his sons will have hemophilia. His wife is healthy and has no family history of the condition. What do you tell him? His children's risk is no higher than that of the general population (close to 0%). Fathers cannot pass X-linked conditions on to their sons.

Polygenic disorders: relatives are more likely to have disease, but there is no obvious heritable pattern (yet).

- Pyloric stenosis
- Cleft lip/palate
- Type II diabetes
- Obesity
- Neural tube defects
- Schizophrenia
- Bipolar disorder
- Ischemic heart disease
- Alcoholism

> ➤ ***CASE SCENARIO:*** Assuming that the parent is an alcoholic, which child has the highest risk of alcoholism—the daughter of an alcoholic father, the son of an alcoholic father, the daughter of an alcoholic mother, or the son of an alcoholic mother? The son of an alcoholic father.

Chromosomal disorders

1. **Down syndrome** (trisomy 21): the most common known cause of mental retardation. The major risk factor is the age of the mother (1/1500 offspring of 16-year-old mothers, 1/25 offspring of 45-year-old mothers). At birth look for hypotonia, transverse palmar crease, and characteristic facies. **Congenital cardiac defects** (especially ventricular septal defect) are common and often affect prognosis. Patients also have an increased risk for **leukemia, duodenal atresia,** and **early Alzheimer disease.**
2. **Edward syndrome** (trisomy 18): more common in females than males; mental retardation, small size for age, small head, hypoplastic mandible, low-set ears, **clenched fist with index finger overlapping third and fourth fingers** (almost pathognomonic).
3. **Patau syndrome** (trisomy 13): mental retardation, apnea, deafness, **holoprosencephaly** (fusion of cerebral hemispheres), myelomeningocele, **cleft lip/palate,** cardiovascular abnormalities, rocker-bottom feet.
4. **Turner syndrome** (females with XO instead of XX): nuchal lymphedema at birth, short stature, webbed neck, widely spaced nipples, amenorrhea, and lack of breast development (due to primary ovarian failure). **Coarctation of the aorta** is common. Patients also may have horseshoe kidneys or **cystic hygroma.**
5. **Cri-du-chat:** due to a deletion on the short arm of chromosome 5. Look for high-pitched cry like a cat, along with severe mental retardation.

> ➤ ***CASE SCENARIO:*** A 33-year-old man comes to you because he and his wife have been unable to conceive. He is tall and thin. On exam, you note gynecomastia, sparse body hair, and small testicles. What is the patient's most likely karyotype? XXY. Infertility is the classic presentation of **Klinefelter syndrome.** Patients are tall with microtestes (< 2 cm in length), gynecomastia, sterility, and mildly decreased IQ.

PHARMACOLOGY

Side effects: bizarre, unique, and fatal side effects are typically tested as well as common side effects of common drugs.

DRUG	SIDE EFFECT(S)	DRUG	SIDE EFFECT(S)
Trazodone	Priapism	Chloramphenicol	Aplastic anemia, gray-baby syndrome
Aspirin	GI bleeding, hypersensitivity	Doxorubicin	Cardiomyopathy
Bleomycin	Pulmonary fibrosis	Busulfan	Pulmonary fibrosis, adrenal failure
Cyclophosphamide	Hemorrhagic cystitis	MAO inhibitors	Tyramine crisis (cheese, wine)
Buproprion	Seizures	Hydralazine	Lupus
Isoniazid	Vitamin B_6 deficiency, lupus, liver toxicity	Procainamide	Lupus
Cyclosporine	Renal toxicity	Minoxidil	Hirsutism
Penicillins	Anaphylaxis, rash with Epstein-Barr virus	Aminoglycoside	Hearing loss, renal toxicity
ACE inhibitors	Cough	Acetaminophen	Liver toxicity (in high doses)
Demeclocycline	Diabetes insipidus	Chlorpropamide	SIADH
Lithium	Diabetes insipidus, thyroid dysfunction	Oxytocin	SIADH
Methoxyflurane	Diabetes insipidus	Opiates	SIADH
Sulfa drugs	Allergies, kernicterus in neonates	DDI	Pancreatitis, peripheral neuropathy
Halothane	Liver necrosis, malignant hyperthermia		
Local anesthetic	Seizures	Succinylcholine	Malignant hyperthermia
Phenytoin	Folate deficiency, teratogen, hirsutism	Zidovudine	Bone marrow suppression
Vincristine	Peripheral neuropathy	Digitalis	GI and vision changes, arrhythmias
Amiodarone	Thyroid dysfunction	Acetazolamide	Metabolic acidosis
Valproic acid	Neural tube defects in offspring	Trimethadione	Terrible teratogen
Isotretinoin	Terrible teratogen	Clozapine	Agranulocytosis
Thioridazine	Retinal deposits, cardiac toxicity	SSRIs	Anxiety, agitation, insomnia
Heparin	Thrombocytopenia, thrombosis	Warfarin	Necrosis, teratogen
Vancomycin	Red man syndrome	Niacin	Skin flushing, pruritus
Clofibrate	Increased GI neoplasms	HMG CoA reductase inhibitors	Liver and muscle toxicity
Tetracylcines	Photosensitivity, teeth staining in children	Ethambutol	Optic neuritis
Quinolones	Teratogens (cartilage damage)	Metronidazole	Disulfiram-like reaction with alcohol
Quinine	Cinchonism (tinnitus, vertigo)	Cisplatin	Nephrotoxicity
Morphine	Sphincter of Oddi spasm	Methyldopa	Hemolytic anemia (Coombs positive)
Clindamycin	Pseudomembranous colitis*		

ACE = angiotensin-converting enzyme, MAO = monoamine oxidase, SIADH = syndrome of inappropriate antidiuretic hormone, DDI = dideoxyinosine, SSRIs = selective serotonin reuptake inhibitors, HMA CoA = 3-hydroxy-3-methylglutaryl coenzyme A.

*May be caused by any broad-spectrum antibiotic.

Side effects of diuretics: thiazides cause hyperglycemia, hyperuricemia, hyperlipidemia, hyponatremia, hypokalemic metabolic alkalosis, and hypovolemia; thiazides are sulfa drugs (be careful with sulfa allergy). Loop diuretics cause **hypokalemic metabolic alkalosis,** hypovolemia, and ototoxicity. All are also sulfa drugs except ethacrynic acid. Carbonic anhydrase inhibitors cause **metabolic acidosis.**

> **CASE SCENARIO:** What is the difference between loop diuretics and thiazides in terms of their effects on calcium? Thiazides cause calcium retention and should be avoided in patients with hypercalcemia, whereas loop diuretics cause calcium excretion and are used as one of the treatments for hypercalcemia.

Side effects of antihypertensive drugs: sedation, depression (worst is methyldopa), and sexual dysfunction. Beta blockers, verapamil, and diltiazem can cause bradycardia or heart block in susceptible patients. Beta blockers can also precipitate attacks in **asthmatics** (who should not take them) and **mask the symptoms of hypoglycemia** in diabetic patients (though the benefits may outweigh the risks, such as in a person with a prior myocardial infarction). Alpha$_1$ antagonists classically cause **first-dose orthostatic hypotension.**

Antidotes for acute poisoning or overdose:

POISON OR MEDICATION	ANTIDOTE
Cholinesterase inhibitors	Atropine, pralidoxime
Quinidine or tricylcic antidepressants	Sodium bicarbonate (cardioprotective)
Iron	Deferoxamine
Digoxin	Normalize potassium/other electrolytes, digoxin antibodies
Methanol/ethylene glycol	Ethanol
Benzodiazepines	Flumazenil
Beta blockers	Glucagon
Lead	EDTA (edetate)
Copper/gold	Penicillamine
Opioids	Naloxone
Carbon monoxide	Oxygen (hyperbaric if severe)
Muscarinic blockers	Physostigmine

Combinations of drugs to avoid:

1. Monoamine oxidase (MAO) inhibitors and meperidine can produce coma.
2. MAO inhibitors and serotonin-specific reuptake inhibitors can produce serotonin syndrome (hyperthermia, rigidity, myoclonus, autonomic instability)
3. Aminoglycosides and loop diuretics can result in enhanced ototoxicity.
4. Thiazides and lithium can produce lithium toxicity.

Note: Barbiturates, antiepileptics, and rifampin are classic inducers of hepatic enzymes; cimetidine and ketoconazole are classic inhibitors of hepatic enzymes (important for drug-drug interactions).

> **CASE SCENARIO:** A 27-year-old woman with chronic complaints of abdominal pain is given sugar tablets and told that they are a great new medicine. She improves. Is her condition psychosomatic? Not necessarily. Normal people with real diseases often have an improvement in symptoms with placebo. It is unethical to give a placebo and lie to the patient about it.

Estrogen/Hormone Replacement Therapy

Hormone replacement therapy (HRT) is no longer thought to be beneficial for all postmenopausal and post-hysterectomy women. The patient must decide whether she wants HRT after you discuss with her the risks and benefits, but the risks are now thought to outweigh the benefits and HRT is thus prescribed for symptom relief only. Observation during therapy is necessary, because estrogen and progesterone are far from harmless. The main reason to give progesterone with estrogen is to eliminate the increased risk of endometrial cancer. If a woman has no uterus, give estrogen only (without progesterone).

Known benefits of estrogen therapy: decreased osteoporosis and fractures (especially hip fractures), possible decrease in coronary heart disease (controversial; if true, probably because estrogen increases HDL cholesterol; this benefit is reduced or negated by coadministration of progesterone), reduced hot flashes, and reduced genitourinary symptoms (helps with dryness, urgency, atrophy-induced incontinence, urinary frequency).

Known risks of estrogen therapy: increased risk of endometrial cancer (eliminated by coadministration of progesterones), increased risk of venous thromboembolism, probable increased risk of breast cancer (controversial), increased risk of gallbladder disease.

Other side effects of estrogen thearpy: endometrial bleeding, breast tenderness, nausea, bloating, and headaches.

Absolute contraindications to estrogen therapy: unexplained vaginal bleeding, active liver disease, history of thrombophlebitis or thromboembolism, history of endometrial or breast cancer.

Relative contraindications to estrogen therapy: seizure disorder, hypertension, uterine leiomyomas, familial hyperlipidemia, migraines, thrombophlebitis, endometriosis, gallbladder disease.

Consider endometrial biopsy and dilatation and curettage at the onset of treatment to rule out hyperplasia and/or cancer and an evaluation of any unexplained bleeding while the patient is on therapy unless she has had a normal evaluation in the past 6 months.

Birth Control Pills/Oral Contraceptive Pills

Oral contraceptive pills (OCPs) are the **most common cause of secondary hypertension** in women, and any woman taking OCPs who is noted have increased blood pressure (BP) should stop the OCPs, then have her blood pressure rechecked at a later date.

Absolute contraindications to OCPs: smoking after age 35 (increased risk of sudden death), pregnancy (do pregnancy test before prescribing), breast-feeding, active liver disease, hyperlipidemia, uncontrolled hypertension, diabetes with vascular changes, prolonged immobilization of an extremity, history of thromboembolism or thrombophlebitis, coronary artery disease, stroke, sickle cell disease, estrogen-dependent neoplasm (breast, endometrium), liver adenoma, history of cholestatic jaundice of pregnancy.

Relative contraindications to OCPs: depression, migraine headaches (may trigger attacks), oligomenorrhea, undiagnosed amenorrhea, gallbladder disease, and heavy cigarette smoking under age 35.

Side effects of OCPs: glucose intolerance (check for diabetes mellitus annually in women at high risk), depression, edema (bloating), weight gain, cholelithiasis, benign **liver adenomas,** melasma ("mask of pregnancy"), nausea and vomiting, headache, **hypertension,** and drug interactions (drugs such as rifampin and antiepileptics may induce metabolism of OCPs and reduce their effectiveness).

Because of the **risks of thromboembolism,** OCPs should be stopped 1 month before elective surgery and not restarted until 1 month after surgery.

The risk of breast cancer does not seem to be increased in most women who take OCPs (although the issue is controversial). Cervical neoplasia may be increased (perhaps due to the confounding factor of increased sexual relations or number of partners). OCP users should have **at least annual Pap smears.**

Benefits of OCPs: reduce ovarian cancer by up to 50% and decrease the risk of endometrial cancer; decrease the incidence of the following: menorrhagia, dysmenorrhea, benign breast disease, functional ovarian cysts (often prescribed for the previous four effects), premenstrual tension, iron deficiency anemia, salpingitis, and ectopic pregnancy.

Aspirin, NSAIDs, COX-II Inhibitors, Acetaminophen

Effects: aspirin and NSAIDs inhibit cyclo-oxygenase (COX) centrally and peripherally, giving them ***anti-inflammatory, antipyretic, analgesic,*** and ***antiplatelet*** effects. Aspirin inhibits COX irreversibly, and thus for the life of the platelet, whereas other NSAIDs reversibly inhibit COX. Acetaminophen is mostly central-acting; thus, it is only an analgesic and antipyretic with no platelet or anti-inflammatory effects.

Toxicity: aspirin may cause GI upset, ***GI bleeding, gastric ulcers,*** and gout; very high doses cause **tinnitus,** vertigo, **respiratory alkalosis and metabolic acidosis,** hyperthermia, coma, and death. Aspirin can be removed by dialysis in severe overdose. NSAIDs also may cause **renal insufficiency or damage** (e.g., interstitial nephritis, papillary necrosis or acute tubular necrosis), especially in patients who take high doses chronically and have preexisting renal disease.

> **Note:** COX-II inhibitors (rofecoxib, celecoxib) or an NSAID/prostaglandin E_1 combination may help prevent GI damage. This approach, however, does not prevent kidney damage.

Do *not* give aspirin to the following patients:

1. Patients with allergies or asthma and **nasal polyps** (hypersensitivity reactions are extremely common in this group). Even in the absence of nasal polyps, patients with asthma may have an attack after taking aspirin.
2. Children < 15 years old. Aspirin may cause **Reye syndrome,** typically in the setting of a viral infection or fever; look for **encephalopathy** and **liver dysfunction** in affected children.

Aspirin has been proved to reduce the risk of stroke in patients with a transient ischemic attack (TIA) or previous stroke as well as the risk of myocardial infarction (MI) in patients who have had a previous MI and patients with stable or unstable angina and no previous MI. Many physicians also recommend daily aspirin for patients with known coronary artery disease. The use of aspirin for primary prevention of MI or stroke in patients with no definite history of MI, angina, or coronary artery disease is controversial. Studies have not shown a clear benefit, and the risk of hemorrhagic stroke and/or sudden death may be increased.

- Always weigh the risk and benefits of aspirin therapy. If the patient has a history of liver or kidney disease, peptic ulcers, GI bleeding, poorly controlled hypertension or bleeding disorder, the risks of aspirin may outweigh the benefits.

Stop aspirin 1 week before elective surgery; other NSAIDs should be stopped on the day before surgery.

Acetaminophen can cause liver toxicity and failure in high doses due to depletion of glutathione and hepatic necrosis. Treat with **acetylcysteine.**

RADIOLOGY

Screening and/or confirmatory radiologic tests for different diseases:

CONDITION	SCREENING (OR ONLY) TEST TO ORDER	CONFIRMATORY TEST	COMMENTS
Skull fracture (depressed)	CT scan		
Head trauma	CT without contrast		
Intracranial hemorrhage	CT without contrast		
Acute stroke	CT without contrast	MRI of brain without contrast	
Multiple sclerosis	MRI of brain with contrast		
Brain tumor	CT or MRI with contrast		
Pneumonia	Chest x-ray		
Chest trauma	Chest x-ray	CT scan with contrast	
Chest mass	Chest x-ray	CT scan with contrast	
Hemoptysis	Chest x-ray	Bronchoscopy or CT scan with contrast	
Pulmonary embolism	Ventilation/perfusion scan (nuclear scan)	Pulmonary arteriogram or CT with contrast	
Aortic aneurysm/dissection	CT with contrast	Angiogram	
Aortic tear (trauma)	CT with contrast	Angiogram	
Carotid stenosis	Duplex ultrasound or MRA	Angiogram	
Esophageal obstruction	Barium x-ray or endoscopy	Endoscopy	
Esophageal tear	Gastrografin x-ray or endoscopy	Endoscopy	
Bowel perforation	Abdominal x-ray	CT scan or laparoscopy	
Hematemesis	Endoscopy		
Peptic ulcer disease	Upper GI series or endoscopy	Endoscopy	
Abdominal trauma	CT scan with contrast	Laparoscopy	
Abdominal abscess	CT scan with contrast		
Cholelithiasis	Ultrasound (US)		
Choledocholithiasis	US	ERCP or MRCP	
Cholecystitis	US	Nuclear hepatobiliary study (HIDA scan)	
Intestinal obstruction	Abdominal x-ray (AXR)	CT scan with contrast	
Appendicitis	AXR, then US or CT with contrast	Laparoscopy	
Nephrolithiasis	AXR, then intravenous pyelogram (IVP) or CT scan without contrast		
Ovarian pathology	US		
Diverticulitis	CT scan with contrast		No endoscopy or barium enema acutely
Upper GI bleeding*	Upper GI series or endoscopy	Endoscopy	
Lower GI bleeding*	Barium enema or endoscopy	Endoscopy	

(Table continued on next page.)

CONDITION	SCREENING (OR ONLY) TEST TO ORDER	CONFIRMATORY TEST	COMMENTS
Unknown GI bleeding*	Nuclear medicine bleeding study		For brisk bleed, angiography or laparotomy
Hydronephrosis	US or CT scan		
Hematuria (persistent)	CT scan	Cystoscopy or CT scan with contrast	
Fibroid uterus	US		
Pelvic mass (female)	US	CT with contrast or laparoscopy	
Bone metastases	Bone scan		Plain x-rays for multiple myeloma
Pregnancy evaluation	US (transvaginal detects sooner than transabdominal)		First get beta-HCG
Fracture	X-ray		CT scan without contrast can help evaluate complex fractures
Osteomyelitis	X-ray	Bone scan and/or MRI with contrast	
Arthritis	X-ray		
Pyloric stenosis	US, upper GI series second choice		
Meckel's diverticulum	Meckel's scan (nuclear medicine)		

MRA = magnetic resonance angiogram (an MRI test), ERCP = endoscopic retrograde cholangiopancreatography, MRCP = magnetic resonance cholangiopancreatography, HIDA = hepato-iminodiacetic acid, HCG = human chorionic gonadotropin.

*For brisk bleeds, endoscopy is preferred. For occult bleeding, barium study or endoscopy can be used. An "unknown" GI bleed means that initial tests failed to localize the bleed and that the patient is still actively bleeding.

NOTE: With suspected GI perforation, do not use barium (it may cause a chemical peritonitis); use water-soluble contrast (e.g.., Gastrografin).

LABORATORY MEDICINE

Isosthenuria/hyposthenuria is the inability to concentrate urine. Think of **diabetes insipidus** or **sickle cell disease/trait.**

The erythrocyte sedimentation rate is practically a worthless test in pregnant women because it is elevated from pregnancy itself. A high-normal blood urea nitrogen or creatinine may mean renal disease in pregnancy.

High amylase may result from sources besides the pancreas (**salivary glands, GI tract, renal failure, ruptured tubal pregnancy**), but elevation of both amylase and lipase in a patient with abdominal pain is almost always due to pancreatitis.

Elevated creatine kinase (CK), which is essentially the same thing as creatine phosphokinase (CPK), is typically due to **muscle injury** (striated or myocardial) or rhabdomyolysis from drugs (**HMG-CoA reductase inhibitors**), **exercise, alcoholism, myocardial infarction** or **burns.** The CK-MB fraction is more specific for cardiac muscle.

- **CASE SCENARIO:** What lab tests can tell you that an elevated alkaline phosphatase is due to biliary disease and not bone disease? If it is due to biliary disease, **gamma-glutamyltranspeptidase (GGT)** and/or **5-nucleotidase** also should be elevated.
- **CASE SCENARIO:** What can cause spurious (i.e. false) hyperkalemia? Hemolysis.
- **CASE SCENARIO:** What do you have to remember if hyponatremia is present in a diabetic patient? The sodium level is artificially low in the setting of hyperglycemia. In addition, **chlorpropamide** (now rarely used) can cause the syndrome of inappropriate antidiuretic hormone secretion (SIADH).
- **CASE SCENARIO:** What is the relationship between pH and potassium and calcium? Alkalosis may cause hypokalemia and symptoms of hypocalcemia due to cellular shift—and acidosis may cause hyperkalemia by the same mechanism. Thus, **bicarbonate** helps to treat severe hyperkalemia.
- **CASE SCENARIO:** What electrolyte disturbance can make hypokalemia and hypocalcemia almost impossible to correct? **Hypomagnesemia.** You cannot usually correct low potassium or calcium levels until you correct magnesium.
- **CASE SCENARIO:** How can the BUN:creatinine ratio help you to determine whether a patient is dehydrated or has prerenal renal insufficiency? A BUN:creatinine ratio $>$ 15 usually implies dehydration.

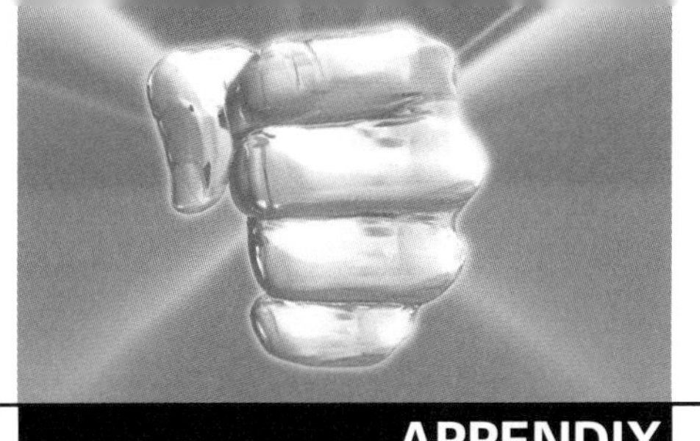

APPENDIX

Abbreviations

AAA	abdominal aortic aneurysm
Ab	antibody
ABC, ABCD, ABCDE	**a**irway, **b**reathing, **c**irculation, **d**isability, **e**xposure (trauma protocol)
ABG	arterial blood gas
ABO	blood types (A, B, AB or O)
ACE	angiotensin-converting enzyme
ACE-I	angiotensin-converting enzyme inhibitor
ACL	anterior cruciate ligament
ACTH	adrenocorticotropic hormone
ADH	antidiuretic hormone
ADHD	attention-deficit hyperactivity disorder
AFP	alpha-fetoprotein
AIDS	acquired immunodeficiency syndrome
ALL	acute lymphoblastic leukemia
ALS	amyotrophic lateral sclerosis (aka Lou Gehrig's disease)
ALT	alanine aminotransferase
AML	acute myeloid leukemia
ANA	antinuclear antibody
ANCA	antineutrophil cytoplasmic antibody
ANOVA	analysis of variance
ARDS	adult respiratory distress syndrome
ARF	acute renal failure
ASA	acetylsalicylic acid (aspirin)
ASD	atrial septal defect
AST	aspartate aminotransferase
ATG	antithymocyte globulin
AVM	arteriovenous malformation
AXR	abdominal x-ray
AZT	azidothymidine (zidovudine)
B, β	beta

BP	blood pressure
BPH	benign prostatic hyperplasia/hypertrophy
BPP	biophysical profile
BT	bleeding time
BUN	blood urea nitrogen
C	centigrade (e.g., 37° C), complement (e.g., C1, C3, C4) or cervical (e.g., C5 vertebral body
c-section	cesarean section
C of A	coarctation of the aorta
CA	cancer antigen (e.g., CA-125)
CAD	coronary artery disease
CBC	complete blood count
CD	cluster of differentiation (e.g., CD4, CD8)
CEA	carcinoembryonic antigen
CHD	coronary heart disease or congenital hip dysplasia
CHF	congestive heart failure
CK	creatine kinase
CLL	chronic lymphocytic leukemia
cm	centimeter
CML	chronic myelocytic (or myelogenous) leukemia
CMV	cytomegalovirus
CN	cranial nerve
CNS	central nervous system
CO	carbon monoxide or cardiac output
CO_2	carbon dioxide
COPD	chronic obstructive pulmonary disease
COX	cyclo-oxygenase
CPD	cephalopelvic disproportion
CPK	creatine phosphokinase
Cr	creatinine
CRF	chronic renal failure
CSF	cerebrospinal fluid
CT	computed tomography scan
CVA	cerebrovascular accident (stroke)
CXR	chest x-ray
D&C	dilation and curettage
DDI	dideoxyinosine (HIV medication)
DES	diethylstilbestrol
DI	diabetes insipidus

DIC disseminated intravascular coagulation
DIP distal interphalangeal (joint)
DKA diabetic ketoacidosis
dl deciliter
DM diabetes mellitus
DMSA 2,3-dimercaptosuccinic acid, succimer
DNA deoxyribonucleic acid
DTP diptheria, tetanus, pertussis (trivalent vaccine)
DUB dysfunctional uterine bleeding
DVT deep venous thrombosis
EBV Epstein-Barr virus
ECG electrocardiogram
EDTA edetate
EEG electroencephalogram
EKG electrocardiogram
ELISA enzyme-linked immunosorbent assay
ELS Eaton-Lambert syndrome
EMG electromyogram
ERCP endoscopic retrograde cholangiopancreatography
ESR erythrocyte sedimentation rate
F fluoride or female
FDP fibrin degradation product
Fe iron
FEV forced expiratory volume
FEV_1 forced expiratory volume in 1 second
FFP fresh frozen plasma
FSH follicle-stimulating hormone
FTA-ABS fluorescent treponemal antibody-absorption test (for syphilis)
FVC forced vital capacity
g, gm gram
G6PD glucose-6-phosphatase deficiency
GERD gastroesophageal reflux disease
GGT gamma-glutamyltranspeptidase
GI gastrointestinal
GnRH gonadotropin-releasing hormone
GU genitourinary
GYN gynecology or gynecologic
H2 histamine type 2 receptor

H&P	history and physical examination
HAV	hepatitis A virus
HbA1c	glycosylated hemoglobin
HBcAb/Ag	hepatitis B core antibody/antigen
HBeAb/Ag	hepatitis B "e" antibody/antigen
HBsAb/Ag	hepatitis B surface antibody/antigen
HBV	hepatitis B virus
HC	head circumference
HCG	human chorionic gonadotropin
HCV	hepatitis C virus
HDL	high-density lipoproteins
HELLP	**h**emolysis, **e**levated **l**iver enzymes, **l**ow **p**latelets (syndrome)
5-HIAA	5-hydroxyindoleacetic acid
HIV	human immunodeficiency virus
HLA	human leukocyte antigen
HPV	human papilloma virus
hr	hour/hours
HRT	hormone replacement therapy
HSP	Henoch-Schönlein purpura
HSV	herpes simplex virus
HTN	hypertension
HUS	hemolytic uremic syndrome
IBD	inflammatory bowel disease
IBS	irritable bowel syndrome
ICP	intracranial pressure
ICU	intensive care unit
Ig, IG	immunoglobulin (e.g., IgA, IgM, IgG, IgE)
IL	interleukin (e.g., IL-2)
IM	intramuscular
IPV	inactivated poliovirus vaccine
IQ	intelligence quotient
IU	international units
IUD	intrauterine device
IUGR	intrauterine growth retardation
ITP	idiopathic thrombocytopenic purpura
IV	intravenous
IVC	inferior vena cava
IVDA	intravenous drug abuse

IVF	intravenous fluids
IVP	intravenous pyelogram
K	potassium
kg	kilogram
KOH	potassium hydroxide
L	liter or lumbar (e.g., L5 nerve root)
LA	left atrium
LAE	left atrial enlargement
lb	pound
LCP	Legg-Calvé-Perthes disease
LDH	lactate dehydrogenase
LDL	low-density lipoproteins
LES	lower esophageal sphincter
LFT(s)	liver function test(s)
LGI	lower gastrointestinal (below the ligament of Treitz)
LH	luteinizing hormone
LLQ	left lower quadrant
LMN	lower motor neuron
LMP	last menstrual period
LR	lactated Ringer's solution
L:S	lecithin:sphingomyelin ratio
LSD	lysergic acid diethylamide
LUQ	left upper quadrant
LV	left ventricle
LVH	left ventricular hypertrophy
M	male
MAI	*Mycobacterium avium-intracellulare* complex
MAOI	monoamine oxidase inhibitor
MCHC	mean corpuscular hemoglobin concentration
MCL	medial collateral ligament
MCP	metacarpophalangeal (hand joint)
MCV	mean corpuscular volume
MEN	multiple endocrine neoplasia
mg	milligram
MG	myasthenia gravis
MHA-TP	microhemagglutination assay for antibodies to *Treponema pallidum* (for syphilis)
MI	myocardial infarct
ml	milliliter

mm	millimeter
MMR	measles, mumps, rubella (vaccine)
mo	month/months
MRA	magnetic resonance angiogram
MRI	magnetic resonance imaging scan
MRSA	methicillin-resistant *Staphylococcus aureus*
Na	sodium
NPH	isophane insulin suspension
NPO	nothing by mouth
NPV	negative predictive value
NS	normal saline
NSAID	nonsteroidal anti-inflammatory drug
O_2	oxygen
OA	osteoarthritis
OCP	oral contraceptive pill
OPV	oral poliovirus vaccine
P1, P2	heart sounds made by the pulmonary valve
PCN	penicillin
PCOS	polycystic ovary syndrome
PCP	phencyclidine or *Pneumocystis carinii* pneumonia
PCWP	pulmonary capillary wedge pressure
PDA	patent ductus arteriosus
PE	pulmonary embolus
PEEP	positive end-expiratory pressure
PG	prostaglandin (e.g., PGE2, PGF) or phosphatidylglycerol
pH	hydrogen ion concentration scale (measures acidity)
PH	pulmonary hypertension
PID	pelvic inflammatory disease
PIP	proximal interphalangeal (joint)
PMN	polymorphonuclear leukocyte
PMS	premenstrual syndrome
PO_4	phosphate
PPD	purified protein derivative (tuberculosis skin test)
PPV	positive predictive value
prn	as needed
PROM	premature rupture of the membranes
PSA	prostate-specific antigen
PT	prothrombin time

PTH	parathyroid hormone
PTT	partial thromboplastin time
PUD	peptic ulcer disease
PVC	premature ventricular contraction
PVD	peripheral vascular disease
RA	right atrium or rheumatoid arthritis
RAE	right atrial enlargement
RAI	radioactive iodine
RBC	red blood cells
RDW	red blood cell distribution width
REM	rapid eye movement (dream sleep)
RF	rheumatic fever
Rh	Rhesus blood-group antigen
RI	reticulocyte index
RLQ	right lower quadrant
RNA	ribonucleic acid
RPR	rapid plasma reagin test (for syphilis)
RSV	respiratory syncytial virus
RUQ	right upper quadrant
RV	right ventricle
RVH	right ventricular hypertrophy
S	sacral (e.g., S1 nerve root)
S1, S2, S3, S4	heart sounds 1–4
SBO	small bowel obstruction
SCD	sickle cell disease
SCFE	slipped capital femoral epiphysis
SD	standard deviation
SIADH	syndrome of inappropriate antidiuretic hormone secretion
SIDS	sudden infant death syndrome
spp.	species
SSRI	serotonin-selective reuptake inhibitors
STD	sexually transmitted disease
SVC	superior vena cava
SvO_2	systemic venous oxygen saturation
SVR	systemic vascular resistance
T_3	triiodothyronine
T_4	thyroxine
Tb	tuberculosis

TCA	tricyclic antidepressant
Td	tetanus-diphtheria booster vaccine
TE	tracheoesophageal
TIA	transient ischemic attack
TIBC	total iron-binding capacity
TIPS	transjugular intrahepatic portosystemic shunt
TMP/SMZ	trimethoprim-sulfamethoxazole
TOF	tetralogy of Fallot
TORCH	**t**oxoplasma, **o**ther, **r**ubella, **c**ytomegalovirus, **h**erpes
tPA	tissue plasminogen activator
TRH	thyroid-releasing hormone
TSH	thyroid-stimulating hormone
TTP	thrombotic thrombocytopenic purpura
TURP	**t**rans**u**rethral **r**esection of the **p**rostate
UGI	upper gastrointestinal (proximal to the ligament of Treitz)
UMN	upper motor neuron
URI	upper respiratory infection
US	ultrasound
UTI	urinary tract infection
VACTERL	**v**ertebral, **a**nal, **c**ardiac, **t**racheo**e**sophageal, **r**enal, **l**imb (malformations)
VDRL	**V**enereal **D**isease **R**esearch **L**aboratory test (for syphilis)
VFib or Vfib	ventricular fibrillation
VIPoma	pancreatic tumor that secretes vasoactive intestinal peptide
VMA	vanillylmandelic acid
V/Q	ventilation/perfusion (ratio)
VSD	ventricular septal defect
VTach or Vtach	ventricular tachycardia
vWF	von Willebrand's factor
WBC	white blood cells
wk	week/weeks
WPW	Wolff-Parkinson-White syndrome
yr	year/years

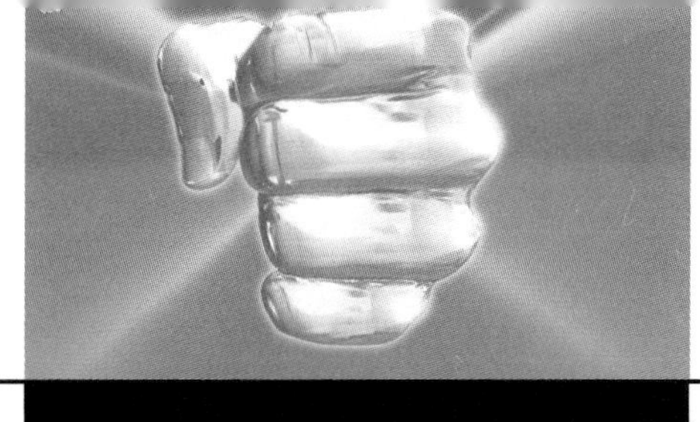

Index

Page numbers in **boldface type** indicate complete chapters.